Diabetic Adolescents and Their Families

Stress, Coping, and Adaptation

A chronic illness in adolescence complicates the developmental problems faced by adolescents and makes it difficult for parents to give up their parental role. Illness may jeopardize adolescents' autonomous development and may place them in danger of becoming fixed in the role of the child. *Diabetic Adolescents and Their Families* presents an innovative approach to the study of coping with chronic illness by focusing on the developmental context in its description of a longitudinal study of families with a diabetic or a healthy adolescent. Inge Seiffge-Krenke considers perspectives of the ill adolescents, their parents, and the physicians treating them. Highlighted topics include typical stressors, individual and family coping strategies, and psychosocial consequences associated with diabetes. The author also examines the changes that occur in adolescents' self-concept and body image and analyzes their relationships with parents, physicians, friends, and romantic partners as sources of support and of stress. Numerous case studies illustrate the difficulty of balancing normative development and adherence to the therapeutic regimen. By integrating clinical concerns with fundamental findings of developmental psychology, this book provides a significant contribution to the study of adolescent health psychology.

CAMBRIDGE STUDIES ON CHILD AND ADOLESCENT HEALTH

Steering Committee:

Klaus Hurrelmann, *University of Bielefeld, Germany*

Candace Currie, *University of Edinburgh, Great Britain*

Vivian B. Rasmussen, *WHO Regional Office for Europe, Copenhagen, Denmark*

The series ISCAH aims at publishing books on the health and disease status of children, adolescents, and young adults and on intervention strategies in medicine, psychology, sociology, public health, and political science. The series is supported by the international research network Health Behavior in School Children (HBSC) and is sponsored by the World Health Organization (WHO) Regional Office for Europe.

Diabetic Adolescents and Their Families

Stress, Coping, and Adaptation

Inge Seiffge-Krenke
University of Mainz, Germany

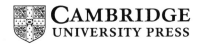

PUBLISHED BY THE PRESS SYNDICATE OF THE UNIVERSITY OF CAMBRIDGE
The Pitt Building, Trumpington Street, Cambridge, United Kingdom

CAMBRIDGE UNIVERSITY PRESS
The Edinburgh Building, Cambridge CB2 2RU, UK
40 West 20th Street, New York, NY 10011-4211, USA
10 Stamford Road, Oakleigh, Melbourne 3166, Australia
Ruiz de Alarcón 13, 28014 Madrid, Spain
Dock House, The Waterfront, Cape Town 8001, South Africa

http://www.cambridge.org

First published 2001

Printed in the United States of America

Typeface Times Ten 10/13 pts. *System* QuarkXPress™ [HT]

A catalog record for this book is available from the British Library

Library of Congress Cataloging-in-Publication Data

Seiffge-Krenke, Inge.
Diabetic adolescents and their families : Stress, coping, and adaptation / Inge Seiffge-Krenke.
    p.   cm.
Includes bibliographical references and index.
ISBN 0-521-79200-2
1. Diabetes in adolescence. 2. Diabetes – Patients – Family relationships. 3. Diabetes in
adolescence – Psychological aspects. 4. Diabetics – Family relationships.   I. Title.
RJ420.D5 S45 2001
362.1′96462′00835—dc21   00-068949

ISBN 0 521 79200 2 hardback

Contents

Foreword

Stuart T. Hauser

Several years ago, I was astonished and delighted to discover a European colleague directing a research project which had striking parallels with our longitudinal study of adolescents with a chronic illness. Since the mid-1970s, our research group had been tracking intersections between insulin-dependent diabetes mellitus and adolescent development (Hauser et al., 1997). Begun within the context of a Diabetes Research and Training Center at the Joslin Diabetes Center, we were examining how adolescents and their families coped with the onset and continued presence of this most common adolescent metabolic illness.

Besides the similar questions being asked by both groups, there were the shared assumptions. We assumed it was improbable that all teenagers with diabetes coped in the same ways. Nor did we expect to find that adolescents with diabetes took the same pathway through the complex teenage years. Dr. Seiffge-Krenke's project and ours also recognized that the lives of these adolescents could not be properly studied unless adolescents' contexts – family, school, medical setting – were also included. When we first started, most studies in this area had been based on special samples, those children and adolescents who were having serious difficulties adjusting to their illness. Consequently, prominent findings in these earlier studies pointed to psychiatric symptoms and disorders. To consider the possibility of multiple developmental pathways, reflecting varied coping processes, we designed our longitudinal studies to include all boys and girls with adolescent-onset diabetes, assessing competence and dysfunction of the adolescents and their families.

The importance of understanding how individual adolescents and their families are first touched and then "shaped" by the onset of an unexpected chronic illness cannot be underestimated. Studies of chronic illness from a developmental and psychosocial perspective are so urgently needed because: 1. health care providers cannot offer optimal services to chronically ill children and their families unless they know as much as possible about the experience of similar adolescents and families dealing with a serious chronic illness in one of their children; 2. along similar lines, preventive efforts for those families and children at risk for becoming impaired must rely on understanding when, where, and how the chronic illness and psychopathology become linked; 3. the unfolding of a chronic illness in the life of an adolescent and his or her family provides an incredibly strong opportunity for observing the spectrum of coping processes, family processes, and parent-to-child communications that emerge as a new illness strikes a younger family member; 4. intensive contextual studies of developing adolescents simultaneously experiencing chronic illness can lead to new insights about other adolescent-relevant contexts – school, peer, and close relationship ones; and, 5. the doctor-patient relationship is yet another context that likely influences the coping and meaning of chronic illness for adolescents and their families. Further understanding of this relationship, from a *developmental* perspective, can spark significant alterations in the treatment of adolescent patients.

Over the past 25 years we have witnessed an increasing number of thoughtful and rigorous studies in this area. In her remarkably comprehensive and well written book, Inge Seiffge-Krenke has given the fields of pediatrics, developmental psychology, and family psychology a major gift. She deftly reports on her own longitudinal study of German adolescents with diabetes, which has consistently included a control group of nondiabetic patients and their families. Preceding reports of her findings, and often woven into discussions of their meaning, she draws upon previous relevant studies of other adolescent chronic illness as well as research targeting specific adolescent dimensions of diabetes. The scholarliness of her work is clear from the book's bibliography of over 500 entries. She correctly recognizes one can only with caution generalize from diabetes to other chronic illness. She is thus careful to point out the ways in which diabetes resembles and differs from other adolescent chronic illness. Prominent amongst its unique aspects is the fact that diabetes is an almost "silent" illness, making it almost possible for teenagers to completely mask its presence in their lives. Other key features of diabetes, shared with chronic adolescent illnesses, are its need for regular attention to regulating self-care, thereby intensifying central adolescent conflicts surrounding independence, peer relationships, and intimacy.

Embedded in this thoughtful and gracefully written book are several major themes weaving through most chapters, providing important continuity from beginning to end of this rich and inclusive volume.

1. *Categorical and generic views of chronic medical illness.* Many medical colleagues, and perhaps many afflicted families, will be understandably cautious about thinking of all childhood or adolescent chronic illnesses as being comparable. Dr. Seiffge-Krenke expresses a balanced perspective about this issue from the very start of the book. As I allude to above, there are ways in which adolescent medical chronic illnesses can be grouped together, and special characteristics that separate a chronic blood illness from a life-threatening tumor from asthma, seizure disorders, and diabetes. One welcome strength of the book is its excellent recognition and use of multiple contexts in presenting diabetes findings. Discussion of adolescents with diabetes are always preceded by considerations of what is known about a given dimension (for example, adolescent coping) and then by what is known about the dimension with respect to other chronic illnesses.

2. *The importance of a developmental perspective when thinking about adolescent illness.* Many studies of psychosocial aspects of diabetes and other chronic illnesses have been taken from either a psychopathology framework or in terms of behavior management (often assessing and modifying the compliance of family or child in treating the illness). Dr. Seiffge-Krenke convincingly argues for the importance of needing to know the age and other developmental characteristics of a child when trying to make sense of his or her experience, responses, and overall illness management. Across all of the chapters, developmental considerations abound, whether it be about knowledge of the illness, coping with diabetes, or the very complicated question of psychopathology versus successful adaptation.

3. *The place of context.* Beside development, a second theme pervading nearly every chapter is the multifaceted significance of social context. Developmental psychologists, particularly those studying developmental psychopathology, recognize how vital it is to view development "within a continuously unfolding, dynamic, and everchanging context. Increased recognition of the effects of social contexts not only on psychological but also on biological structures and processes has emerged." Through these comments Dante Cicchetti recently introduced *Developmental Psychopathology and Family Process* (2000), a book targeting many issues dealt with in this volume.

Dr. Cicchetti also recognizes what a challenging endeavor it is to fully incorporate contextual considerations into empirical research concentrating on families and child development. It is to Dr. Seiffge-Krenke's credit that she steadily maintains an eye on contexts – family, peer, medical – throughout all of the chapters. Context is an especially important idea in her reflections, in the final chapter, on implications of her work for prevention and intervention initiatives. Although the primary context addressed throughout the book is the family, no context is left untouched. Most ambitious is the fact that peer relations ranging from peers to close friends to romantic relationships are considered from conceptual and empirical perspectives.

4. *Person-centered versus variable-centered analyses.* When collecting and analyzing longitudinal data, a persistent dilemma is whether to organize data around individual people and their unfolding lives (person-centered) or through aggregates of many individuals with respect to one or more dimensions (for instance, coping, friendship formation, characteristics of friendships). Posing this question in such an either-or way is clearly oversimplifying and runs the risk of losing the benefits of each approach. Once again, it is a credit to Dr. Seiffge-Krenke's balanced approach that we see strong examples of both approaches. To the clinically minded individual, it is almost reflexive to focus on one individual over time – the trajectory of his or her overall adjustment, strengths, self-esteem, peer network indices. Yet, from a social science perspective, even with longitudinal data, there is often a strong inclination to aggregate many individuals together comparing them with contrasting individuals (for example, nondiabetic adolescents versus diabetic adolescents, boys and girls) in terms of a single key variable, such as romantic relationship development or body image. Almost all of the chapters present and discuss analyses based on both approaches. The significance of using a person-centered approach, and the challenge of carrying out such analyses, are well illustrated in two ways in this book. First, we see poignant case examples, summarizing observed specific changes in individuals (and at times their families too). These examples are very inform-

way to pursue the problematic fundamental question that has lingered over the years in psychiatric and clinical studies of children with diabetes mellitus: Does the onset of diabetes and/or its course lead to psychopathology for all or most children with diabetes? Posed in such a bald and global way, this question has not been readily resolvable. Not surprisingly, answers depend on measurement approaches and samples. Different studies have provided different answers to the question. Through the organizing idea of multiple pathways and contexts, it becomes easier to think about patterns of events (and mechanisms) that can lead to psychopathology, and then think about prevention interventions that may reduce the incidence of unfavorable outcomes.

5. *Internal narratives and external observations.* Not surprisingly, we view a spectrum of approaches to observing adolescents during the four-year longitudinal study. There are semistructured interviews through which Dr. Seiffge-Krenke obtains internal narrative data about the experience of individual patients and their families. In addition, the research team watched and analyzed families and children communicating with one another. Finally, through repeated use of psychometrically rigorous observations, the research group collected evidence of specific psychological and social processes and their change over a four-year interval. Given the multifaceted nature of diabetes mellitus, individual development, and contextual processes, it was surely a wise decision to use such a theoretically-driven and demanding measurement plan. The reader is helped in all instances by careful diagrams and summaries in each of the chapters.

One more overarching theme characterizes this remarkable book, integrating a vast array of knowledge about chronic illness and adolescent development. Dr. Seiffge-Krenke reminds us, throughout the chapters, of the resilient adolescents – those showing unmistakable signs of competent development, despite the many "anti-adolescent" challenges posed by diabetes. The self-care demands of diabetes often run directly counter to the experiences of adolescence: new autonomy striving, coming to grips with bodily changes of puberty, an expanding social life of parties, outings, and spontaneous adventures. Norman Garmezy (1982) underlines the tremendous benefits associated with understanding resilient children:

... These "invulnerable" children remain the "keepers of the dream." Were we to study the forces that move such children to survival and to adaptation, the long-range benefits to our society might be far more significant than are the many efforts to construct models of primary prevention to curtail the incidents of vulnerability.

This important volume, through its dual focus on adaptation and problematic adjustment, will take us a long way toward providing more outstanding care, and to informing families of how they may care for their vulnerable adolescents. The most rewarding benefit may be to adolescents carrying a new illness burden, through the conveying of a message about their agency (Bandura, 2001) – that they can construct pathways to well being despite the challenge of a new vulnerability that has arisen within their own bodies.

References

Bandura, A. (2001). Social cognitive theory: An agentic perspective. *Annual Review of Psychology, 52:* 1–26.

Cicchetti, D. (2000). Foreword. *Developmental psychopathology and family process* (by E. M. Cummings, P. T. Davies, & S. B. Campbell), pp. ix–xi. New York: The Guilford Press.

Cummings, E. M., Davies, P. T., & Campbell, S. B. (2000). *Developmental psychopathology and family process.* New York: The Guilford Press.

Garmezy, N. (1982). Foreword. *Vulnerable but invincible: A study of resilient children* (by M. E. Werner & Ruth S. Smith), pp. xix. New York: McGraw-Hill.

Hauser, S. T., Jacobson, A. M., Benes, K. A., & Anderson, B. J. (1997). Psychological aspects of diabetes mellitus in children and adolescents: Implications and interventions. In N. E. Alessi (Ed.), *Handbook of child and adolescent psychiatry, Vol.* 4, (pp. 340–354). New York: Wiley.

Preface

From a statistical standpoint, chronic illness is uncommon in adolescence. According to German, other European, and other international overviews, only about 10% of all adolescents are afflicted with a chronic illness. In the individual case, however, the onset of a chronic illness in adolescence can become a major stressor, which requires extraordinary coping efforts on the part of the adolescent. Similarly, the additional responsibilities involved in caring for a chronically ill adolescent may become a burden for the parents. Epidemiological surveys have shown that adolescents with a chronic illness are at significantly greater risk than their healthy peers for developing behavioral and emotional problems. Indeed, the onset and progression of a chronic illness exert many negative effects on the developmental processes occurring in adolescence. For example, chronic illness may jeopardize an adolescent's autonomous development, often to the point that he or she becomes fixed in the role of a child. All adolescents afflicted with a chronic illness, irrespective of severity and duration of the illness, must negotiate a delicate balance between adhering to the medical treatment regimen and following the normal course of developmental progression.

This book is largely based on the results of a longitudinal study of coping processes in chronically ill adolescents that I initiated and led at the University of Bonn, Germany. Although the study focused on one particular illness, juvenile diabetes, the findings are applicable to other chronic illnesses showing similar characteristics and long-term stress. This has been borne out in our efforts to discover which parallels and contrasts might exist between our findings and those obtained through research on other chronic illnesses. In this research, great emphasis was placed on assessing important information about the psychologically relevant aspects of coping processes as garnered from the perspectives of those individuals most involved in or affected by the adolescent's management of the illness, that is, those of the adolescents themselves as well as of their parents, siblings, and physicians. Furthermore, we endeavored to compare these perspectives with those of healthy controls and their families. Consequently, not only do our findings yield much insight into normative development but they also may be considered as paradigmatic for describing adolescent development under illness conditions or even for coping with any severe chronic stressor.

This longitudinal study is ongoing. Here I report the results obtained from four surveys conducted during the adolescent years of our sample, starting in 1991, when the participants were about 13.9 years old, and continuing until 1994, when they were about 16.9 years old.

This intensive research project was supported for over 4 years, from 1991 to 1995, by a grant from the Bundesminister für Forschung und Technologie (BFT Grant No. 0706567) and for 2 years, from 1995 to 1997, by the Deutsche Forschungsgemeinschaft (DFG Grant No. Se 408/10-1). The adolescents belonging to the original sample are currently being investigated as they make the transition to young adulthood (DFG Grant No. Se 408/10-4). It is my pleasure to thank my former research team in Bonn, Annette Boeger, Frank Kollmar, Sonja Fentner, Judith Hanl, Carina Schmidt, and Marcus Roth, who worked with me on this project from 1991 to 1997. They interviewed and tested the adolescents and their families, and Frank Kollmar was particularly helpful in analyzing the rich longitudinal data. During this time, Anette Floss helped greatly with the organization of the study and the management of data. On assuming a new academic position at the University of Mainz, Gerd Nummer helped in completing data collection on the attachment styles of the participants as young adults. Markus Sonntag, Carola Kirchheim, and Martina Hertel helped us to code and analyze the attachment and family coping interviews. Falk Berger, of the Sigmund Freud Institute in Frankfurt, advised us on all clinical and therapeutic matters. Rachel Bond competently assisted me in translating the manuscript, and Linda S. Lewis corrected this updated revision. Hiltrud Kirsch and Tanja Nieder worked through the final version and checked the references. Nicole Wollmerstedt prepared the figures.

Above all, thanks are due to all of the adolescents and their families who gave us so much of their time and energy. Their intensive and continuous cooperation made this research project possible and gave us valuable insight into the processes not only of coping with illness but also into parent-adolescent relationships and developmental processes in general. The low dropout rate indicates that our study offered the participants valuable insights as well. The project was an arduous yet extraordinarily worthwhile undertaking, and I am glad we were able to guide so many families through one stretch of their journey. With my new research team in Mainz, I have continued this project and hope to accompany our subjects during their transition to young adulthood.

Inge Seiffge-Krenke
Mainz, March, 2001

1

Epidemiology of Chronic Illnesses in Adolescence

Since the beginning of the 20th century, the relative distribution of somatic illnesses in the population has changed. Acute illnesses such as infectious diseases and deficiencies such as malnutrition have lost much of their significance; today, chronic illnesses predominate. Progress in medical knowledge and improvements in living conditions have been responsible for this change. In this chapter, data on causes of death and rates of mortality are presented first, followed by rates of incidence (frequency of newly appearing cases within a certain time period) and rates of prevalence (frequency of an illness in a special population at a certain point in time or over a particular period of time) for chronic physical diseases in adolescence. Finally, an approach to categorizing chronic physical illnesses is presented.

Changes in the Spectrum of Illnesses and Causes of Death

Chronic diseases are the main cause of death in the population today. However, the mortality rates for chronic illness are not as high for adolescent populations as for adult populations. According to the German Federal Bureau of Statistics (Statistisches Bundesamt, 1994), 10- to 20-year-olds show the lowest mortality rates of all age groups. The likelihood of dying in this age range is therefore relatively low, compared with other age groups. In Germany, accidents, particularly those involving motor vehicles, are the major cause of death in this age group, not illness as in adults. Similar trends have been documented for other European countries (Seiffge-Krenke, 1998a). According to the National Center for Health Statistics (1993), accident-related injuries are also the leading causes of death in young people aged 15 to 24 years old in the United States; 78% of all deaths caused by motor vehicle accidents are suffered by adolescents under 19 years old (National Safety Council, 1993). Sells and Blum (1996) have pointed out that accidents, together with violent injuries, homicides, and suicides, account for 77% of adolescent deaths in the United States.

The leading causes of death in adulthood, such as cancer and cardiovascular disease, also rank among the leading causes of death in adolescence, although the prevalence rates are comparatively lower. In Germany, 1 in 100,000 15- to 20-year-old adolescents dies from cancer or heart disease (Bundesminister für Gesundheit, 1991). Comparable rates have been reported in Scandinavian countries (Westbom & Kornfält, 1987). Similarly, in 1991, cancer and heart disease were the fourth and fifth leading causes of death among American adolescents, followed by the acquired immunodefiency syndrome (AIDS). Thus, chronic illness in adolescents rarely becomes life-threatening. It is important, however, to take note of the morbidity rates for chronic illness in this age group. Various studies have reported incidence rates of chronic disease ranging from 5% to over 30% (Newacheck & Taylor, 1992; Westbrook & Stein, 1994). Underlying this large variation in estimates is a lack of consensus as to which forms of illness should be included in the category of chronic illnesses. It is therefore necessary to define chronic illness precisely before epidemiological studies can be presented.

Epidemiology of Chronic Illnesses in Adolescence

Chronic physical illnesses must be distinguished from acute illnesses on the one hand, and various forms of disability on the other. Both distinctions have been made by Petermann, Noecker, and Bode (1987b), who defined chronic illnesses exclusively as "…physical illnesses … that determine the planning, actions, and feelings of the child and his family in a more or less threatening way over the space of several years or a lifetime" (p. 5). The aspect of chronicity ("several years or a lifetime") in this definition allows sufficient distinction from acute forms of illness. In contrast, other definitions typically set a lower limit for the illness duration, for example, at around 3 months (Pless, Cripps, Davies, & Wadsworth, 1989; Westbom & Kornfält, 1987). A second element of this definition, referring to the ominous course of the illness, is appropriate for excluding the more static disabilities that are often equated with chronic diseases. Such a distinction is necessary, since a definition that encompasses both types of illness could lead to prevalence values of up to 30% in children and adolescents. This definition does not imply that chronic disease necessarily follows a threatening course; rather, it states that this possibility always exists. For example, the development of life-threatening complications due to diabetes mellitus can never be ruled out. Some authors' definitions also refer to the onset of chronic illnesses to distinguish them from acute illnesses. For example, Schulz and Hellhammer (1991) have stated that "chronic illnesses as a rule develop slowly, last a long time, and have an unpredictable course" (p. 421). The reference to the slow onset, however, is not characteristic of all chronic physical illnesses.

The following section deals with the statistical distribution of chronic diseases in adolescence. In epidemiological studies, children and adolescents are frequently grouped together. Owing to this common practice, most of the epidemiological data presented here are based on groups of mixed ages. As compared with adults, children and adolescents are seldom affected by chronic physical illnesses (La Vecchia, Decarli, Negri, Ferraroni, & Pagno, 1992; Rakonen & Lahelma, 1992; Schellevis, van der Velden, van der Lisdonk, van Eijk, & van Weel, 1993). Nevertheless, even in this age group, the prevalence is considerable, amounting to about 10% in various countries (Eiser, 1990a; Offord, Boyle, & Racine, 1989; Seiffge-Krenke, 1998a); this indicates a significant increase since earlier decades. Results of the National Health Interview Survey in the United States (Newacheck, Budetti, & McManus, 1984) showed that rates of chronic illness and disability in children and youth under 17 doubled between 1960 and 1980. Similarly, Hurrelmann (1991) reported that since 1960, an increasing number of German adolescents have been affected by chronic disease.

These structural changes in pediatric epidemiology, marked by a relatively sharp increase in chronic illnesses in children and adolescents, cannot be fully explained by rising incidence rates for these age groups (Gortmaker, 1985; Perrin, 1985). Moreover, progress in medical treatment and diagnostics has contributed greatly to the decrease in childhood mortality rates. Nowadays, many children with life-threatening diseases survive, or at least reach adulthood (Newacheck, Stoddard, & McManus, 1993). Some formerly fatal illnesses have, consequently, become chronic illnesses.

Table 1.1. *Prevalence Rates of Chronic Illnesses in Childhood and Adolescence*

| Illness | Prevalence Rate (%) | |
	Gortmaker et al. (1990) (0–15 Years)	Newacheck & Taylor (1992) (10–17 Years)
Asthma	2.93	4.68
Epilepsy	0.30	0.33
Gastrointestinal diseases	0.16	—
Diabetes mellitus	0.10	0.15
Sickle cell anemia	0.09	—
Cerebral palsy	0.09	0.12
Heart disease	0.07	1.74
Cancers and tumors	0.06	—
Cystic fibrosis	0.03	—

only a few frequently occurring illnesses and a large assortment of different diseases with low prevalence rates.

Prevalence rates for children and adolescents in the United States, estimated by Gortmaker, Walker, Weitzman, and Sobol (1990), are reproduced in Table 1.1, along with the results of the National Health Interview Survey (Newacheck & Taylor, 1992). Only the most common types of illness are recorded here. Table 1.2 displays estimates for the Federal Republic of Germany, taken from Petermann et al. (1987b).

Table 1.2. *Estimated Frequencies of Chronic Illnesses in Childhood and Adolescence in the Federal Republic of Germany (Petermann et al., 1987b)*

Illness	Approximate Incidence (Cases per Year)	Approximate Prevalence
Chronic bronchitis/asthma	30,000	500,000 children
Congenital heart defects	4,000–5,000	30,000 children
Epilepsy	3,000	47,000 children
Diabetes mellitus		6,000 children
Cancers	1,200	4,000 children
Celiac disease	280	6,000 children
Hypothyroidism	280	6,000 children
Cystic fibrosis	120	2,350 children
Muscular diseases	110	1,750 children

According to these results, bronchial asthma is the most widespread chronic disease of childhood and adolescence, with a prevalence of about 3 to 5%. All the other forms of illness show considerably lower prevalence rates of about 0.03 to 1.7%. Gender ratios for the entire group of chronic illnesses are balanced in adolescence (Cadman, Boyle, Szatmari, & Offord, 1987). The remainder of this section will discuss, in some detail, those diseases that have been studied more frequently in psychological research.

The course of bronchial asthma, along with the high likelihood of its occurrence, appears typical of childhood and adolescence. Most patients become ill within the first 5 years of life. If asthma begins in childhood, the prognosis for its further course is favorable, as one-third of the afflicted patients lose their symptoms spontaneously during puberty. Of the remaining patients, only about 10% suffer from severe or lasting asthma. Spontaneous remission occurs largely among boys. While the male-to-female ratio in childhood is 2:1 – figures may also range from 4:1 to 3:2 (Reinhardt, 1993) – the relation evens out to 1:1 after puberty.

Unlike asthma, cancer seldom occurs in childhood and adolescence. Only 1% of all cancer manifestations occur in these age groups. Cancer ranks second after accidents as the principal cause of death among German adolescents; nevertheless, its morbidity rate in this age group is relatively low. According to Niethammer (1993), 14 new cases occur annually in every 100,000 children and adolescents up to the age of 15. Older children and adolescents show the lowest prevalence rate (10 in 100,000), whereas babies (23 in 100,000) and infants under 4 years (19 in 100,000) have the highest. In addition, large differences in the types of cancer manifested in childhood and adolescence are apparent as compared with adulthood. Whereas various types of carcinomas predominate among the adult population, the most frequent type of cancer in children and adolescents is acute lymphoblastic leukemia (ALL), which accounts for 27% of all cancer diagnoses in this population, followed by tumors of the central nervous system. Nowadays about half of all children suffering from cancer can expect to recover in the long term, although prognoses vary with the specific type. In the case of the most widespread form, ALL, the survival rate is generally estimated at about 70%.

Juvenile diabetes is the most common metabolic disease of childhood and adolescence (Struwe, 1991). Findings differ, however, with regard to the age of onset. The first manifestation is most frequently diagnosed in late childhood or early adolescence (Bremer, 1990). In contrast, Weber (1993) has proposed two peaks of first manifestation: the first between 3 and 6 years of age, the second between 9 and 13. The National Health Interview

Survey (Newacheck & Taylor, 1992) of a representative sample of the American population revealed a prevalence of 150 cases in 100,000 children and adolescents between the ages of 10 and 17 years. A much lower prevalence rate, 60 per 100,000 was reported for younger children in this study. Similar statistics are available for other countries. For example, Petermann (1994) reported that an estimated 17,000 children and adolescents under the age of 20 with diabetes live in Germany, of whom about 6,000 are no older than 15 years. It is well known that a north–south incline can be established in Europe, although its causes have not yet been adequately explained. According to Seiffge-Krenke (1998a), annual incidence rates vary considerably, ranging from 35 new cases per 100,000 children and adolescents in Finland to 6 in France and 8 in Germany.

Psychological Perspectives on Chronic Illness: From the Biomedical to the Categorical Approach

In this section, chronic disease will be examined from a primarily psychological perspective, with biomedical aspects only of incidental interest. From a medical standpoint, different forms of chronic illness would obviously have to be viewed separately, owing to their different etiologies. In contrast, a psychological discussion can identify many specific characteristics common to most forms of disease, as Pless and Pinkerton (1975, p. 52) have emphasized:

> The chronicity of the illness and the impact that it has on the child, his parents, and his siblings is more significant than the specific character of the disorder, be it diabetes, cerebral palsy, hemophilia, etc. In other words there are certain problems common to all illnesses over and above particular challenges posed by individual needs.

Perrin (1985) has highlighted several characteristics common to chronic illness, namely, the necessity for expensive treatment, the intermittent need for medical intervention, the experience of pain and physical complaints, and the possibilities of slow degeneration or premature death. In fact, for a range of psychological parameters, Stein and Jessop (1982; 1984) and Jessop and Stein (1985) found no significant differences between children with asthma, spina bifida, hemoglobinopathies, and various forms of disability. Rather, they identified much larger differences within the individual illness groups. Hence they have argued for what they term a noncategorical approach, which sees chronically ill children and adolescents as a more or less homogeneous group. Stein and Jessop (1982) have asserted that above all, the advantage of this approach lies in its practical contribution to the health care system. In this regard they state:

> When chronic illness is viewed noncategorically, it is possible to begin to learn more about characteristics, attitudes, and behaviors of the affected children in relation to the total child population in given communities. Additionally, since local communities are more likely to contain children with a range of conditions, but only a small number within each disease category, the noncategorical approach facilitates the creation and evaluation of service programs targeted to meet the needs of those with diverse conditions. (p. 361)

As Stein and Jessop (1984) have argued, whether long hospital stays result from asthma or from sickle cell anemia, their psychological consequences are much the same. Moreover, since some universal features in coping with various kinds of chronic illnesses appear to exist (see chapter 3), it is reasonable to assume that there may be certain aspects of stress that are generic to most chronic illnesses.

However, in emphasizing the similarities among different illnesses, their differences should not be overlooked. Apart from biomedical distinctions, important psychosocial differences exist. It would be inappropriate to subsume all the many and varied illnesses under the global category of chronic illness. The expected outcome of an illness may illustrate this point: The cognitive developments that generally occur in adolescence allow the youth to reflect about the facts in an abstract manner (Piaget, 1970). In this way, a potentially fatal illness would affect the adolescent differently from an illness that as a rule is not life-threatening. A more appropriate view is the partial categorical approach (Pless & Perrin, 1985, p. 45). In contrast to the noncategorical approach, this perspective does distinguish between individual diseases, but along psychological rather than biomedical lines. Rolland (1984; 1987) has offered one interpretation of this approach. According to his categorization of illnesses in childhood and adolescence, chronic diseases can be described and classified according to four dimensions: (1) their onset, which may be acute or gradual; (1) their course (progressive, recurrent, or stable); (3) the expected outcome; and (4) whether a disability is present.

This perspective stands on intermediate grounds between a biomedical approach, which views each illness in isolation, and a noncategorical approach, which subsumes the different disorders under the global concept of chronic disease. On the one hand, this allows many sorts of illness to be drawn together; on the other hand, there is still the flexibility to adopt certain medically and psychologically driven distinctions.

This book focuses on insulin-dependent diabetes mellitus, a relatively common chronic illness in adolescence. In terms of Pless and Perrin's (1985, p. 45) partial categorical approach, this illness is characterized by a gradual beginning and a progressive, possibly life-shortening course, which poses no severe impairments for the affected adolescent. After a more labile initial phase, most patients with diabetes show a relatively stable course.

2

Coping with Illness in Adolescence: An Overview of Research from the Past 25 Years

As mentioned in chapter 1, adolescents assume a middle position in morbidity rates in comparison with other age groups. Problems with health and illness rarely crop up in adolescents' spontaneous remarks, although – or perhaps precisely because – adolescents are so concerned with their physical development and want to be "as normal as possible." One should not forget, of course, that at least 10% of all families in Germany care for a chronically ill adolescent (Seiffge-Krenke, 1998a); comparable surveys in the United States and Great Britain have documented rates of 7 to 12% (Eiser, 1992; Gortmaker et al., 1990). Thus, chronic illness in adolescence is not a rare occurrence. In this chapter, research on adolescent coping with chronic illness will be reviewed. Thereby it will become evident that interest is growing in understanding the psychological processes and outcomes that are linked with chronic illness in this particular age group.

Current State of Research: Results of Two Meta-analyses

This chapter provides a brief overview of the current state of research on adolescents' coping with chronic illness, based on two meta-analyses. In the first meta-analysis, the period from 1970 to 1988 was studied. A literature search of the databases Psychinfo and Psyndex retrieved 249 publications on the topic of coping with illness in adolescence (for a summary, see Seiffge-Krenke & Brath, 1990). In a subsequent meta-analysis, Hanl (1995) found 85 studies published between 1989 and 1995. Generally, both analyses revealed a growing interest in theoretical and conceptual approaches as well as an increase in empirical studies. However, the proportion of empirical studies was meager in both analyses, amounting to 25% and 35%, respectively. Most articles were overviews, descriptions of therapies, or works of a conceptual nature.

Adolescence was defined in the first meta-analysis as the age span of 12 to 18 years. However, only 30% of the 249 publications analyzed by Seiffge-Krenke and Brath (1990) were strictly confined to this age range; most studies included a broader range, lumping together children, adolescents, and young adults. This reflects the tendency to select mixed groups covering a wide age range, thereby neglecting to differentiate further within the phases of adolescence. In the following discussion the findings pertaining to adolescent population samples will be dealt with more specifically.

Early research on adolescents characteristically focused on rare, extremely burdensome illnesses, for which no suitable treatment was available and which often had serious, unavoidable outcomes, such as death or serious physical damage. Besides illnesses with high mortality rates, diseases that are associated with crises or life-threatening phases have also been researched (e.g., acute renal failure, asthma attacks, diabetic coma, and hypoglycemic shock). The larger volume of research in more recent years has devoted more attention to illnesses that are less often fatal, more easily treated, and in principle, more readily managed by the patient. Lately this approach has included diabetes and some types of cancer, which nowadays are not necessarily fatal but rather chronic, very stressful illnesses.

The studies analyzed varied with respect to their definitions, operationalizations, and assessments of coping with illness. In the first meta-analysis, 42% of the studies employed a very broad definition of coping with chronic illness and explored the ill person's general adaptation; 27% of these studies employed a very narrow definition, equating coping with compliance with physicians' instructions or adherence to a therapeutic regimen and only 31% of the studies listed under the entry "coping with chronic illness in adolescence" employed an adequate definition of coping or defense. The measures for assessing coping tended to vary with age. Whereas in children, predominantly family coping was examined, the focus for adolescents was on individual coping (see chapter 6).

Most studies were based on samples of individuals suffering from similar types of illnesses or belonging to the more undifferentiated group of "chronically ill," without including control groups. Because the illnesses studied were quite rare, most studies were based on small samples (from individual case studies to $N = 50$). A minority of studies incorporated samples greater than $N = 100$. Only 12% of the studies included a healthy control group, and 10% included a control group consisting of patients with another type of illness. Most studies were cross-sectional; longitudinal studies were rare and amounted to 8% of all studies published.

According to Hanl's (1995) more recent meta-analysis of 85 studies published between 1989 and 1995, the situation has changed little. Over 75% of the studies analyzed were based on samples that mixed children, adolescents, and young adults. Only 21% of the studies used samples of adolescents between the ages of 12 and 18 years. Accordingly, the two meta-analyses demonstrated that it is still common practice to examine convenience samples with a broad variance in age. Even in more recent research, 60% of studies on coping with illness omitted a control group. As far as the concepts under investigation are concerned, Hanl's analysis showed that conceptual clarity has, if anything, decreased. Over 70% of the analyzed studies looked at adjustment or psychosocial functioning, whereas a mere 11% addressed the issue of adaptation from a purely medical standpoint, that is, compliance and adherence. Only 14% of the studies investigated coping as a well-defined construct. The proportion of longitudinal studies had diminished even further to 8% since the publication of Seiffge-Krenke and Brath's (1990) analysis. A shift in the range of illnesses being researched was already evident in the 1990 overview of literature. This became even more apparent in Hanl's analysis, in which 62% of all studies focused on diabetes. As can be seen in Figure 2.1, chronic illnesses with a high prevalence, such as asthma (see chapter 1), were considered in only a small percentage of the studies.

In summary, both meta-analyses revealed similar results. In general, chronic illnesses have not been studied in proportion to their prevalence and incidence. The lack of conceptual clarity in questions of coping stands out against the significantly more frequently researched areas of general adaptation and compliance with physicians' instructions. Another problem is that the majority of studies were carried out on groups with wide age spans. It is also noteworthy that although interest in coping with illness rose continually between 1970 and 1995, distinctly more theoretical than empirical works were published during this time. Considering the substantial methodological shortcomings discovered in the two meta-analyses, it is dif-

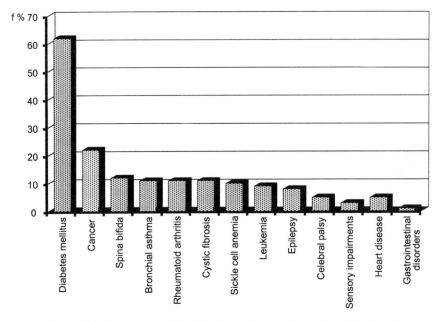

Figure 2.1. Frequencies of studies, depending on illness type. Results of a meta-analysis by Hanl (1995, p. 56).

since the life situations and developmental tasks of a 12 year old differ substantially from those of an 18 year old.

Factors That Influence Coping Processes and Coping Resources

As mentioned in the previous section, most investigators have studied general aspects of dealing with illness, whereas only a fraction of them have specifically examined coping. In the following sections, findings on the developmental, social, and illness-specific factors that play a role in shaping a person's coping resources and abilities are reviewed. The findings summarized in the meta-analyses conducted by Seiffge-Krenke and Brath (1990) and Hanl (1995) form the basis for this discussion. Although the focus here is on diabetic adolescents, findings on adolescent coping in cases of other illnesses will also be covered.

Type of Illness

In their noncategorical approach, Stein and Jessop (1982) emphasized that the specific type of chronic illness does not determine the course of coping and adjustment. Instead, they maintained that any chronic illness represents an existential burden for the adolescent and his or her family. Nevertheless, apart from general stressors resulting from a chronic disease, there appear to be additional burdens for special illness groups. For example, illnesses involving neurological impairments (e.g., cerebral palsy, brain tumors, various forms of epilepsy, and spina bifida) restrict the possibilities for cognitive coping as well as for emotion management strategies, thereby leading to problems in dealing with the illness and achieving a good quality of life. Consequently, it is reasonable to expect that coping behavior may indeed be influenced by the type of illness. This question, however, has not been directly addressed in research. At best, different illness groups have been compared with respect to variables related to coping, such as self-concept or overall symptomatology.

Several studies have failed to find any differences in personality variables and self-concept between illness groups. For example, no differences in emotional sensitivity were found by Howe, Feinstein, Reiss, Molock, and Berger (1993), by Sanger, Copeland, and Davidson (1991), or by Seigel, Golden, Gough, Lashley, and Sacker (1990), nor were Howe et al. (1993) able to distinguish groups on the basis of self-concept. With respect to psychological symptoms and psychiatric illnesses, adolescents with a neurological impairment are at a higher risk than those with cystic fibrosis for developing internalizing as well as externalizing symptoms (Pumariega, Pearson, & Seilheimer, 1993). The study by Howe et al. (1993), which compared adolescents with neurological diseases to those suffering from cystic fibrosis, diabetes, and juvenile arthritis, also revealed that adolescents with neurological illnesses exhibit more problem behavior than healthy adolescents or those with nonneurological illnesses. Nevertheless, the role of illnesses of the central nervous system in developing psychopathological symptomatology is disputed. Sanger et al. (1991) showed that more problem behavior was displayed in adolescents with cancers or brain tumors than in healthy control groups, but no differences between illness groups emerged. Adolescents with orthopedic illnesses, such as juvenile arthritis, appear to be better, or at least as well, adjusted as healthy adolescents and those without overt signs of illness (Wallander et al., 1988). Perrin, Ayoub, and Willett (1993) have suggested that these adolescents may even profit from the fact that their illness is visible to themselves and others because they are not troubled by having to conceal their illness. Indeed, patients seem to have more trouble adjusting to an illness that does not manifest itself in an overt manner. This point has been discussed more frequently with regard to adolescents suffering from diabetes.

Illness Severity

One of the most important illness-specific variables is the severity of the illness. Research has generated quite heterogeneous findings. Some studies have shown that psychological adjustment worsens with increased illness severity (O'Malley, Koocher, Foster, & Slavin, 1979). Other studies comparing different illness groups have also indicated that poor psychological adjustment may be associated with severity of the illness; however, after physical recovery, emotional health can improve (Orr, Weller, Satterwhite, & Pless, 1984). As already mentioned, the visibility of the illness is a particularly important determinant of coping processes. Overt stigmata (e.g., dermatological reactions, bodily disfigurations, or amputated limbs) are frequently accompanied by feelings of insecurity and behavioral disorders, but invisible physical impairments or illnesses may similarly be associated with significant problems (Wallander et al., 1988). Sometimes it can be socially and psychologically easier to come to terms with an openly visible stigma.

From a clinical perspective, it is obvious that illness severity accounts for a certain proportion of variance in psychosocial adaptation and coping with illness. Studies testing this assumption face the problem of defining and operationalizing illness severity. For this task, most studies rely on objective medical data that characterize the respective illness and/or the number of absences from school due to the illness.

Parental descriptions, in contrast, suffer from inconsistencies in reporting, such as a tendency to exaggerate the severity of an illness (Pumariega et al., 1993). For instance, the parents of adolescents with bronchial asthma tend to describe the illness as being more serious than is indicated by objective criteria, such as use of medication, frequency of asthma attacks, and absences from school in the past year (Perrin, 1985). Despite such methodological weaknesses, several studies have found a link between the severity of various illnesses and maladaptation or poor coping (Brown et al., 1992; Billings, Moos, Miller, & Gottlieb, 1987; Greenberg, Kazak, & Meadows, 1989; MacLean, Perrin, Gortmaker, & Pierr, 1992; Patterson, Budd, Goetz, & Warwick, 1993). Billings et al. (1987), for example, analyzed the adjustment of adolescents with arthritis and rheumatoid illnesses. As compared with patients with milder forms of the illnesses, seriously ill patients reported considerably more physical as well as emotional problems (such as increased anxiety and depression). Such patients also reported more absences from school and more performance problems, and their participation in social activities with friends and family was limited. A positive relationship has also been found to exist between illness severity and poor psychological adjustment or poor coping in asthma patients (MacLean et al., 1992).

Illness Duration

The duration of the illness represents an additional factor that may influence coping behavior. One might expect that the longer an illness has played a role in an adolescent's life, the better he or she learns to cope with it. Unfortunately, because of the lack of longitudinal studies, this claim cannot be unequivocally confirmed. In this regard, however, it is surprising that recent research suggests that illness duration exerts no direct effect on the success of psychological or medical adaptation (Malhotra & Malhotra, 1990; Patterson, McCubbin, & Warwick, 1990; Smith, Mauseth, Palmer, Pecoraro, & Wenet, 1991). Although medical adaptation has frequently been assessed by using measures of illness severity (for example, the frequency of asthma attacks in asthma patients or the quality of metabolic control in diabetic patients), most studies have not considered illness duration. La Greca, Follansbee, and Skyler (1990) found no correlation between the duration of an illness and adolescents' overall adjustment, but metabolic control, that is, physiological adaptation, tended to worsen with increased illness duration. In the special case of diabetes, most investigators agree that although physiological adaptation is not necessarily impaired by increased duration of the illness per se, it may be worsened in combination with additional factors, such as age-related hormonal changes (Kager & Holden, 1992) or lower levels of patient compliance with therapeutic recommendations (Hanson et al., 1989). Similar relationships probably also apply for other chronic illnesses, although there are still no studies relating medical parameters to the duration of other illnesses.

Developmental Factors

Developmental factors have been largely neglected in research on coping with chronic illness in adolescence. The variable of age is one exception. Although its influence on coping behavior has been repeatedly demonstrated, few published studies have adequately differentiated samples on the basis of age. Even for adults, the phase of life in which an illness occurs is important. However, a 14 year old is affected by the onset of a severe chronic illness in a very different manner than a 24-year-old adult, who has already achieved most of the developmental tasks that the 14 year old is still confronting. Empirical studies do, in fact, suggest that chronic illness can delay or prevent adolescents from achieving important developmental tasks. Additional problems arise from the specific developmental dynamics of the adolescent age group. Among these are adolescents' increased tendency to daydream and fantasize (Giambra, 1974), their decreasing willingness to disclose personal information to adults (Norell, 1984), and their general inclination to distance themselves from adults and orient themselves more strongly to their peer groups. Participating in peer activities and engaging in risk-taking behaviors, which are specific to this phase of life, can have deleterious consequences for the adolescent's diagnosis, treatment, and compliance.

From a developmental point of view, the age of illness onset is especially relevant because of the close association between cognitive development and coping. A study conducted by Rovet, Ehrlich, and Hoppe (1988) represents one of the few studies to consider this important aspect. In their investigation of 51 children with diabetes, aged 6 to 13 years, younger male patients were found to be particularly psychologically vulnerable. Among the age-related changes described in other studies was an increase with age in intropunitivity (a tendency to blame oneself when anything goes wrong). Control-related and cognitive coping strategies were more frequently used by 13- to 17-year-old cancer patients than by 7- to 12-year-old patients (see, for example, Worchel, Copeland, & Barker, 1988; Grey, Cameron, & Thurber, 1991), and 13- to 15-year-olds showed poorer compliance with physicians' instructions than did younger diabetic patients (Eiser, 1990b). This suggests that compliance can worsen despite increased age and that an increase in cognitive understanding is not always accompanied by improved coping (Hanson et al., 1989; Joy, 1987).

Several studies have confirmed that the burden on chronically ill adolescents increases with age, leading to poorer adaptation to the illness. Kager and Holden (1992) showed that among diabetic adolescents, increasing age was associated with a greater number of negative life events, which in turn corresponded to poorer metabolic control. Adolescents with other chronic illnesses also suffer from more stress or poorer adaptation as they grow older. In adolescents with sickle cell anemia, for example, age is associated with more internalizing problems (Brown et al., 1993b) as well as with more school problems (Hurtig, Koepke, & Park, 1989). In older adolescent rheumatic patients with severe forms of the illness, social problems are multiplied, as may be seen in their frequent absences from school and their participation in fewer social activities. Compliance, too, appears to decrease with age. However, in studies of adolescents with various chronic illnesses including diabetes, other authors have found no relationship between age and maladaptation (Perrin et al., 1993; Sanger et al., 1991; Smith et al., 1991; Wallander et al., 1988; Worchel et al., 1988).

Gender

Gender differences in coping with chronic illness and physical impairments have been confirmed by a series of findings. Male adolescents, for example, find it particularly difficult to come to terms with impairments in strength and physical abilities (Hofmann & Becker, 1973), whereas female adolescents, as they grow older, suffer increasingly from any changes that make them less physically attractive. Studies on healthy adolescents have frequently demonstrated that girls tend to work out tensions and conflicts internally and to develop psychosomatic complaints more frequently than boys, whose reactions are characteristically more overt. These findings are mirrored in studies of chronically ill adolescents. Research has demonstrated that diabetes mellitus and eating disorders (e.g., anorexia nervosa, bulimia nervosa) are comorbid at above chance levels in female adolescents (Rodin et al., 1985). Diabetic adolescent boys are more prone to developing problem behavior, such as antisocial tendencies or aggression (Rovet et al., 1988).

Several studies on diabetic adolescents have shown that girls have better metabolic control (Kager & Holden, 1992; Niemcryk, Speers, Travis, & Gray, 1990). Similar gender differences in adaptation to illness have been found in studies of adolescents with cancer (Sanger et al., 1991). However, the evaluations were quite often made by mothers and teachers and thus could be biased. The finding that girls adapt more positively to some illnesses may be related to their socialization, which encourages them to be part of and maintain social networks. Girls may thus find it easier to find and make use of social structures for dealing with their chronic illness (Kager & Holden, 1992). Nevertheless, the results of gender effects on coping with illness are not uniform, because there are also studies that have revealed no association between gender and adaptation to the illness. For example, in their studies of diabetic adolescents, Smith et al. (1991) and La Greca et al. (1990), as well as Sayer, Hauser, Jacobson, and Bliss (1993), found no link between gender and level of metabolic control.

Personality and Self-Concept

It is difficult to make a general statement about the influence of personality on adolescents' coping with illness, in as much as personality variables fulfill different functions. As a result, they have been analyzed partly as dependent and partly as independent variables and have been operationalized in several ways, including psychosocial adaptation, psychological adjustment, and personality adaptation. The conceptualizations of personality variables as state, trait, and process variables have been analyzed repeatedly in association with coping processes since the research work of Lazarus, Averill, and Opton (1974). Still, very few studies have focused on the relationship between personality variables and coping with illness in adolescent population samples. Koski (1982), for example, showed that alexithymic personality characteristics (an inability to express emotion openly) are accompanied by immature defense and splitting mechanisms in diabetic adolescents. However, research has been inconclusive as to whether the personality construct of extraversion represents a particular risk for diabetic control. As mentioned already in the section on type of illness, a number of studies have failed to find any differences in personality variables between illness groups.

Self-concept takes on an especially meaningful role among the many other personality variables that influence coping. Positive self-esteem is associated with better cooperation with therapy in rheumatoid arthritis (Litt, Cuskey, & Rosenberg, 1982) and in those diabetic adolescents who show good metabolic control (Jacobson et al., 1990). Howe et al. (1993) studied groups of adolescents suffering from a variety of chronic illnesses including neurological diseases, diabetes, cystic fibrosis, and juvenile arthritis. They found no significant differences in self-concept between the different groups, although self-concept was generally poor for all illness types. The observed phenomenon that adolescents with a chronic illness have lower self-esteem than healthy control subjects has been empirically confirmed in several studies (for a summary, see Hanl, 1995).

Social Support

The constant burdens imposed by a chronic illness deplete adolescents' personal resources and abilities to cope if they are unable to tap resources of social support, in particular those provided by the family. The family, however, is not only a social resource. Instead, the family members, the family as a unit, and members of the adolescent's extended social environment are all affected by and react to the illness. In the classic study conducted by Minuchin, Rosman, and Baker (1978), it was shown that unclear role definitions and a lack of problem-solving competence in the family impaired adolescent patients' abilities to cope with the illness. A high degree of conflict in the family also seems to negatively influence psychosocial adjustment in chronic illnesses (Hanson et al., 1992a; Patterson et al., 1993; Wertlieb, Hauser, & Jacobson, 1986). In contrast, families that experience little conflict and exhibit high levels of cohesion, moderate levels of organization, and open expression of feelings contribute to successful coping (Anderson, Auslander, Jung, Miller, & Santiago, 1990; Marteau, Bloch, & Baum, 1987; Murch & Cohen, 1989).

The social support provided by the family must be viewed in the context of a particular family's life circumstances. Several authors therefore distinguish between the family's material resources (e.g., income) and psychological resources (e.g., family climate dimensions of cohesion, conflict, and organization). Family income can be a good predictor of the family's competence in coping (Wallander et al., 1988). The positive influence on psychosocial adjustment in families with ample material resources at their disposal results largely from the family's ability to exhaustively exploit all possibilities of medical treatment.

As far as the family's psychological resources are concerned, most studies have rather uniformly described the positive effects of high family cohesion, open expression of emotions, and low conflict as factors that help to protect the patient from developing problem behavior and psychological symptoms. This has been demonstrated in studies of adolescents with different chronic illnesses, for example, diabetes (Hanson et al., 1992a; Anderson et al., 1990; Wysocki, 1993), cystic fibrosis (Patterson et al., 1993), and sickle cell anemia (Hurtig et al., 1989). However, research has neglected the supportive family's function as a model for coping with illness-specific problems.

In contrast to the large volume of research investigating how family factors influence chronically ill adolescents' coping, only a few studies have explored the role of nonfamilial sources of social support. Outside the family, the adolescent's most important relationships are those with peers and close friends. Having a chronic illness often makes it impossible for the adolescent to attend school regularly and maintain previous levels of school performance. The absences from school due to hospital stays and operations can sometimes be compensated for by exercising an uncommon self-discipline and by relinquishing leisure activities. In the long run, deterioration of health coupled with overt, often unattractive changes in physical appearance, as well as the necessity of being subjected to prolonged medical procedures, can consolidate the sick role and lead to a painful loss of status in peer groups.

These important features have, however, barely been researched. Johnson (1980) showed that only a handful of studies in the previous 20 years had investigated the friendships of chronically ill adolescents. More recent studies have found that chronically ill adolescents feel isolated and shut out (Toeller, 1990); others have reported conflicts with friends (Wallander et al., 1988). From a developmental perspective, the deficit of research on support from outside the family is hard to understand, since gradually separating from the parents and turning to the peer group are as much important developmental goals for the chronically ill as they are for healthy adolescents.

Critical Life Events and Normative Stressors

A chronic illness, because of the stress and demands it imposes, represents a massive intrusion into an individual's life. More and more studies on individuals' everyday burdens and more recent critical life events have shown that these are relevant to the individual's state of physical health (e.g., Brand, Johnson, & Johnson, 1986). Some studies have found an association between stressful life events and metabolic control in diabetes (e.g., Smith et al., 1991; Kager & Holden, 1992; Hanson, Henggeler, & Burghen, 1987), whereas others have failed to find a substantial relationship (e.g., Gilbert, 1992; Niemcryk et al., 1990). To some extent, these contradictory findings result from the failure to distinguish stressful everyday events from critical life events. Furthermore, a stressor might not affect the medical course of an illness or coping directly; rather, the effects may be mediated by other variables (such as the patient's age) or buffered (as by social support). A study by Delamater, Kurtz, Bubb, White, and Santiago (1987) demonstrated the mediating role of coping mechanisms. Their results showed that diabetic adolescents with good, medium, or poor metabolic control did not differ on measures of stress. However, there were differences in coping styles. Adolescents with poor metabolic control displayed far more wishful thinking and avoidance but also sought help more often. All in all, research still excludes too many considerations of how coping processes can vary with different life events and stressful everyday situations.

Universal and Illness-Specific Coping Strategies

As detailed already, only a fraction of the studies published on the topic of coping with chronic illness in adolescence have examined the specific coping strategies that individuals apply in dealing with chronic illness. It is noteworthy that defensive mechanisms were frequently found in these studies. The most common defensive mechanisms in chronically physically ill adolescents are denial and rationalization (Jacobson et al., 1986), which have also been found in psychiatric patients and physically healthy adolescents. The widespread use of denial strategies by chronically ill adolescents has been documented in many studies and has also been found to exist on the interpersonal level, for example, in the collaboration between patient, family, and physician (Reiser, 1987; Erlich, 1987). Aside from these relatively common defensive strategies, uniform coping strategies, such as cognitive and emotional coping efforts, have been found for different types of illnesses. In view of the enormous social and biographical variation among adolescents with different illnesses, along with their differing levels of competence in coping, this is an astonishing result.

While some aspects of coping behavior appear to be universal, there are also indications of illness-specific coping strategies. Controlled comparative studies of physically healthy adolescents and those with various illnesses have found, for example, that asthmatic adolescents are less willing to express emotions, adolescents with hypopituitarism have difficulty dealing adequately with frustrating situations, and adolescents with severe acne display extremely restricted social contact (Drotar, Owens, & Gotthold, 1981; Hanl, 1995). This suggests that coping processes are determined by the stressors associated with particular illnesses as well as by more general burdens and conditions. There are only isolated examples of comparative studies among different illness groups, and these have mostly focused on psychosocial adjustment and compliance; ill adolescents' coping was not in the foreground (Berman, 1983).

This section has summarized research on coping with illness in adolescence, based on two meta-analyses of published studies. The focus of interest here has been on coping processes and resources. Many conceptual and methodological problems were uncovered. For example, most of the studies included adolescents belonging to a narrow age range. This and the practice of combining a variety of illness groups into convenience samples, along with the absence of control groups and longitudinal designs, make it difficult to assess the outcome of research. Although there are many findings related to illness-specific and universal effects on coping, overall they are most heterogeneous. Different aspects (coping, compliance, and adaptation) were often intermixed. Aspects of general adaptation, such as adjustment or psychopathology, were most prominent. Maladjustment was frequently equated with poor coping. Among those studies assessing specific coping strategies, defense mechanisms were frequently reported. Since the studies seldom followed the illness process longitudinally, many of the contradictory findings could be related to differences in the time points of assessment. Furthermore, developmental factors were rarely examined. In addition, the fact that illness severity was not always appropriately considered could be responsible for some of the controversial findings.

Psychopathology

As mentioned already, a considerable number of studies on coping with illness in adolescence have looked at psychosocial adjustment. Again, the focus has largely been on the negative outcome of psychopathology. In the past two decades, over 168 studies have been conducted to test whether adolescents afflicted with a chronic illness are at higher risk for developing psychopathology. The results, however, are inconclusive. Some epidemiological overviews (Gortmaker et al., 1990) have documented greater psychosocial morbidity in the chronically ill. Psychological symptoms and problem behavior have been found, for example, in adolescents with sickle cell anemia (Hurtig et al., 1989), bronchial asthma (MacLean et al., 1992), cancer (Olson et al., 1983a), cystic fibrosis (Pumariega et al., 1993), various neurological diseases (Howe et al., 1993), spina bifida (Wallander et al., 1988), diabetes mellitus (Rovet et al., 1988), and juvenile rheumatoid arthritis (Daniels, Moos, Billings, & Miller, 1987). The majority of these studies compared symptomatologies of ill and healthy adolescents. These results seem to support Stein and Jessop's (1982) noncategorical approach, which assumes that the mere presence of a chronic illness places certain burdens on the afflicted adolescents and their families. Still, it is important to consider how prevalence rates vary across illness groups. For example, while 31% of neurological patients display problem behavior on a clinical level, the rate is only 4% in patients with cystic fibrosis (Pumariega et al., 1993).

While externalizing symptoms, such as problem behavior, can be operationalized quite well, internalizing symptoms are considerably more difficult to assess. This is partly because of the high comorbidity of internalizing symptoms, such as anxiety disorders or depression. As Grey et al. (1991) showed, emotional disturbances, such as anxiety and depression, are closely intertwined and linked with poor coping behavior and unsatisfactory adjustment to a chronic disease. The pessimistic, anxious style of attribution that accompanies depression can hamper effective coping with an illness (Brown, Doepke, & Kaslow, 1993a; Schoenherr, Brown, Baldwin, & Kaslow, 1992). For example, severe anxiety can interfere with metabolic control in patients with diabetes, because the production of stress hormones raises blood sugar levels, thereby affecting adjustment. As Niemcryk et al. (1990) demonstrated, 75% of the variance in blood sugar levels can be explained by the interaction of anxiety, gender, and prior hemoglobin A_1c (HbA_1c) values.

It is often expected that adolescents with chronic diseases will be more vulnerable to developing emotional disturbances on both subclinical and clinical levels. In a study by Pumariega et al. (1993), adolescents with cystic fibrosis were above the clinical cutoff point for depression and anxiety. A comparison between adolescents with cystic fibrosis and adolescents with diagnosed psychiatric disorders revealed both considerable differences and considerable similarities between the groups with respect to the amount of expressed fear and anxiety (Thompson, Hodges, & Hamlett, 1990). As compared with healthy adolescents, subclinical yet elevated levels of psychopathology have also been found in adolescents with bronchial asthma, rheumatic heart disease, and various kinds of cancer (Malhotra & Malhotra, 1990). Another study conducted by Engström (1992) on adolescents with Crohn's disease and ulcerative colitis showed that 60% of the sample population had emotional disturbances.

Other authors have failed to demonstrate higher rates of internalizing symptoms. Niemcryk et al. (1990) found no increase in the depression and anxiety ratings of diabetic adolescents, in contrast to the previously mentioned study by Seigel et al. (1990). Similarly, Greenberg et al. (1989) reported no differences between healthy adolescents and those who had survived serious cancer with respect to the frequency and severity of depressive symptoms or the occurrence of anxiety. Even in comparisons between healthy adolescents and those who had experienced acute cancer, no significant differences in anxiety were evident (Goertzel & Goertzel, 1991). Another study (Fife, Norton, & Groom, 1987) found that patients with various types of cancer were in comparatively good emotional condition, despite the life-threatening nature of the illness. However, this finding has not been consistently replicated in other studies.

Altogether, these findings suggest that the relationship between chronic illness and psychopathology is far from understood. While some studies have revealed clearly increased levels of symptoms, others have reported an increase of symptoms only on a subclinical level. Other studies found no differences at all between chronically ill adolescents and physically healthy control subjects. These contradictory results are probably related to the fact that most studies did not control for the duration and severity of illness. Moreover, they rarely took the time phases of the illness into account. The time around diagnosis, the chronic phase, the time after successful treatment or recovery, and the terminal period all involve different stressors, along with different amounts of social support that might buffer the adverse effects of stress. Although comparisons with healthy control subjects might be considered appropriate for some time phases (e.g., around the time of first diagnosis), for others they are certainly not. This has already been recognized by Koocher and O'Malley (1981, p. 48), who asked:

> How does the survivor of childhood cancer compare with a matched person in the street who is not a survivor of cancer?

A further issue pertains to whether outcomes are measured globally or specifically. Nearly half of the studies used a global measure of psychopathology, whereas roughly one third assessed specific disorders. Internalizing symptoms were found most often.

In summary, studies on the links between chronic physical illness and psychopathology suffer from major limitations and thus have produced contradictory results. An explanation of these links would be highly relevant to the understanding of coping. It is well known that adolescents with clinical disorders show poorer coping skills than normal adolescents (Seiffge-Krenke, 1993a). The coping style of chronically ill adolescents could be impaired if behavioral or emotional problems existed alongside the chronic illness.

3

Coping with Diabetes:
A Longitudinal Study

In this book the challenges of coping with chronic illness are examined, with the focus on one illness in particular, namely, insulin-dependent diabetes mellitus (IDDM), which is also known as diabetes mellitus type I or juvenile-onset diabetes. Diabetes is a comparatively frequently occurring chronic disease in adolescence and exhibits the typical aspects of a chronic illness as detailed in chapter 1. The manifestation of diabetes confronts patients and their families with a flood of questions, and the demands on the adolescent's understanding, self-discipline, and responsibilities are very high. The medical treatment regimen is relatively burdensome, and the consequences of not following physicians' instructions may be severe and even life-threatening. Consequently, compliance and adherence are highly relevant aspects to be considered in assessing the coping process. An analysis of coping processes, however, must be embedded in the context of the adolescent's family and extended social environment. Furthermore, the adolescent's overall developmental progression needs to be taken into account.

After the main medical features of diabetes have been described, a preliminary model for understanding the relationships among variables involved in the process of coping with a chronic illness is outlined. This model may serve as a guide in the discussions of the theoretical questions related to coping. Then, a 4-year longitudinal study of diabetic adolescents and their families, which aimed to integrate medical, developmental, psychosocial, and family dynamics perspectives, is presented. Finally, a broader model of coping with diabetes in adolescence is put forth, which will serve as a framework for discussion of the specific topics to be dealt with in the following chapters.

Insulin-Dependent Diabetes Mellitus

Medical Characteristics

Insulin-dependent diabetes mellitus is a complex metabolic disorder. It is characterized by an absolute or relative lack of circulating insulin. It develops as a consequence of an imbalance between insulin production and release on the one hand and hormonal or tissue factors modifying the insulin requirement on the other hand. Insulin, a hormone produced by beta cells of the pancreas and secreted into the blood, facilitates entry of glucose to body cells. Without insulin, excess glucose accumulates in the blood. The cells, deprived of their main source of energy, turn to the body's energy reserves, beginning with glycogen, then proceeding to protein and ultimately fat, for sustenance. The burning of fat leads to the formation of highly acidic ketones, which also accumulate in the blood. The kidneys work overtime in an effort to clear the blood of both excess glucose and ketones, resulting in frequent urination. This leads to dehydration and concurrent losses of essential substances such as sodium.

The diagnosis of diabetes is frequently suggested by a history of polydipsia (excessive thirst), polyuria (excessive urination), and polyphagia (excessive food intake), associated with weight loss. A clinical suggestion of diabetes is confirmed by finding glucose in the urine and by detecting an abnormally elevated blood glucose level. Left untreated, insulin-dependent diabetes leads inevitably to death caused by the metabolic consequences of insulin insufficiency. In essence, the cells "starve" in the presence of sufficient foodstuffs (Hauser, Jacobson, Benes, & Anderson, 1997).

Insulin-dependent diabetes mainly strikes children and adolescents and accounts for 10% of all known cases of diabetes. It is the most frequently occurring endocrine disorder in American and European adolescents. Although the exact cause of the disorder is not known, several factors, including heredity and viral infections, are thought to play a role.

Medical treatment of diabetes primarily strives to maintain blood glucose levels within a range that avoids wide swings, which may lead to severe hyperglycemia or hypoglycemia. The status of a diabetic patient's metabolic adaptation may be assessed by monitoring certain physiological parameters at regular intervals, for example, by regularly testing blood and urine sugar levels. Most physicians use glycosylated hemoglobin (HbA_1 or HbA_1c) values. The HbA_1 or HbA_1c value, that is, the fraction of glycosylated hemoglobin in the blood, provides information about the average state of the metabolism over the preceding 4 to 8 weeks.

Insulin replacement is only possible by injection. Most diabetics are therefore required to perform daily injections of insulin at specific intervals. The timing of insulin injections must be balanced with food intake and energy expenditure on a daily basis. Inability to maintain sufficient metabolic control can result in long-term physical damage, such as retinopathy, nephropathy, cardiovascular disease, and peripheral vascular problems leading to gangrene of the limbs.

Impact on the Afflicted Adolescents and Their Families

The course of diabetes is characterized by several phases related to dealing with the first diagnosis, hospitalization for initial treatment, and the corresponding curative procedures. Diabetes is not a static illness. While the need for insulin replacement in the first weeks following diagnosis typically decreases, it usually increases and remains at a stable level a year or two after onset of the illness. Generally, a critical time takes place around the start of puberty, when hormonal changes interfere with therapeutic efforts to maintain metabolic control.

The management of diabetes places a variety of complex demands on both the patient and the family. For example, insulin injections must be performed at specified times, blood and urine glucose levels must be tested, and dietary regulations must be followed. Successful therapy will first depend on how well the patient and the patient's family have been instructed about and understood the treatment. Obviously, successful therapy requires that the patient be conscientious about following instructions. In this regard, the burden of illness management is largely placed on the adolescents themselves. The adolescent has to live by the clock and to administer insulin at predetermined times during the day. Adhering to diet and checking blood and urine glucose levels are also important daily activities. Yet, these are not necessarily matters that concern the adolescent alone. Although it is essentially up to the diabetic adolescent patient to carry out the procedures belonging to the treatment regimen and to maintain adequate blood glucose levels, the parents still need to monitor their adolescent on a continual basis. In addition, numerous family activities are interrupted or impaired by diabetes management, including mealtimes and leisure time activities. Thus, it is obvious that the onset of diabetes leads to quite radical changes in the adolescent's and the family's life-styles. Finally, the chronicity of the stressor has a major impact on the adolescent's ongoing life and future, and in part, on those of the family as well. The threat of long-term physical damage poses additional burdens on adolescents with diabetes and their families.

A Preliminary Model

Diabetes is the most common metabolic illness in adolescence both in Europe and in the United States (Newacheck & Taylor, 1992; Seiffge-Krenke, 1998a). As detailed in chapter 2, it is one of the most frequently occurring illnesses in adolescence and has recently received increased attention in research. In 1995, 62% of all published studies on coping with chronic illness in adolescence were concerned with diabetes. Seiffge-Krenke and Brath's (1990) and Hanl's (1995) overviews unanimously revealed that coping processes were typically neglected in research. Instead, the majority of studies focused on global indices of adaptation or maladaptation. At best, investigators typically elected to study several psychological variables that might be associated with metabolic control or compliance. Among these were the patient's knowledge of the illness, developmental age, and various stressors, as well as social support systems. Most studies were cross-sectional and produced weak to moderate correlations.

In addition, many results were contradictory, as seen in the controversy over the mental health of diabetic adolescents (see chapter 2). Another critical point was that many studies employed a univariate approach (or "shotgun approach" as La Greca [1988, p. 156] ironically described it) in analyzing a range of variables. Such an approach cannot do justice to the complexity of the events and processes involved with the illness. What is truly lacking is a theoretical framework on the basis of which previous and further research work in this field can be compared and assessed and that would permit hypotheses to be appropriately and reliably tested. Above all, in creating such a theoretical model, the complexity and interrelatedness of the variables outlined above must be taken into consideration. La Greca's (1988) model, presented in Figure 3.1, is restricted to the control of diabetes and as such reflects only one aspect of coping with illness; nevertheless, it does offer a useful starting point.

According to the model, psychosocial factors are organized into levels of increasing complexity. Factors on one level can interact with those on another and thus mask or potentiate their effects. Nevertheless, although the factors included in the model are important for diabetic control, the selection is not exhaustive. A more complete model must also contain the diachronic perspective because coping is a complex process spread out across a long time span, which affects individuals in particular ways depend-

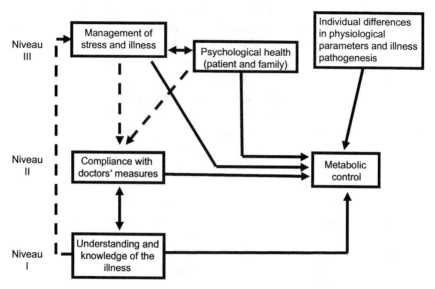

Figure 3.1. Psychosocial factors related to diabetic control (modified from La Greca, 1988).

ing on their current situations and psychosocial histories. Consequently, the developmental perspective must also be considered, along with interactions between individual and environment. Such interactions are, for example, apparent in the ways parents influence their ill child's coping processes. When an adolescent family member falls ill, changes may occur in the parents' and siblings' life situations and psychosocial conditions, which may in turn affect the adolescent patient. Such changes have barely been studied to date.

A Longitudinal Approach to Studying Coping with Diabetes in Adolescence

In the following, findings from the first 4 years of an ongoing longitudinal investigation[1] of coping with diabetes from a developmental perspective will be presented. A general aim of the study has been to describe adolescent adaptation to the illness, especially in relation to developmental pro-

---

[1] The research project was supported by the Bundesminister für Forschung und Technologie (BFT Grant No. 0706567) from 1991 to 1995 and the Deutsche Forschungsgemeinschaft (DFG Grant No. Se 408/10-1) from 1995 to 1997 and in 2000 (DFG Grant No. Se 408/10-4).

gression and psychological health. Another important aim of this study has been to identify the specific stressors related to this disease. Furthermore, this study has endeavored to systematically observe and document how diabetic adolescents and their families cope with this illness over time. In particular, attempts have been made to identify which coping strategies adolescents employ in each phase of the illness. In this regard, it has been important to learn what kind of assistance is offered by the adolescents' social support network (friends and family) and the medical system (e.g., physicians) and to what extent such assistance is utilized. Another point of interest has been to learn if and how adolescents' personal resources (e.g., self-concept) affect how they deal with this burden. Changes in family dynamics and parental roles as a result of an adolescent developing a severe chronic illness have also been important aspects. The significance of these changes becomes especially apparent when one considers that the onset of a chronic illness around the time when adolescents are normally beginning to distance themselves from the parents might delay their mastery of certain developmental tasks.

Due to the low incidence of the disease, diabetic adolescents were recruited from a total of 17 hospitals in Germany. Every effort was made to ensure that the sample population closely matched healthy adolescents. It was especially important to study adolescents who had only recently been diagnosed with diabetes. A total of 109 diabetic adolescents participated in the study, as well as 119 healthy adolescents and their families. The majority of families in the sample were intact, with both parents married to each other or living together. The diabetic adolescents' physicians also participated in the study. The study began when the adolescents were about 13 years old. As indicated above, this study is still in progress, and the participants in the original sample are currently being followed up as they make the transition to early adulthood.

The results of four longitudinal surveys, conducted from 1991 until 1994, are reported here. Adolescents, their parents, and their physicians participated in each of the annual surveys, which included extensive questionnaires as well as interviews concerning stress, coping, and interpersonal relationships. Adaptation to the illness was measured according to three criteria: the realization of the developmental tasks typical of this age group, the frequency of behavior and emotional problems, and the level of metabolic control. After this general overview of the study, its important features, such as the sample population, its representativeness, and the instruments used, will be described. Further details can be found under the individual section headings elsewhere in this book.

Sample Characteristics

Adolescents. A total of 228 early adolescents (M = 13.9 years, SD = 1.28) participated in the first survey in 1991. At the time of the fourth survey in 1994, the sample consisted of 198 adolescents (M = 16.9 years, SD = 1.25). The gender ratio was balanced in each survey. About half of the participants suffered from diabetes (first survey, 109 diabetic and 119 healthy control subjects; second survey, 99 diabetic and 111 healthy control subjects; third survey, 93 diabetic and 109 healthy control subjects; fourth survey, 91 diabetic and 107 healthy control subjects). The dropout rate over four annual surveys was low, with 198 of the original 228 adolescents continuing their participation to the end of the fourth year. Somewhat more diabetic adolescents (16%) dropped out than healthy peers (10%); however, the difference was not significant.

Parents. A total of 387 parents participated in the first survey (218 mothers and 169 fathers). These included 100 mothers and 79 fathers of adolescents in the diabetic group, along with 118 mothers and 90 fathers of healthy adolescents. Here, too, the dropout rate was low, ranging from 8 to 16%. By the time of the fourth survey, a total of 336 parents were still participating, including 152 parents of diabetics (86 mothers and 66 fathers) and 184 parents of healthy adolescents (103 mothers and 81 fathers).

Physicians. The diabetic adolescents' physicians were also asked to participate in the study. Of 103 physicians who took part in the first survey, 82 continued their participation to the fourth survey, which corresponds to a dropout rate of 21%. The gender ratio remained even across time.

Demographic and Socioeconomic Characteristics of the Sample. All participants resided in Germany. Of the adolescent sample, 89% were German nationals. The remaining 11% did not have German citizenship; they and their families were of Turkish, Italian, or Greek origin but had lived and/or worked in Germany for over 10 years and had a good command of German. Altogether, 81% of the adolescents were raised in two-parent families; 19% were raised in single-parent or divorced families. The percentage of families with both parents present was 84% for the group of diabetic adolescents and 76% for the healthy group. The families had an average of 2.3 children. All of the fathers and 65% of the mothers were employed. Most of the diabetic adolescents were middle-class, and 25% belonged to the upper socioeconomic class. The comparatively high percentage of upper-class youths in the group of healthy adolescents (39%) is worth mentioning. The parents' levels of education differed correspondingly between groups, with parents of diabetic adolescents having somewhat lower levels of education than parents of healthy adolescents. However, adolescents' educational levels did not differ between groups, as 74% of the diabetic adolescents and 79% of the healthy adolescents attended the same type of secondary school (*Gymnasium,* a type of German high school).

Medical Data of the Diabetic Sample. Glycosylated hemoglobin (HbA$_1$ or HbA$_1$c) values served as criteria for metabolic control in the group of diabetic adolescents. These laboratory values were determined immediately before the research project team members visited the families at home. At the beginning of the study, the sample was divided into three groups according to their status of metabolic control. Based on the physicians' reports, 25% of the adolescents had good metabolic control (HbA$_1$ < 7.6, HbA$_1$c < 6.5); 48% had satisfactory metabolic control (HbA$_1$ from 7.6 to 9.5, HbA$_1$c from 6.6 to 8.5); and only 27% displayed poor control (HbA$_1$ > 9.5, HbA$_1$c > 8.6). Gender differences were insignificant. Thus on the whole, the adolescents showed a positive physiological adjustment. The mean duration of illness at the first survey was 5.4 years: 10% of the diabetic adolescents had been ill for less than 1 year, 22% for 1 to 2 years, 22% for 3 to 5 years, and the remaining 46% for over 5 years. At the beginning of the study, more than 90% of the adolescents injected themselves with insulin and were responsible for adhering to their diets as well as for performing their daily blood sugar and urine tests.

Representativeness. The representativeness of the diabetic sample was checked by comparing biographical and social data with the distributions provided by the German Federal Bureau of Statistics for a sample of German adolescents of the same age (Statistisches Bundesamt, 1991). The variables examined were gender and schooling of the adolescents, along with the parent's age, nationality, type of employment, level of education, marital status, and number of children. The sample of diabetic adolescents was found to be representative of adolescents of the same age for most age-relevant variables. However, the sample did differ from other research samples of diabetic adolescents (Roth, Neuper, & Borkenstein, 1988; Hanson et al., 1987; Kulzer, 1992) by having a shorter average illness duration and showing slightly better metabolic control at the beginning of the study.

Altogether, the diabetic sample in this study may be considered to be largely representative in terms of the variables analyzed. An attempt was made to select participants for the healthy control group so that a "research twin" existed for each ill adolescent, and this was largely achieved. Age and gender distributions did not differ between groups, nor did variables associated with family structure (intactness of the family, number of siblings) or educational levels. As already mentioned, there was a small difference in socioeconomic status, with slightly more adolescents in the healthy sample belonging to the upper socioeconomic classes. This difference was statistically controlled for in all further analyses. No statistical differences were found between the characteristics of those families that participated in all four surveys and those who dropped out. The remaining sample was still representative with respect to the selection criteria.

Procedure: Recruitment of the Sample, Annual Survey, Care and Maintenance of the Sample

Recruiting the Participants. Adolescents diagnosed with insulin-dependent diabetes mellitus were recruited from hospitals offering outpatient care. During a 9-month period, all adolescents and parents who had made appointments in 17 different hospitals and specialized clinics were asked to participate in the study. These hospitals and clinics provided primary treatment facilities for children and adolescents with IDDM in Germany and offered standard care for adolescents, such as regular blood and urine tests or dietary assistance. The centers typically recommended that the adolescents participate in annual summer camps for diabetes education. Of the families that were approached in these hospitals, 88% agreed to participate in the study. Families that had early adolescents (aged 12 to 14 years) and that were largely representative with respect to the criteria mentioned in the previous section were selected for participation in the study. The healthy adolescents and their families were recruited by written requests distributed in various schools. Of these families, 79% agreed to participate. In the sample of healthy adolescents, the age range was fixed from 12 to 14 years, and their families were selected to match the families with a diabetic adolescent according to parents' marital status, number of siblings, and adolescent's educational level.

In the individual requests to participate, it was made clear to all potential participants that a longitudinal study about coping with chronic illness in the context of adolescent development was planned. It was explained that it involved annual interviews with ill as well as healthy adolescents together with their families at home. Parents were requested to complete a letter of consent. It is worth mentioning that the recruited diabetic adolescents and their families were highly motivated to participate in the study. Also, it was surprising to experience so few difficulties in recruiting healthy controls. It appeared that the adolescents and their families agreed to participate because they themselves were genuinely interested in the developmentally relevant questions to be examined, such as self-concept, body image, relationships with friends, and family interactions. The ease with which the sample was recruited, with the exception of the very recently diagnosed diabetics (see the explanations of seasonal variation in chapter 4), and the high rate of continued participation over the years indicate that the study contained interesting and motivating aspects for the families with healthy and ill adolescents alike.

Procedure for the Annual Surveys. After the initials contacts were made and the research plan explained to the families in more detail, appointments for further meetings were made for each family. From 1991 to 1994, the research project team members visited the families at home each summer and carried out interviews first with the adolescent, then with the parents, and finally with the entire family. Each individual interview covered aspects of the adolescent's development over the previous year (e.g., leisure activities, academic achievements, family relations, friendships, romantic relationships, and career plans). In interviews with the parents, the parents were asked to give their perspectives on their child's development and answer specific questions about family development, family stress, and family interaction. In families with a diabetic adolescent, inquiries were made about individual and family coping with the illness. This included reaction to the diagnosis, attitude to diabetes, compliance with physicians' instructions, diabetes-specific problems, and coping strategies. Because of the range of topics covered, interviews took place during an entire afternoon; the average interview duration in families with healthy adolescents (2 hours) was shorter than that with the ill adolescents' families (3 hours).

After the interviews, adolescents and their parents were requested to fill out a set of questionnaires. In designing the layout and organization of the questionnaires, every possible attempt was made to use ideas appropriate to the age groups. For example, a dwarflike cartoon character guided the adolescents through the test booklet, and numerous comics commented on and illustrated the contents. The questionnaire packets, divided into three separate parts, were to be completed within 3 weeks and sent back to the research project team members. The families each received 50 German marks per survey as compensation for their time.

The physicians responsible for the diabetic adolescents' treatment were sent a two-page questionnaire requesting information about their patients' metabolic control, cooperation, and compliance as well as an evaluation of their patients' development relative to their ages. Questionnaire packets from the families were sent back quite quickly, whereas the physicians tended to need more prompting to return the materials.

Care and Maintenance of the Survey Sample. Close contact was maintained with all the families that took part in the study. Each project team member was assigned responsibility for specific families, the ratio of families with a healthy adolescent to families with a diabetic adolescent being kept even. This team member was responsible for interviewing those families over the entire 4 years, so that each family always met with the same interviewer. A short profile of each family was prepared containing significant data, such as family structure, living conditions, special incidents, and stressors as well as degree of cooperation with the research team members. Before each new round of house visits, the interviewer would read the relevant profile to prepare for meeting the family again. Following the interview, the team member wrote up a short summary of the interview, and the profile was updated accordingly.

In general, one or two telephone calls were necessary to remind families to return their test packets. This was quite understandable in view of the volume of questions and tasks assigned to them. The fact that so many families participated in all the surveys suggests that not merely the contents of the questions but also the form of contact with the project team members and the continuity of the relationship were important to them.

The contact between a family and the responsible project team member was often very close. Sometimes a team member would receive telephone calls between interviews, usually when something special had happened or if a question needed explanation. Aside from this, each adolescent was sent amusing Christmas and birthday cards each year, which were well received. Not infrequently, the adolescents called to thank the research project team for the greetings and congratulations. Brief annual reports about the progress of the project were prepared for the adolescents and their families and were mailed or brought to them on the occasion of the following interview. The physicians also received these reports.

Cooperation with Physicians and Psychotherapists

All members of the research project team believed that it would be beneficial to the participants and the project team members to encourage the professionals involved in the study to share their expertise and opinions in matters pertaining to specific problems the participants might have during the study. Thus, in addition to seminars held for the purpose of reviewing individual cases, regular meetings with the attending physicians and psychotherapists were planned to exchange pertinent information related to the progress of the study as well as to discuss any questions related to medical problems or psychological disturbances that the participants might show.

Case Discussions during Project Team Meetings. In the framework of meetings relating to the progress of the study, individual families were discussed in regular case seminars. About two families were reviewed in each meeting. Analysis of the families' longitudinal profiles was one objective of these discussions. Additional aims of the case discussions were to understand what caused particular problems as well as to determine which concrete measures might be suggested to assist the family in solving the problems. For example, should counseling or psychotherapy be suggested to an adolescent who had developed an eating disorder? Although the cases usually involved families with poorly adjusted diabetics, problems needing discussion also arose in families with healthy adolescents. It is worth mentioning that the case seminars were exceptionally productive. Above all, they profited greatly from the contributions of the project team members, whose extensive clinical experience and training in psychoanalysis and other forms of psychotherapy proved to be highly useful in understanding the nature of the participants' and their families' problems.

Supervision by Psychotherapists. In parallel to the case seminars, all members of the project team participated twice annually in a consultation with a trained psychoanalyst. One central aim of these consultations was to better understand the psychodynamics of some problem families; another aim was to be advised about the possible preventive or therapeutic measures. The collaboration with an external expert was very fruitful, and new insights into the participating families were often gained.

Colloquium with the Physicians. All physicians were regularly informed about the progress of the research project. The contact with a few of the participating physicians was more extensive. The idea of discussing questions in a joint medical-psychological colloquium arose from this close contact. The study's results were reviewed in biannual seminars, with various themes, such as "Developmental Factors Contributing to Metabolic Instability," "Coping with Illness: The Viewpoint of Adolescents and Their Parents," and "Developmental Delay through Chronic Illness?" The ideas and contributions of medical experts assisted the research project team in important ways, for example, in defining the objective boundaries for good and poor metabolic control.

Methods: Interviews, Questionnaires, and Family Tasks

Interviews. As mentioned, several interviews were carried out in each annual round of surveys. These interviews were semistructured and dealt with a general set of questions (concerning the adolescent generally and the family generally), which were employed in both samples. In the adolescent generally interviews, adolescents were asked about experiences in school, friendships, dating, and romantic relationships. These topics were also touched on from the families' perspectives in the family generally interviews and supplemented by family-related questions about unusual stressors in the family, family dynamics, sibling relationships, etc. In families with a diabetic adolescent, the standard, general questions were supplemented by additional questions pertaining to individual coping and family coping. In the interviews about individual coping, the adolescents were asked about illness-specific stress and coping ability. Similar questions were also posed in the interviews about family coping, in which the interview guide developed by Hauser et al. (1988a) was largely adhered to. Interviews were carried out both with parents and with the adolescent alone. Finally, there was a common interview session with the adolescent and his or her family together to discuss family coping with illness and to solve a problem together, the Family Interaction Task (FIT) (Condon, Cooper, & Grotevant, 1984). This task concluded the session.

Questionnaires. Corresponding to the format of the interviews (division into general and illness-specific aspects) and the topics discussed (stressors, coping strategies, social support, family climate), the test packages contained two sections. The first part measured general variables relevant to both groups of adolescents (for example, self-concept, stressors, coping strategies, achievement of developmental tasks, body image, perceived health, and psychopathology); the second, administered only to the diabetic subjects, concerned illness-specific aspects (for example, knowledge of the illness, attitude to diabetes, compliance, illness-specific stressors, and coping strategies). The parents of both adolescent groups received the same test sections containing questions pertaining to general stressors and family coping strategies along with estimates of their child's psychological health. The parents of diabetic adolescents filled out an additional questionnaire about how the family coped with the illness. Physicians only filled out a short questionnaire.

The selection and application of test procedures was carried out following a "funnel principle." In total, 25 instruments were applied consistently across all surveys. A large number of variables were assessed in the adolescents, considerably fewer in their parents, and the least in the physicians. This funnel principle followed from the idea that the adolescent should be the focus of the study.

In summary, this was a process–outcome study, which followed healthy and diabetic adolescents, starting in early adolescence, and their families over a course of 4 years. The overall developmental changes in families with a diabetic adolescent were compared with those in families with a healthy adolescent. In the group of diabetic adolescents, emphasis was placed on examining the interaction between adaptation to the illness and developmental progression. In this regard, great importance was assigned to eliciting the different perspectives of the adolescents themselves, along with the views of their parents, siblings, and physicians, and integrating these perspectives into the analysis.

A Developmentally Oriented Model of Coping with Diabetes in Adolescence

The overview of research results on coping with chronic illness in adolescence in chapter 2 has made it clear that previous research has suffered from many methodological and conceptual weaknesses. One significant methodological problem common to most of the studies reviewed in both meta-analyses was the absence of control groups. The conceptual weaknesses have been many. For one, too many studies have focused on the aspects of general adaptation, compliance with medical advice, or the pattern of symptoms in the chronically ill. The strongly clinical orientation of previous research is particularly noticeable in the dominance of studies investigating chronically ill adolescents' symptomatology and defensive processes in dealing with the illness. Too few studies have attempted to identify adaptive coping strategies used in dealing with the illness.

Furthermore, although an adolescent's chronic illness is inevitably treated in the context of the family and can lead to massive changes in family roles and responsibilities, most investigators have not considered the family's perspective on coping processes. Only 9% of the studies examined in the first meta-analysis of studies on the subject (Seiffge-Krenke & Brath, 1990) dealt with family coping strategies. The perspectives of the physicians treating the patients have remained almost entirely unknown.

Above all, the developmental aspect has hardly been addressed. In this regard, the scarcity of longitudinal studies represents a major deficit. Seiffge-Krenke and Brath (1990) found that only 11% of the studies published between 1970 and 1988 were longitudinal; Hanl (1995) found a rate of merely 8% from 1989 to 1995. Because the majority of studies used a cross-sectional design, no appropriate conclusions can be drawn about general progress in coping and adaptation. At best, extrapolating statements have been made, based on a summation of means taken from a sample with a large range of ages. A developmental orientation for examining the specific influences and conditional factors in a more homogeneous group (in terms of age) is clearly lacking. Such a developmental orientation would, of course, encourage the use of longitudinal experimental designs to explain development and change. In any case, this kind of approach is especially suitable for this age group, because it is generally important to understand how adolescents deal with the abundance of various normative developmental stressors occurring during this time. If a chronic illness should occur in this phase, then the adolescent is doubly confronted with a nonnormative and highly demanding stressor in addition to normative developmental stressors. The combination of these stressors might overtax the adolescent's coping competence, particularly immediately after diagnosis.

Social support systems may be most decisive for ensuring positive adaptation, as they can help the adolescent to cope with the illness or other developmental tasks. Owing to the changing quality of the parent–child relationship at this age, friends and romantic partners become increasingly important. However, although the family represents a significant source of social support, the parents themselves may be worried and burdened by the illness and its course. In addition, their adaptive and maladaptive forms of coping with problems can serve as a model for the adolescent. In the phase of separation from the parents, other adults take on a significant role for the adolescent. This phenomenon, although frequently described in the literature (Blos, 1973), has not received enough attention in research. The close, long-standing relationship a chronically ill adolescent develops with his or her physician deserves similar consideration.

This chapter began by presenting La Greca's (1988) model of psychosocial factors related to diabetic control. Then, a 4-year longitudinal study of healthy and diabetic adolescents and their families, which aimed to integrate medical, developmental, psychosocial, and family dynamics perspectives, was briefly outlined. This study encouraged the development of a broader model for understanding the process of coping with chronic illness in adolescence. Figure 3.2 provides a general outline of this developmental model of coping with diabetes, which may serve as a guide for understanding the relationships among the complex questions to be explored in the following chapters.

The following chapters, which are oriented toward the results of the longitudinal study introduced in this chapter, will examine these associations in detail. Adaptation to the illness and overall development was assessed in a longitudinal study of early adolescents with diabetes and compared with the development of healthy adolescents until both groups approached late adolescence. Illness-specific factors, such as the duration and severity of the illness, played an important role in that they represented additional, objective terms of reference with which a comparison of coping processes could be made. Furthermore, numerous developmental variables, such as self-

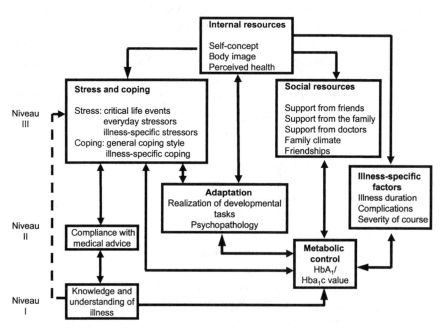

Figure 3.2. Developmental model of coping with diabetes in adolescence.

concept, body image, relationships with parents and friends, normative and illness-specific stressors, and general and illness-specific coping abilities, were assessed in both groups. Symptomatology and the realization of developmental tasks were selected for both groups as measures of general adaptation. In the group of diabetic adolescents, HbA_1 or HbA_1c values were additionally used to assess medical adaptation. Although the focus of this study was on the adolescents in the entire context of their development, parental and sibling perspectives and details about the entire family situation were considered to be important aspects related to the coping process. In addition, the viewpoints of the physicians involved in the medical care of the diabetic adolescents were included. Thus, information was obtained about coping with illness in the context of development from three different sources: the adolescents, their parents, and the physicians responsible for treatment. Furthermore, the psychological data were linked to the "hard" medical facts, such as quality of metabolic control.

As shown in Figure 3.2, medical and psychological variables are closely intertwined. Attitudes and knowledge about the illness are necessary but not sufficient conditions for good adjustment to diabetes in terms of metabolic control. It is reasonable to assume that stressors in general, as well as illness-specific stressors, have an impact on knowledge of the illness, attitudes about the illness, and compliance. They can lead to the use of certain illness-specific coping strategies, which are embedded in the general coping register available to the adolescent in dealing with everyday stressors. Since coping skills are dependent on social relationships, many coping strategies are supported by the use of social resources, advice, and help from parents and friends. Indeed, people close to the adolescent, including physicians, could also represent important coping models. Yet, even when parents and friends are not used as models for coping, the qualities of an adolescent's relationship with them can influence that adolescent's appraisal of stress as well as metabolic control. The same applies to internal resources, such as self-concept and body image. They not only directly influence the perception of stress and coping style but also are closely linked to the use of social resources and can affect both medical and psychological adjustment to the illness.

4

Knowledge of the Illness, Compliance, and Patient–Physician Relationships

As detailed in previous chapters, insulin-dependent diabetes mellitus displays several typical features of a chronic illness. Medical adaptation can be clearly ascertained through metabolic control, as determined by HbA_1 and HbA_1c values, and the quality of metabolic control is directly related to short- and long-term complications. The therapeutic demands on patients and their parents are complex and involve injecting insulin, monitoring glucose levels in the blood and urine, and attending to dietary regulations on a daily basis. Obviously, diabetes therapy can only be successful if both the adolescent and the parents understand the treatment. For the attending physician, the goals of diabetes therapy include reducing or eliminating clinical symptoms and helping the patient to achieve normal growth, correctly timed maturation, and physical efficiency. Certainly, the most important aim is to minimize the danger of long-term damage. Long-term optimization of metabolism can only be based on acceptance of the illness by the adolescents and on their readiness to act independently and responsibly. Accordingly, because adolescents must receive intensive and adequate medical treatment, the quality of the patient–physician relationship will also decisively influence their motivation to follow physicians' instructions.

This chapter examines the medical parameters and the course of diabetes, based on the results of the longitudinal study presented in chapter 3. The adolescents' acceptance of medical assistance will also be explored, as well as the effects of diabetes-related knowledge and attitudes on metabolic control. In particular, compliance with medical instructions and patient–physician relationships are analyzed longitudinally over the course of 4 years.

Medical Parameters

Patient Age at Diagnosis, Seasonal Course of Diabetes

As indicated earlier in this book, diabetes is the most common metabolic illness in adolescence both in Europe and in the United States. However, strong regional variations in prevalence rates exist in Europe. Germany holds a median position between northern Europe (Finland), with the highest rates of new diagnoses, and southern Europe (France, Italy), with the lowest. The constant increase in incidences of diabetes over recent years is of particular concern (Struwe, 1991). Findings on age at first manifestation for German populations are inconclusive but suggest a peak in late childhood or early adolescence (9 to 13 years). Epidemiological studies in the United States have documented a steady increase in the age of onset. Most diabetics fall ill in early adolescence (12 to 14 years), with onset occurring earlier in girls than in boys. This gender difference is often related to hormonal changes, in particular as reflected in the accelerated development of female adolescents. A later onset of the illness could also be documented in our sample: Most of the adolescents had become ill between the ages of 8 and 13 years.

A seasonal dependence for the onset of juvenile diabetes has been observed since as early as 1926 (Ahmed & Ahmed, 1985). The frequency of manifestation is much higher in winter than in summer. This association has been repeatedly confirmed in diabetes research (Gamble, 1980; Joner & Sovik, 1989) and was also apparent in our study. At the time of the first survey in the summer of 1991, it was difficult to find any newly diagnosed adolescents, whereas in fall and winter, the number of cases rose. The 10% of diabetics who had been ill for less than a year at the first survey had become ill only in the months from October to December. This seasonal variation is particularly evident during puberty (Fishbein et al., 1982), which seems to suggest a common etiology.

Etiological Factors, Manifestation, and Course of the Illness

Epidemiological studies have found differences in the frequency of the illness, depending on race and climatic zone, yet the significance of environmental influences, genetic factors, viral infections, and premorbid personality factors is still unclear (Tuomilehto et al., 1991). Low socioeconomic status, along with the number of stressors at the outbreak of illness, can largely be ruled out as risk factors (Ahmed & Ahmed, 1985). Even if they are not considered to be etiological factors, psychological and physical stressors, such as banal infections, can accelerate the manifestation of diabetes. The importance of genetic markers has been intensively researched for some time (Rotter, 1981) and has stimulated analysis of the long-term risk for siblings who are not yet ill. Although viral infections occurred along with 5% of first manifestations analyzed by Ahmed & Ahmed (1985), seasonal effects must also be considered; for example, viral infections are more common during the winter months. An autoimmune disturbance has also been proposed. The hypothesis is that viral infection leads to the production of antibodies, which not only attack the virus but also damage the pancreas.

Unlike the adult form of diabetes, the manifestation of juvenile diabetes is sudden, and the illness progresses rapidly. Within a few weeks, patients display excessive thirst (polydipsia), abnormally frequent urination (polyuria), weight loss, and overall deterioration in physical health and mental efficiency (Struwe, 1991). If these symptoms are not recognized and correctly diagnosed in the early stages of the disease, metabolic breakdown and diabetic coma may occur. Within our sample, the time between onset of first symptoms and diagnosis of diabetes varied in length; in some cases even the most obvious manifestations of the disease had been denied for some time (see chapter 6).

The typical course displays a series of distinct phases. With appropriate therapy, an initial remission is achieved, and the need for insulin therapy decreases. A second phase of relative metabolic stability follows; however, should the body's own insulin production become exhausted, a full phase of diabetes ensues. As a rule, the need for insulin increases again during puberty (termed the "labile pubertal phase" by Struwe, 1991, p. 280), and adjustment becomes difficult. As puberty draws to a close, a condition of relative metabolic stability gradually emerges, with a constant but high need for insulin (termed the "postpubertal stabilization phase" by Struwe, 1991, p. 281). The adolescents in our sample showed this sequence of phases precisely as described in the literature.

Generally, the course of the illness depends on the time of manifestation and the building of humoral antibodies. In patients with a very early onset, diabetes can remain very mild for many years, with insulin secretion remaining constant. In contrast, diabetes that manifests itself in puberty often progresses quickly, thereby creating additional difficulties. Among the complications of diabetes are diabetic coma (a direct consequence of an insulin deficit), further delays in growth due to chronic lack of insulin, and finally long-term damage to certain organs, especially the eyes (retinopathy) and kidneys (nephropathy). The development of this long-term dam-

Table 4.1. *Illness Duration*

Duration (Years)	Percent of Sample
< 1	10
1 to 2	22
3 to 5	22
> 5	46

age is more closely associated with the level of metabolic control than with illness duration. The frequency and severity of vascular changes are disproportionately smaller in well-adjusted patients than in patients with poor or fluctuating metabolic control. According to Schernthaner (1994), HbA_1 values above 9 are associated with a rapid increase of up to 30% in risk for long-term damage.

Illness Duration and Quality of Metabolic Control

In this section the medical parameters of the diabetic sample of our longitudinal study are examined more closely. As mentioned in chapter 3, 109 diabetic adolescents (51 girls, 58 boys; mean age 13.9 years) took part in the study during the first year. Table 4.1 and Figure 4.1 illustrate two important parameters in this sample, the duration of the illness and the quality of metabolic control at the beginning of our study. It was important to include not only adolescents who had recently become ill and were only just coming to terms with illness management but also those who had been ill as children, yet were having to deal with a sudden deterioration in their meta-

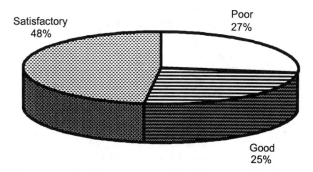

Figure 4.1. Quality of metabolic control (HbA_1) in diabetic adolescents ($N = 109$). Good, < 7.6; satisfactory, 7.6 to 9.5; poor > 9.5.

bolic control as they entered puberty. At the time of the first measurement, 32% of the adolescents had only been ill for a relatively short time, and 46% of the sample had been ill for over 5 years.

The HbA$_1$ or HbA$_1$c values were used as a measure of the level of adaptation. The HbA$_1$ value, the fraction of glycosylated hemoglobin in the blood, provides information about the average state of the metabolism over the preceding 4 to 8 weeks. Most of the physicians in our study used this measure; a small number (11%) used the HbA$_1$c value, which can be compared with the HbA$_1$ value through a conversion factor. The level of metabolic control was classified as good, satisfactory, and poor according to Blanz, Rensch-Riemann, Fritz-Sigmund, and Schmidt's (1993) standards for adolescent samples. At the time of the first measurement, 25% of the adolescents were classed as well adjusted, 48% as satisfactorily adjusted, and 27% as poorly adjusted.

Instability of Metabolic Control over Time

The quality of metabolic control in our sample changed over time. Table 4.2 presents the levels of metabolic control in the longitudinal sample of 91 diabetic adolescents (46 boys, 45 girls). As can be seen in Table 4.2, the number of well adjusted adolescents declined noticeably between the first and third surveys, whereas the proportion of poorly adjusted diabetics increased. This phenomenon is probably linked to the progress of puberty in our sample. In the first and second surveys, when most adolescents had just entered puberty, the proportions of adolescents with good, satisfactory, or poor metabolic control did not differ significantly. In the third survey, when most adolescents had matured, metabolic control worsened considerably. An analysis of the fourth survey showed that metabolic control had improved again but did not reach levels documented in the first survey. The average female adolescent suffered deterioration in metabolic control 1 to

Table 4.2. *Changes in Metabolic Control over Time^a (N = 91)*

	Mean Age of Adolescents (Years)			
	13.9	14.9	15.9	16.9
Good	25 (25.3%)	24 (24.5%)	13 (14.6%)	17 (21.8%)
Satisfactory	47 (47.5%)	46 (46.9%)	41 (46.1%)	30 (38.5%)
Poor	27 (27.2%)	28 (28.6%)	35 (39.3%)	31 (39.7%)

^{a} Columns may not add up to 91, due to missing values.

2 years earlier than the average male, corresponding to their accelerated physical development. Adolescent girls also displayed greater fluctuations in metabolic adaptation, which might be related to effects of premenstrual or menstrual-related hormonal changes.

An analysis of the HbA_1 and HbA_1c "wanderers" revealed that most adolescents' metabolic control levels were unstable over the adolescent years. Overall, metabolic control improved in 28%, deteriorated in 30%, and varied unsystematically in 13% of the adolescents we studied. A mere 29% of the diabetic adolescents displayed stable, satisfactory metabolic control over time.

For the longitudinal analysis it was necessary to convert these process-based diagnoses to status diagnoses. Therefore, a mean value was determined for each adolescent's metabolic control values over the 4 years, and the adolescents were classified into three groups according to these means. Based on these longitudinal metabolic control values, 20% of the diabetic adolescents were categorized as well adjusted, 40% as satisfactorily adjusted, and 39% as poorly adjusted.

Type of Insulin Therapy, Complications

The goal of treatment in the diabetic patient is to maintain insulin–glucose homeostasis. This typically entails maintaining a careful balance of the following therapeutic interventions: administration of insulin, control of diet, and physical exercise. Struwe (1991) pointed out that the need for insulin rises with the patient's age and the duration of diabetes; as a rule, younger children with recent onset of diabetes need only a morning injection of intermediary insulin, whereas older children require morning and evening injections. During the labile pubertal phase, satisfactory insulin compensation typically requires about three injections daily. Easy methods of monitoring blood glucose levels at home, such as are used with intensive therapy, enable considerable freedom in scheduling of activities and diet planning provided that levels are checked several times daily. This type of therapy is, in general, most suitable for adolescents. The same is true of insulin pumps.

In our study, the attending physicians advised their patients about the most appropriate type of therapy, and changes in therapy were usually made following consultation with the physician. An analysis of the types of insulin therapy used in our sample at each of the four surveys revealed that the percentage of adolescents relying on the conventional form of insulin therapy decreased over the course of the study (from 35% to 12%), whereas the percentage using intensive therapy rose (from 47% to 72%). The insulin pump was only used by a fraction of the adolescents in the sample (between 1% and 4%). The ratios of conventional to intensive therapy in our study, especially in the later surveys, reflect the distributions reported by Blanz, Rensch-Riemann, Fritz-Sigmund, and Schmidt (1993) for 17- to 19-year-olds. These authors described intensive therapy as the form of treatment most suited to the patients' needs but also requiring more patient responsibility and cooperation.

As parameters for the course of illness, the number and severity of hypo- and hyperglycemic episodes were determined. In the first survey, the adolescents experienced an average of two to three instances of hypoglycemia or severe hyperglycemia annually. By the second survey, the number of annual episodes of hypoglycemia had increased to three and four, whereas the number of severe hyperglycemic episodes remained constant. By the third survey, the number of hypoglycemic episodes had risen to seven or eight, and the number of episodes of severe hyperglycemia had increased slightly. The physicians further reported that at the beginning of our study, 28% of the adolescents required hospitalization because of severe imbalances in glucose–insulin levels. The number of hospital admissions associated with diabetes remained largely constant in the second and third surveys. Finally, in the fourth survey, the numbers of hypoglycemic episodes and diabetes-related hospital admissions decreased, signifying improved metabolic control.

Use of Medical Facilities

Adolescents' Acceptance of Medical Care

Aside from the social support system, the ill adolescent has the opportunity to utilize the support offered by the medical system. The relationship between physician and patient is recognized as essential for the patient's compliance and ability to deal with the illness. Patients consider the investment of trust in their physicians as being particularly helpful in dealing with their health problems (Freund & McGuire, 1991). However, findings from studies on adult populations cannot be generalized to adolescents, who can be unmotivated patients owing to their strong wish for independence (Seiffge-Krenke, 1998a). Further barriers to using health care lie in developmental changes in self-disclosure behavior and dealing with nudity. Privacy is very important to adolescents, who are extremely concerned about issues of confidentiality. In a study conducted by Ginsburg et al. (1995), adolescents considered a physician's honesty, confidentiality, competence, knowledge, and carefulness to be the most important personal characteristics necessary for ensuring a positive patient–physician relationship.

Recent studies have shown the proportion of adolescents who consult physicians to be below the mean of all other age groups in the population (Kerek-Bodden, 1989). In comparison with childhood, the utilization of medical care services decreases sharply between the ages of 10 and 20 years but rises again in adulthood. Palentien, Settertobulte, and Hurrelmann (1994) explored the reasons for this deficit in a research project on health risks and medical and psychosocial care facilities available for children and adolescents. They investigated over 2,000 adolescents and about 900 physicians who provided medical care for children and adolescents. The authors found that less than half of the adolescents had consulted a physician within the previous 3 months, although the adolescents had been ill significantly more often. Only one in three adolescents between the ages of 13 and 16 reported having consulted a physician when ill. Although the physicians seldom reported problems of acceptance by adolescent patients, they did not allocate much time for these patients' appointments. They believed that the adolescents' reluctance to use medical facilities was mostly due to lack of knowledge (64%), embarrassment (59%), and uncertainty (58%). Fear (49%) and ambivalence (48%) were also mentioned. Less than one third of the physicians mentioned other barriers, such as long waiting times or considerable travel distances.

Relationships Between Physicians and Diabetic Adolescents

In contrast to the healthy adolescent's tendency to avoid physicians, the diabetic adolescents in our sample had good relationships with their physicians at the beginning of the study, when they were about 13.9 years old. In some cases, the diabetic adolescents even preferred to talk to their physicians about problems rather than to discuss them with parents and friends. Several features were named by the adolescents as playing an important role in creating a positive patient–physician relationship: when the physician knew them well and was aware of their individual living conditions; when they could speak openly with the physician without fearing sanctions for not adhering to the diabetes regimen; when the physician allowed plenty of time for the consultation and explained everything understandably and in detail; and when the patients felt that the physician's suggestions were beneficial. A physician's medical competence was stressed. Only a small proportion of the adolescents reported having truly poor relationships with their physicians, and most of these had experienced frequent changes of physicians at the hospitals and clinics. Indeed, continuity of medical care was reported by less than half of the adolescents. It was established that 49% of the families had changed clinics, with 29% having changed clinics or physicians more than once. This is regrettable, because continuity in care is necessary for adaptation to any type of chronic illness (Freeman & Richards, 1994).

The importance of the patient–physician relationship is supported by the results on coping with illness-specific problems (see chapter 6). For example, 70 to 83% of the adolescents cited the strategy of "trusting the physician" in relation to coping with the problems of hospital stays, metabolic instability, injections, diet, and long-term damage. Surprisingly, 51 to 59% of ill adolescents also employed this strategy in dealing with diabetes-related problems in the family context or with friends. Adolescents with good, satisfactory, and poor metabolic control did not differ significantly in the frequency of using this strategy. However, if problems arose with physicians and medical care personnel, the adolescents, especially those with poor metabolic control, reacted by retreating or adopting the attitude that they had to cope with the problem alone. In other problem areas (e.g., family, friends, injections, and diet), adolescents with poor metabolic control could be distinguished by the attitude "I have to cope with this myself." This finding is of concern in that it relates mainly to patients who are at a higher risk of later complications and need intensive, continual medical supervision.

In the course of the longitudinal study, it became evident that the patient–physician relationship changed over time. First of all, fewer and fewer diabetic adolescents reported close and continuous contact with their physicians. Second, contact between physician and patient decreased drastically, particularly from the third survey onward, when the adolescents were about 15.9 years old. It became difficult to obtain HbA_1 and HbA_1c values from the physicians, who reported that the adolescents had rarely, if at all, contacted them or made appointments with them in the previous few months. In addition to this problem, which was most likely related to the adolescents' increasing independence, were the problems created by the switch from the family's pediatrician to another specialist. For example, adolescents frequently failed to visit any physician at all during this transition time. Requests to the adolescents to have the medical tests performed for the purposes of the research project were often met with a lack of understanding or even outright refusal. Thus, in the third year of the study, it appeared that the diabetic adolescents had begun entering a phase of reluctance to accept medical care, which, as already described, is typical for healthy adolescents.

The Physician's Evaluation of Cooperation and Compliance

At the beginning of the study, a total of 103 physicians were responsible for treating the 109 diabetic adolescents. These physicians predominantly saw the adolescents in children's clinics or other medical centers with pediatric units. In the second and third surveys, the number of cooperating physicians decreased (see chapter 3), which was partly the result of the adolescents' growing avoidance of physicians. The attending physicians were asked to fill out a short two-page questionnaire about their patients. The questionnaires included requests for medical data (level of metabolic control, duration of illness, patient's age and weight, characteristics of the illness course, and complications) and for other types of information, such as cooperation with the family, compliance, and the patient's coping with illness. The physicians generally found it difficult to return the questionnaires promptly. While this was party due to their heavy workloads, in later surveys they simply could not fill out the questionnaires because some adolescents, owing to their increasing independence, did not visit them. Furthermore, it is likely that the physicians' interactions with their adolescent patients might have become so limited in scope that the physicians were simply unable to provide the information requested. Indeed, it is unfortunate that in some cases, the physician's main duties may have become limited to supervising insulin intake and prescribing dietary restrictions. Thus, as Bowman (1985) correctly noted, although psychological factors and the patient's compliance are seen as very important, the patient–physician relationship is often reduced to mere supervision.

The opinion that good metabolic control depends on the patient's willingness to adhere to the suggested treatment is prominent among physicians who treat diabetic adolescents (Rapoff, 1998). Without question, some patients, particularly adolescent ones, adjust poorly, partly because of their lack of compliance. As Amon (1989, p. 68) remarked:

> The sugar levels could easily be brought under control, if only the patients would let themselves be brought under control.

It may happen that the diabetic adolescent may react to poor adjustment by finding dissatisfaction with the physician, which in turn creates a poor basis for further compliance. Sensible medical treatment should not focus too much on blood sugar levels; it must take the patient's entire psychosocial situation into consideration (Sayer et al., 1995). Even when a patient follows instructions very closely, good metabolic control may be difficult to obtain because of the marked hormonal changes that take place during adolescence. The analysis of diabetic adolescents' ratings of patient–physician relationships in the previous section revealed that the physicians initially experienced a great deal of patient trust and that they displayed a genuine (and desirable) interest in the adolescents' life situations and everyday problems. Although much competence in helping the adolescents to solve their problems was often ascribed to the physicians, it is not unreasonable to assume that the physicians might have been overtaxed in helping adolescents to deal with too many problems of a nonmedical nature. The question remains unanswered as to whether the adolescents' retreat from seeking medical care in the later years of the study, aside from their increasing independence and the typical adolescent aversion to physicians, is associated with disappointment resulting from unrealistic expectations.

According to our observations, most of the physicians in the study took the ill adolescents' problems quite seriously, as shown by their interest and participation in the seminars about the research results (see chapter 3). However, in most physicians' opinions, the sheer number of patients requiring treatment did not allow the physicians to provide the ideally intensive treatment their patients needed. In addition, many physicians were not able to respond to other needs requiring competence outside their field of expertise, for example, when adolescents openly requested psychological assistance. Physicians also reported frequently about the formation of coalitions (adolescent and physician against the parents or physician and parents against the adolescent), which were detrimental to further treatment (Seiffge-Krenke & Kollmar, 1996). In some cases, these coalitions were so strong and so antagonistic that the physician felt compelled to forbid parents' access to the adolescent patient's medical records. However, this was not common; in general, the family's cooperation with the physician was regarded as satisfactory.

In the first survey, the physicians reported that adolescents complied differently with respect to the different areas of treatment (Table 4.3); however, a poor level of adherence to prescribed diet plans was evident among all adolescents. Coping with illness was classified by the physicians as good in about one third of the adolescents, satisfactory in 47%, and poor in 23%.

Interestingly, the attending physicians described their poorly and well adjusted patients as being different in every relevant feature. With respect to adolescents with poor metabolic control, physicians indicated that cooperation with the family was poor; fewer family members were concerned with the adolescent or maintained regular contact with the physician. These adolescents' coping efforts and in particular their compliance were

Table 4.3. *Diabetic Adolescents' Compliance (in percent) Evaluated by Their Physicians (N = 103)*

Compliance	Diet	Use of Insulin	Metabolic Control	Diabetes Diary
Very good	11	22	16	23
Good	37	62	45	36
Moderate	4	4	6	4
Poor	43	10	23	21

Note: Columns do not add up to 100 owing to missing values.

described as highly inadequate. Furthermore, they were less careful about following their diets, failed to precisely adhere to the prescribed insulin dosage, kept their diabetes diaries less conscientiously, and followed the instructions for maintaining metabolic control less strictly than adolescents with good metabolic control. Thus, all relevant psychological parameters, that is, compliance, coping, and cooperation with the family, were described by physicians more negatively in poorly adjusted than in well adjusted adolescents. Most strikingly, the least cooperation and support from the family was reported in precisely those families whose poorly adjusted adolescent surely needed the most support. The physicians also emphasized that it was primarily the mother who took on the responsibility for management of the illness. The close link postulated by the physicians participating in our study between poor metabolic control and inadequate compliance has also been found in other studies (Garrison, Biggs, & Williams, 1990; Kaplan & Chadwick, 1987; Wing et al., 1985; Van Sciver, D'Angelo, Rappaport, & Woolf, 1995).

Physicians were additionally asked to make a global estimate of the adolescents' mental and physical development, general physical health status (e.g., other chronic illnesses, frequency of minor infections), and mental health. According to their reports, the adolescents' physical and mental development was normal for their ages in 75% of cases, and 89% showed no signs of behavioral or emotional disturbances. No differences in these results appeared between adolescents with good and poor metabolic control. Differences were related solely to the treatment regimen and the nature of the cooperation between the adolescents, their families, and their physicians.

The information in the physicians' reports was in accordance with the descriptions of the patient–physician relationships provided by adolescents with good or poor metabolic control. Adolescents with good metabolic control stated that their physicians spent more time on them, were more attentive and more open to questions, and listened more. In contrast, the poorly adjusted adolescents portrayed their relationships with their physicians much more negatively. Poor patient–physician relationships can have a lasting influence on patient compliance. As the study by Aimez, Tutin, Guy-Grand, Desme, and Bour (1971) showed, a good patient–physician relationship is conducive to better acceptance of insulin therapy and closer adherence to dietary measures. In adolescents with poor metabolic control, the converse could contribute to the creation of a vicious cycle: Poor metabolic status might lead to deterioration of the patient–physician relationship, which in turn could result in low compliance and further worsening of metabolic control. The adolescent might thus experience the physician's delivery of stricter instructions, which must be followed in order to remedy the adolescent's poor metabolic state, as authoritative pressure. A troubled patient–physician relationship experienced by patients with poor metabolic control may therefore lead them to change physicians, which may not necessarily be beneficial. Of course, much of the success of a physician's relationship with the patient may be related to the style of interaction between the two. In any case, even if complications arise in the treatment, the best approach is to offer praise, positive encouragement, and constructive criticism rather than scolding and punishment. Positive feedback, according to Blanz et al. (1993), is the basis of a functional patient–physician relationship and stable compliance.

Some studies have looked at the link between the adolescent's satisfaction with his or her physician and the adolescent's compliance (see, for example, Blanz et al., 1993), but none before has simultaneously compared the physicians' and adolescents' views. Our results showed that the adolescents' assessments of their own compliance deviated strongly from the physicians' estimates. All adolescents considered their compliance to be equally good, independently of whether their metabolic control was good or poor. In this respect, our adolescents' reports contradicted those of their physicians, whose ratings of compliance corresponded to the quality of metabolic control.

The Influence of Knowledge of the Illness and Compliance on Metabolic Control

The physicians' viewpoints having been described in the preceding section, the adolescents' perspectives will now be presented in more detail. Becker's

(1974) Health Belief Model allows the adolescents' judgments of dealing with the illness and compliance with physicians' instructions to be operationalized. Until recently, the patient's knowledge of the illness, its origin, and its prognosis has been used to measure the perceived danger associated with the illness. Most investigators have treated knowledge about the causes of diabetes and the treatment regimen, along with attitudes towards the illness, as important determinants of compliance and metabolic control (Johnson, 1980; 1984). According to La Greca's (1988) model, these factors exert a major influence as well; indeed, they encompass two of the model's three levels (see Figure 3.1). Thus, this model suggests that a considerable portion of the variance in poor metabolic control could be explained by these factors. Unfortunately, research findings on the topic have not upheld this view. Nevertheless, many studies have examined cognitive, attitude-related, and treatment-related variables, often as the only ones pertinent to coping. Research on other chronic illnesses has also placed this emphasis on the cognitive aspects of coping with illness (see chapter 2).

Illness-Related Knowledge, Attitudes, and Compliance

One of the central aims of our study was to examine the factors leading to good or poor metabolic control. Therefore it was important to determine which, if any, associations existed among compliance, knowledge of diabetes, and attitudes toward the illness and to do this as specifically as possible, that is, by examining several forms of medical treatment (such as injections, dietary control, urine checks, and physician's instructions). A decisive factor was the clarification of who was responsible for supervising the diabetes treatment regimen. To date, this aspect has received insufficient consideration from a developmental perspective.

Illness-related knowledge was assessed by means of a diabetes knowledge questionnaire designed by Roth, Borkenstein, and Otto (1987a). An analysis of the results showed that the level of knowledge among diabetic adolescents in our study was not substantially related to their metabolic status. Only one of the 11 scales in Roth's questionnaire, physiology and causes of diabetes mellitus, differentiated between well and poorly adjusted subjects with diabetes: Adolescents with poor metabolic control obtained lower scores on this particular scale. A comparison with the mean results reported in the literature revealed that the adolescents in our study had a good overall level of knowledge, achieving values that usually have been reported only for adolescents who attended a diabetes training camp (see Roth et al., 1988). In contrast to the findings of the Graz group (Roth, 1986;

Roth et al., 1988), we found no age or gender differences in illness-related knowledge.

In general, research indicates that theoretical knowledge and skills in practical self-control increase with age-related increases in levels of cognitive development (Roth, Frantal, & Borkenstein, 1987b). From the age of about 9 years onward, most diabetic children are able to inject correct amounts of insulin by themselves, whereas self-performed urine tests are first observed to be reliable at about 12 years. In our sample, the relatively late onset of illness (average illness duration 5.4 years) and the comparatively older age of the patients at the first survey (13.9 years) probably contributed to the high levels of cognitive maturation, good level of understanding of the illness, and large amount of illness self-management. In fact, almost all the adolescents in our study administered insulin themselves and claimed to be involved in decisions about their diet (97%). More than a quarter (27%) of the adolescents believed they had assumed responsibility too early, but half (54%) wished to be even more independent. These results clearly illustrate the disparity between the poles of autonomy and dependence.

The analysis of Sullivan's (1979) Diabetic Adjustment Scale (DAS) also revealed that the diabetic adolescents we studied not only were very independent but also went to some trouble to follow the treatment regimen. Depending on the specific content of each question, 90 to 94% of them approved of following the physician's instructions for the diabetes regimen, although only 78% believed it necessary to obey the physician's directions to the letter. According to the information obtained in the first survey in 1991, almost all of the adolescents (97%) had decided to do all they could to ensure successful treatment, and almost as many (87%) actually observed the restrictions and guidelines belonging to the diabetes treatment regimen. Still, 31% confessed that they sometimes thought it was good to have an episode of hypoglycemia. This finding reflects the adolescents' interest in having new experiences as well as a willingness to take risks despite the knowledge of negative consequences. A comparison between the group with good metabolic control and those with satisfactory or poor metabolic control revealed only minor differences in attitudes toward compliance. Adolescents with satisfactory or poor metabolic control confessed to forgetting to inject insulin more frequently when they were feeling good as well as to falsifying urine test results more often. Later we will see that this group reported a disturbingly negative body image (see chapter 5), that is, the adolescents considered themselves to be unattractive and felt that their bodies had many pockmarks and hardenings at the sites of injection. These adolescents also reported higher everyday stress (see chapter 6) and difficulty in finding romantic partners (see chapter 8).

The relationship between level of knowledge and quality of metabolic control reported in the literature is not strong. Roth et al. (1988), for example, reported a correlation of $r = -.16$. We also found a trivial correlation of $r = .12$ (see Figure 4.2). At first glance it may be surprising that knowledge about the illness is not significantly correlated with the quality of metabolic control, and that even negative correlations, for example, high level of knowledge about diabetes but unsatisfactory metabolic control, have been reported (Hamburg & Inoff, 1985). The equally surprising finding that no significant correlations were found between metabolic control and attitudes toward the illness has also been reported by other investigators (Roth et al., 1988).

Obviously, theoretical understanding or adequate cognitive insight represent necessary but not sufficient conditions for successful coping and especially for compliance. Very little attention has been paid to developmental factors that have a bearing on the understanding of the diagnosis or occurrence of the illness. Eiser's (1985) study demonstrated that misconceptions about physical reactions and false body-related ideas could persist for a very long time despite otherwise age-appropriate cognitive development. Kaufman and Hersher (1971) found that even children and adolescents who were well-informed about the disease believed for a long time that their pancreas was full of holes or that they had an unusually large stomach because they had to eat more often than healthy peers. It appears that for the adolescent, having knowledge is not enough to ensure that it will be used – the patient must want to apply it. Willingness to accept medical offers is often low not only in diabetic adolescents but also in patients with other chronic illnesses. As Schober (1992) showed, over 80% of dialysis patients with chronic kidney illness and asthma patients failed to follow their physicians' instructions. In contrast, our adolescents showed very good compliance on most of the variables we examined.

One may speculate what may cause an adolescent to show low compliance despite having adequate knowledge of the illness and understanding the recommendations for achieving good metabolic control. In some cases it might be that the goal of achieving and continuing to maintain a positive course of the illness and good metabolic control demands too much of the adolescent. Conversely, an adolescent who has failed to achieve satisfactory metabolic control despite having conscientiously adhered to the treatment regimen may consider all the initiatives to be pointless. It has been reported that compliance is diminished by the low perceived severity of the illness, the low perceived benefit of preventive or curative behaviors, and the considerable barriers the adolescent must overcome in order to carry out health-related activities, such as injecting insulin and observing a special diet (Givin, Given, Gallin, & Condon, 1983; Jenny, 1983). These barriers are particularly evident when health-related procedures or restrictions hamper the adolescent in pursuing age-typical behaviors or in sharing in activities with the peer group, for example, in engaging in adolescent patterns of eating and drinking, mobility, and risk-taking behaviors. Such age-typical activities and behaviors present significant temptations for the ill adolescent. Often, the adolescent may feel compelled to withdraw socially or seek contact with other chronically ill adolescents of the same age. An evaluation of the results obtained by using the DAS revealed that 6% of the ill adolescents we studied had a friend with diabetes, 21% believed they would enjoy school more if they were not diabetic, 12% felt that having diabetes hindered their friendships with healthy peers, 36% felt rejected by healthy peers, and 20% thought they were less attractive in the eyes of healthy romantic partners.

Factors That Influence Metabolic Control

According to La Greca's (1988) model, illness-related knowledge and attitudes represent the first and second level of factors connected to diabetes control, with the third level including stress, coping, and the mental health of the patient and family. As explained in chapter 3, we believe that psychosocial factors must assume a larger role in the model for explaining diabetes control. Hence, we have revised and elaborated La Greca's (1988) original model (see Figure 3.2 in chapter 3). In the following chapters we will examine the influence of the various psychosocial factors in more detail. At this point, though, we shall take an initial glance at the importance of the different levels for explaining metabolic adjustment. The correlations between the various factors and the quality of metabolic control in a subsample of our diabetic adolescents, those with a poor level of metabolic control ($HbA_1 > 9.5$), are indicated in Figure 4.2.

As Figure 4.2 shows, data obtained at the time of the first survey already confirmed that knowledge of the illness ($r = .12$) and compliance ($r = -.10$) were only trivially related to poor metabolic control. The correlation between knowledge and compliance also was not high ($r = .21$). Considerably more of the variance was explained by developmental variables, such as a negative body image (too childlike, $r = .62$), everyday stressors (minor stress, $r = .45$), and poor coping skills, that is, low active coping ($r = -.36$). Delays in certain

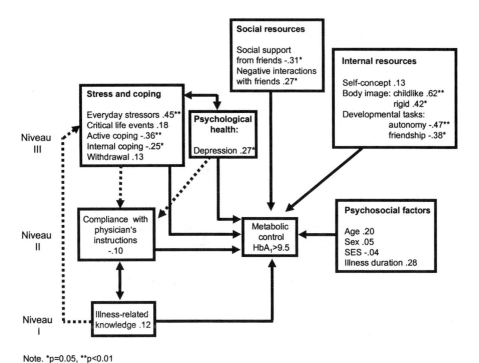

Note. *p=0.05, **p<0.01

Figure 4.2. Psychological factors associated with poor metabolic control in diabetic adolescents (*N* = 31).

developmental tasks were also associated with poor metabolic control.
Another notable feature was the comparatively high correlation between
negative social interactions (a lack of social support, many disagreements
with friends) and poor metabolic control. Depressive mood was similarly
related (*r* = .27) to poor metabolic control. This suggests that in adolescents
with poor metabolic control, psychosocial factors are more highly associated
with metabolic adjustment than are knowledge of the illness and compliance
with the physician's instructions.

Although the relationships between developmental and psychosocial
factors and poor metabolic control are fairly clear, it is considerably more
difficult to isolate those factors that are associated with good metabolic
control. Only a few of the psychosocial and developmental factors correlated substantially with good metabolic control. For example, positive self-
concept correlated significantly *r* = .39 with good metabolic control, as did
the attainment of professional competence *r* = .52. This suggests that the

overall development and psychosocial situations of these adolescents were normal and that protective factors were difficult to identify. Also noteworthy was the finding that in this group of well adjusted adolescents ($N = 23$, $HbA_1 < 7.6$), knowledge of the illness ($r = -.09$) and compliance with the physician's instructions ($r = .04$) were not relevant factors. This corresponds to the finding that well adjusted and poorly adjusted diabetics barely differed in their understanding of diabetes and compliance with their physicians' instructions. However, there were interesting associations between compliance and developmental variables in the group of well adjusted adolescents. Positive compliance in adolescents with good metabolic control was associated with low everyday stress (as perceived by the adolescents), few critical events (as perceived by the parents), and a positive family climate (as perceived by the adolescents). The "classical" medical view is that the quality of metabolic control is a good predictor of compliance (Alvin, Rey, & Frappier, 1995; Garrison et al., 1990; Schafer, Glasgow, McCall, & Dreher, 1983), yet in our study the correlation between good metabolic control and compliance ($r = .04$) was negligible. As already mentioned, however, we found no significant differences between well adjusted and poorly adjusted diabetics in the DAS. The fact that these correlations were found with regard to compliance but not metabolic control suggests that different criteria are relevant to the two different groups of adolescents.

Changes in Illness Management, Attitude Towards the Illness, and Compliance over Time

As mentioned in chapter 3, in our longitudinal study illness-specific data were obtained annually from diabetic adolescents aged 13.9 to 16.9 years. An examination of the level of knowledge revealed no significant changes over time, so a generally high, constant level of knowledge about questions related to diabetes can be assumed. The proportion of adolescents who took part in educational seminars decreased slightly across time (from 36 to 22%); nevertheless, the percentages are substantial enough to indicate how involved and responsible the adolescents were in terms of remaining informed about the illness. As far as illness management is concerned, a great deal of independence was identified as early as the first survey (mean age of adolescents 13.9 years), although the adolescents judged this independence with ambivalence. In subsequent years, illness management remained characterized by a high level of independence. However, about one third of the diabetic adolescents continued to feel that they had been forced to take on too much responsibility, at least before they were ready to do so. The percentage of adolescents who would have preferred more independence was in line with expectations and rose with age (from 53 to 69%). At age 16.9 years, roughly two thirds of the adolescents said that they would have preferred more independence in illness management.

The longitudinal analysis of the DAS revealed only minor differences between poorly and well adjusted diabetics with respect to compliance over time. Overall, compliance decreased significantly over the years. Table 4.4 displays several examples of DAS items, showing the decrease in willingness to follow the physician's instructions, which corresponds to the increasing desire for independence. It is worth mentioning that the majority of adolescents acknowledged the seriousness of the illness (between 62 and 69% at the different times of measurement).

In all adolescents, regardless of the quality of metabolic control, the attitude toward compliance became more negative over time. This corresponded to the small rise in the proportion of adolescents who denied having experienced hypoglycemic incidents (from 9 to 17%) or who gave false statements about glucose levels (from 12 to 16%). A slight decrease occurred in the level of openness with teachers (from 96 to 87%) and with friends and schoolmates (from 92 to 78%). Some authors have suggested that diabetic adolescents' dishonest tendencies (e.g., lying about their health status or being secretive with others) is related to their need for autonomy (see, for example, Ahmed & Ahmed, 1985), a hypothesis that appears quite reasonable in view of our data.

Table 4.4. *Changes in Percentages of Agreement with Selected Compliance Items in Sullivan's Diabetic Adjustment Scale (DAS) Over Time (N = 91 Diabetic Adolescents)*

DAS Items	Mean Age of Adolescents (Years)			
	13.9	14.9	15.9	16.9
7. I feel better if I follow the instructions for managing my diabetes.	91.0	89.9	84.3	82.0
13. Diabetic adolescents should follow the physician's instructions, even when they don't think it helps them much.	92.1	73.0	70.8	67.4
19. I think it's necessary to obey all of the physician's orders precisely.	79.8	61.8	60.7	58.6
25. I have decided to do everything in my power to make the treatment a success.	96.6	92.1	89.9	84.3

It is worth mentioning that the duration of the illness was only associated with a few of the variables we studied. This was the case for metabolic adjustment: There was a small but significant correlation ($r = .22$) between illness duration and quality of metabolic control found in the first survey, signifying that HbA$_1$ values increased with illness duration. In the group of poorly adjusted adolescents, the correlation was higher (see Figure 4.2). However, no significant correlations with compliance were found. Several other developmental variables were associated with illness duration; these will be discussed in separate sections.

5

Self-Concept, Body Image, and Perceived Health

Studies of chronically ill adolescents have typically concentrated too much on social resources as factors that can buffer the effects of stress, while neglecting internal resources, such as self-concept and overall health (Cohen & Wills, 1985; Jamison, Lewis, & Burish, 1986). For a long time, studies on diabetic adolescents only focused on certain aspects of internal resources. Corresponding to studies carried out on adults with diabetes, much research concentrated on understanding the "diabetic personality" (Dunn & Turtle, 1981). It is surprising that so little consideration has been given to examining the role of the self-concept, because it is known that this internal resource is central to the process of restructuring identity during adolescence (Dusek & Flaherty, 1981). Moreover, reference has been made to its protective function in coping with illness (Pearlin & Schooler, 1978; Badura, 1971). The neglect of body image in research on chronically ill adolescents is even more puzzling. If one recognizes that the normal processes of physical maturation that take place during adolescence increase the adolescent's interest in and awareness of his or her body, it is reasonable to assume that the changes due to the effects of illness will have a direct bearing on body image. For this reason it is astounding that so few studies have examined how chronically ill adolescents perceive their bodies. In our longitudinal study, results related to body image, self-concept, and general health proved to be especially conclusive.

The Self-Concept of Ill Adolescents

Developing an independent identity is one of the most important developmental tasks of adolescence (Erikson, 1968). One aspect of identity, the self-concept, represents one of the central variables in research on adolescents. The self-concept is commonly differentiated into an affective component (positive self-esteem) and a cognitive component (self-perception), which includes knowledge of the self and self-perception (Pumariega et al., 1993). It has been suggested that the self-concept of chronically ill adolescents is impaired by the onset or progress of a severe illness. This hypothesis has been supported by various studies that found low self-esteem and a negative self-concept in adolescents afflicted with several different illnesses (Hurtig et al., 1989; Engström, 1992; Greenberg et al., 1989; Thompson et al., 1990). However, other studies found no differences in comparison with healthy control groups, for example, in adolescents with cystic fibrosis (Cappelli et al., 1989), asthma (Hanl, 1995), diabetes (Auslander, Anderson, Bubb, Jung, & Santiago, 1990), and cancer (Goertzel & Goertzel, 1991). How can these divergent results be explained? Perhaps adolescents cope with a severe stressor, such as the onset of a chronic illness, with different levels of success, which in turn differentially affects their self-concepts. Competence in coping could thus lead to specific increases or decreases in self-esteem, regardless of the particular illness involved. Several authors also mention the denial and repression employed by chronically ill adolescents (Fife et al., 1987), as well as their strong desire to be "normal," which was confirmed in our study.

Our study also found that the diabetic adolescents' self-concepts did not differ significantly from that of their healthy peers at the beginning of our study. In the healthy sample, an analysis of the results of a German version of the Offer Self Image Questionnaire (OSIQ, Seiffge-Krenke, 1990) showed gender differences, which were originally identified by Offer, Ostrov, and Howard (1981) and have frequently been replicated in research. Healthy girls generally had lower positive self-esteem and presented themselves as more depressed than boys. Overall, the diabetic adolescents' self-concepts were very similar to those displayed by healthy adolescents; in four of the five self-concept scales, no significant differences emerged between the groups. However, diabetic adolescents had higher means on scale 5, which assessed depressive self-image. This indicates that their self-concepts were similar to the self-concepts of healthy peers but were more negative in nature.

However, diabetics with poor metabolic control differed from those with good metabolic control on several self-concept scales. As compared with diabetic adolescents with good metabolic control, those with poor metabolic control showed generally lower values for self-esteem, their self-image was more depressive, and their mean values for aspects of self-concept related to relationships with parents were also lower. With respect to the stress and coping paradigm, the low self-esteem of diabetic adolescents, particularly those with poor metabolic control, suggests that they may lack internal resources for buffering the effects of stress. A high level of self-esteem, for instance, might help the diabetic adolescent to adjust to the many undesirable changes imposed by the illness and might buffer the painful effects of potentially negative reactions of significant others, such as family members, close friends, and classmates (Hauser et al., 1997). One consequence of a more negative self-concept could be that poorly adapted diabetic adolescents are more inhibited about making use of the social support system available to them (see chapter 6). Our results further illustrate that global comparisons between ill and healthy groups may hide differences within the group of chronically ill adolescents who are at risk.

In the longitudinal analysis, only scale 1 of the OSIQ was included because this scale provides a good estimate of overall positive self-esteem. Annual reviews of the data obtained in the surveys revealed that over the years, both healthy and diabetic groups of adolescents showed typical decreases in positive self-esteem. In their research, Offer et al. (1981) found that a decrease in positive aspects of self-esteem began in early adolescence and continued throughout adolescence. The authors explained this finding in terms of a restructuring of the self and an increasingly realistic self-evaluation. According to these authors, it is not until the transition to adulthood that self-esteem becomes more positive. Figure 5.1 further illustrates gender differences in positive self-esteem across time in the healthy sample, paralleling those described by Offer and co-workers. In contrast, male and female diabetic adolescents did not differ in their overall lower levels and developmental courses of self-esteem.

In summary, healthy and diabetic adolescents in our study showed a similar self-concept with characteristic, developmentally related decreases over time. The clearly more negative self-concepts of diabetic adolescents with poor metabolic control should, however, be stressed. The longitudinal analysis of scale 1 of the OSIQ further revealed that the low self-esteem of adolescents with poor metabolic control remained stable over all four surveys. Over the years, the discrepancy between well adjusted and poorly adjusted adolescents became even larger.

Evaluation of Health Status

The body image is one of the self-relevant cognitions that has particular importance for chronically ill adolescents. Before presenting results on

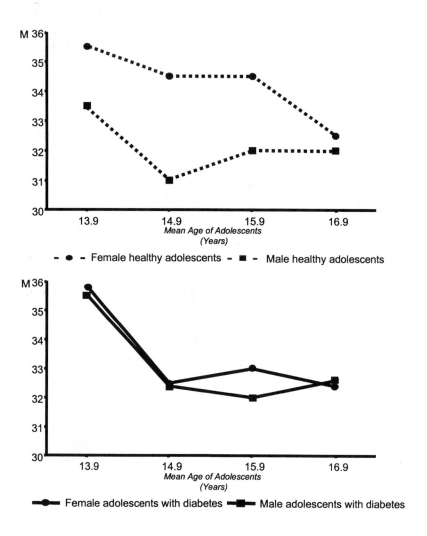

Figure 5.1. Changes in positive self-esteem over time in diabetic adolescents (*N* = 91) and healthy adolescents (*N* = 107).

body image, some findings about the general health status of adolescents will be presented. The comprehensive definition of health set down by the World Health Organization (WHO) (1946) emphasizes that physical, mental, and social aspects contribute to well-being and underlines the fact that health is more than merely the absence of disease. The subjective perception of health does not necessarily parallel objective health status in either the healthy or the ill, as Freund and McGuire (1991) have shown.

How Healthy Are "Healthy" Adolescents?

One distinct characteristic of adolescent individuals is the discrepancy between their objective health status, which is comparatively good, and their assessments about how they feel physically. As detailed in chapter 1, a comparison of mortality and morbidity rates for various populations indicates that adolescents are relatively healthy in comparison with other age groups. Nevertheless, they do have illnesses requiring hospitalization. German adolescents between the ages of 12 and 16 years receive outpatient hospital care for the treatment of illness an average of 1.6 times in this time period, with adolescent boys being admitted to hospitals more frequently than girls (Seiffge-Krenke, 1998a). Similar trends exist in the United States, where boys are 1.3 times more likely to be hospitalized than girls (Centers for Disease Control and Prevention, 1996). Because of the typical adolescent's strong tendency to engage in risky behavior, between 30 and 35% of all adolescent hospital admissions are related to injuries suffered in accidents (Deschamps, 1983). Hospital stays are usually quite short, seldom exceeding 1 to 2 weeks. Although adolescents in the United States, Canada, and Germany generally consult physicians in private practice more often than they seek outpatient hospital care, they generally have the lowest annual rates of physicians' visits (Katz, Hofer, & Manning, 1996; Seiffge-Krenke, 1998a). Mrazek (1987) reported a clear decrease in the regularity of physicians' visits, particularly in 12- to 15-year-olds. The developmental changes that may cause adolescents to avoid physicians are discussed in chapter 4.

When adolescents are asked to estimate their subjective health status, they almost invariably (in 80 to 90% of all cases) describe their health as "good" or "very good" (Bundeszentrale für gesundheitliche Aufklärung [BzgA], 1992; Mrazek, 1987). These sweeping statements contrast sharply with the answers adolescents give when questioned about specific health complaints. Most noticeable are the diffuse symptoms accompanying mild health complaints. Several studies in Europe, including Germany, and in the United States (Brähler, 1988; Bundeszentrale für gesundheitliche Aufklärung [BzgA], 1992; Dubow, Lovko, & Kausch, 1990; Hurrelmann & Lösel, 1990) have shown that the most common somatic health complaints reported by adolescents are colds and influenza, dental problems, headaches, nausea, circulatory complaints, gastrointestinal complaints, lack of appetite and weight loss, allergies, skin problems (acne), back pain, and muscle aches. In addition, female adolescents often suffer from abdominal complaints or menstruation-related pain. Although the relative frequencies of these complaints have varied strongly among these studies, the breadth of symptoms has been comparable. Overall, most studies have found that 30 to 50% of healthy adolescents report health complaints. In addition, most studies have reported that complaints are more frequently made by adolescent girls than by boys.

When adolescents' and adults' reports of physical complaints are compared, it becomes apparent that adolescents make the most somatic health complaints (Brähler, 1988). In German samples, these complaints are largely associated with school-related stressors. Hurrelmann, Engel, Holler, and Nordlohne (1987) showed, for example, that expected or actual failure in school was associated with an increase in psychosomatic symptoms. Similarly, conflicts at home resulting from difficulties in school were related to an increased number of body complaints. In this regard it is worth noting that as compared with children, adolescents show more frequent use of medication, particularly analgesics and prescribed psychoactive drugs (Nordlohne & Hurrelmann, 1990).

Perceived Health in Diabetic Adolescents

In the previous section, the discrepancies between healthy adolescents' objective health status and subjective perceptions of health were discussed. The most outstanding features of this age group are the high complaint rates and the number of diffuse physical complaints, which suggest that the physical health of adolescents is significantly impaired. How healthy, then, do chronically ill adolescents feel?

In our study, self-reports and parental reports were used to arrive at an estimate of the health status of the healthy and diabetic adolescents. Table 5.1 illustrates that at the beginning of the study (mean adolescent age 13.9 years), diabetic adolescents' health status differed from the healthy controls' status in only a few aspects, the majority of which were related specifically to diabetes. The diabetic adolescents stayed in hospitals more often (the most common reason for admission being related to diabetes), went to a hospital for the first time at a younger age, and needed to spend more time in hospitals than did healthy adolescents. Parents assessed their children's health in ways similar to the ways used by the adolescents themselves; however, the profiles provided by the diabetic adolescents' parents were generally less positive.

Table 5.1. *Estimated Health Status (percent agreement)*

	Healthy Adolescents	Diabetic Adolescents
Parents' assessments		
Other chronic illnesses	13.9	12.8
Frequency of banal illnesses		
(once to twice per year)	55.1	53.7
Stability of the adolescent's health	92.5	81.5
Number of hospital stays	0.9	3.9
Causes of hospital stays		
Diabetes	→	55.6
Injuries, fractures	8.4	3.1
Infections	7.9	4.5
Length of hospital stay		
1 week	31.2	15.9
2–3 weeks	15.1	50.2
Adolescents' assessments		
Other chronic illnesses	12.1	14.3
Good health	95.3	89.8
Physical complaints	53.1	30.6
Number of physical complaints		
1 or 2	37.4	24.1
3 to 5	6.5	12.0
Type of complaint		
Headaches	17.8	11.1
Nausea, stomach aches	10.3	8.7
Colds and influenza	7.5	8.3
Allergic complaints	3.9	2.3
Circulatory disturbances	3.0	3.5

The analysis of health complaints revealed that in one aspect diabetic adolescents described their overall health status as better than did the control subjects. Only 31% of the chronically ill adolescents expressed physical complaints, as compared with 53% of the healthy adolescents. The most common complaints were aches or pains (especially in the head area), followed by cold and influenza symptoms, nausea, and stomach aches. These percentages correspond to Hurrelmann and Lösel's (1990) findings. When asked whether they or other family members suffered from other chronic illnesses, both the healthy and the diabetic adolescents reported the same rates. About 13% of the adolescents suffered from another chronic illness, such as asthma or allergies. Thus, in summary, diabetic adolescents reported the same number of health problems, such as additional chronic illnesses, but a lower number of physical complaints than the healthy adolescents did.

In addition, all of the adolescents were asked to describe how much attention they paid to their health, which factors they believed influenced their health, and what they did to maintain good health. The questions were taken from Hurrelmann's (1992) health questionnaire. As compared with the healthy adolescents, the diabetic adolescents claimed more often that they paid very much attention to their health. In addition, they indicated more factors that might influence their health and mentioned more ways of maintaining good health.

Diabetic adolescents were more likely to consider the home situation, including family living arrangements and relationship with parents, as having an important influence on health status. Also, they believed that the family's financial situation had a greater bearing on their health than did the healthy adolescents. Although diabetic adolescents were more content with their weight than were healthy adolescents (61.8% vs. 51.4%, respectively), they checked it more frequently (78.2% vs. 54.3%) and did more to lose weight or maintain ideal weight, for which increased athletic activity (69.5% vs. 36.4%) and dieting (22.5% vs. 7.7%) were the preferred methods. The data relating to dieting in diabetic adolescents are not related to their adherence to the diet created for diabetes control but refer to additional diets aimed at weight loss. It is notable that nearly twice as many diabetic as healthy adolescents (69% vs. 34%) pursued some kind of athletic activity on a regular basis (at least once per week) in addition to participating in school sports and athletics classes. In the group of ill adolescents, very few differences were associated with the quality of metabolic control. As compared with adolescents with better metabolic control, poorly adjusted adolescents were less satisfied with their weight and considered the diabetes to be an impairment in both school and leisure activities.

Overall, our results confirmed the findings of other studies on adolescent samples. As expected, diabetic adolescents were treated in hospitals more often and spent more time there than their healthy peers, but they did not differ from the healthy control group in other relevant features (e.g., frequency of common infections, type of physical complaints, or additional chronic illnesses). Moreover, diabetic adolescents were engaged in considerably more activities to improve their health. A surprising finding, however, was the low number of physical complaints reported. Based on their clinical work with chronically ill adolescents, Reiser (1987) and Erlich (1987) have offered similar explanations for this finding, suggesting that physical complaints and symptoms in the chronically ill are subject to "double repression." Thus, when confronted with their diseased, defective bodies, chronically ill adolescents will tend to ignore symptoms not specifically related to their illness. Among other things, this may result in very few complaints of poor health being mentioned by chronically ill adolescents in medical examinations.

Differences in Body Image of Diabetic and Healthy Adolescents

Adolescence is a time during which dramatic changes to the body take place; this is one of the reasons that adolescents direct so much attention to their bodies. Health, attractiveness, and physical abilities are of enormous importance, not only in self-perception but also in close friendships and romantic relationships. It appears obvious that self-concept and body perception may be negatively affected if adolescents believe that their bodies are defective and deformed (which is, as we shall discuss later, the case for many chronically ill adolescents). In psychology, most relevant research on this question has been published under the concept of body image, which encompasses a variety of emotional, cognitive, and perceptual phenomena (Schonfeld, 1969). As Davies and Furnham (1986a) correctly pointed out, ideas about one's own body also imply evaluations; hence, studies of body image generally also make statements about satisfaction with the body.

The Body Image of Healthy Adolescents

Male and female adolescents differ greatly not only in the value they place on physical attractiveness but also in the way they evaluate their own bodies. All studies on this topic have revealed clear gender effects. Twice as many high school-aged females as males would like to change their appearance (Musa & Roach, 1973), and at college age, many more males (75%) than females (45%) are satisfied with the way they look (Dacey, 1979). Female adolescents also think they are less attractive than their female peers, while male adolescents tend to think they are more attractive than their male peers (Freedman, 1989). The level of satisfaction with the body varies with age as well as gender, with gender differences seeming to decrease toward the end of adolescence (Rauste-von-Wright, 1988). Satisfaction with the body is closely linked to physical maturity. Anglo-American studies have most commonly found that late-maturing girls are more satisfied with their body than early maturers, whereas the opposite is true of male adolescents (Blyth, Simmons, & Zakin, 1985; Petersen &

Crockett, 1985). Tobin-Richards, Boxer, and Petersen (1983) found positive body images among early-maturing male adolescents and a stronger sense of attractiveness than in later maturers. Simply having achieved physical maturity is not what makes the condition so positive for boys; rather, they are pleased with the advantages associated with becoming an adult.

The dissatisfaction with body weight in adolescent girls increases with age and is greater after menarche than before (Davies & Furnham, 1986a; 1986b; Tobin-Richards et al., 1983). This increase in dissatisfaction with age can partly be explained by the proportionally greater weight gain relative to body size in girls during puberty (Davies & Furnham, 1986b). However, the desire to lose weight does not correspond to actual excess weight levels (Davies & Furnham, 1986a).

In addition, several studies have found that adolescent girls' lower satisfaction with their bodies, greater differences in body perception (Rierdan & Koff, 1980), and increased dependence on external measures of value (e.g., sociocultural norms of physical attractiveness) may be accompanied by depressive symptomatology (Rierdan, Koff, & Stubbs, 1987). Rierdan and colleagues found that correlations between depression and negative body image already existed in early puberty; these correlations proved to be stable over time and were unrelated to developmental progress. Overall, studies of healthy adolescents have revealed a variety of interesting and consistent findings about the perception and attractiveness of the body and the consequences of maturational timing. It is remarkable that empirical investigations of physically ill adolescents have not taken these results into account.

The Body Image of Diabetic Adolescents

Body image, body attractiveness, and body perception have been thoroughly researched in adolescents for decades. The lack of studies investigating ill adolescents' body images is therefore all the more surprising. On the basis of the meta-analyses of 334 studies on coping with illness in adolescence (Hanl, 1995; Seiffge-Krenke & Brath, 1990), it was discovered that only a handful of studies had addressed this issue during the period 1970 to 1995. Although much research has been done on ill children's understanding of the body and its functioning, usually concentrating on Piagetian cognitive development of body concepts (e.g., Eiser, 1990a; Geleerd, 1972) the body image of ill adolescents, including their sexual identity, has not received the same attention. Kaufman and Hersher (1971) conducted one of the few studies exploring body image and perceptions of the body based on case studies of diabetic adolescents. They asked five diabetic adolescents to draw their conceptions of the condition of their inner organs. All adolescents, regardless of metabolic control, depicted parts of their bodies as seriously damaged; the organs were presented as deformed or mutilated. Similarly, Fällström (1974) and Hauser and Pollets (1979) found a more severely impaired body perception and a less complex body image in diabetic adolescents than in healthy adolescents. Recently, dissatisfaction with the body among adolescents with chronic illness has been investigated (Neumark-Sztainer et al., 1995), as have been the links between diabetes and bulimia (Neumark-Sztainer et al., 1996).

The striking paucity of research on chronically ill adolescents' perceptions and concepts of their bodies aroused our interest. In our longitudinal study (see chapter 3) we investigated whether the body images of diabetic adolescents differed from those of healthy adolescents, whether the level of metabolic control had any bearing on body image, and whether there was any association between objective indicators of physical maturity and the subjective evaluation of the body. To answer these questions, we employed the Body Experience Scale (BES) (Rierdan et al., 1987) and the Frankfurt Body Concept Scales (FBCS) (Deusinger, 1992). The BES consists of a polarity profile with 14 pairs of attributes related to the body. The FBCS assesses several aspects of the body concept including body competence, body attractiveness, and body feelings. In the interviews with the adolescents and their parents, weight, height, and the age of menarche or of the first nocturnal emission (semenarche) were also documented. In the sample of diabetic adolescents, physicians also provided an estimate of the level of physical maturity according to the Tanner criteria (Tanner, 1972).

The results obtained in the semistructured interviews and on the questionnaires in the first survey revealed that almost all of the diabetic adolescents displayed problems in accepting their own bodies. Diabetic adolescents at age 13.9 years described their bodies considerably more negatively in the BES than healthy adolescents of the same age. They experienced their bodies as being sicker, weaker, less interesting, less mature, less flexible, more childlike, and less changeable than their healthy peers did. In the interview, many diabetic adolescents expressed a strong sense of threat to their physical integrity caused by injuries related to their daily insulin injections (e.g., lesions, hardening of the skin, and bruises). The feelings of having deformed and damaged bodies often caused the diabetic adolescents to feel so ashamed that they avoided participating in certain activities with their peers, such as swimming. This negative view of the body may also have been associated with the difficulty that diabetic adolescents had in realizing certain age-specific developmental tasks, such as establishing romantic relationships, which were only begun after some delay (see chapter 9).

Diabetic adolescents did not view the process of becoming an adult, including physical maturation, as positively as healthy adolescents did. For example, the evaluations of menarche and semenarche made by diabetic adolescents were more negative than those of healthy adolescents. Whereas 25% of healthy girls thought positively of their own menarche, only 13% of the diabetic females had positive attitudes. These differences were also obvious in boys, although their evaluations were overall less negative than those of girls. Of the healthy boys, 62% viewed their semenarche positively, compared with 41% of the diabetic boys. It should be noted that there were no significant differences between both groups in the age of menarche (healthy, 12.6 years; diabetic, 12.7 years) or semenarche (healthy, 13.6 years; diabetic, 13.8 years) or in height and weight. The diabetic adolescents showed the same rates of physical maturation as their healthy peers. In this respect, there was no objective basis for the diabetic adolescents' misperceptions of their own bodies as being more childlike and less mature than normal.

The fact that the diabetic adolescents perceived their bodies as more regular and structured in the BES is probably associated with the strict therapeutic regimen to which they were subjected, a regimen that pushed them behaviorally as well as physically into a strict temporal plan. The negative body image in diabetic adolescents was also marked by their judgments of their bodies as being less competent. On Deusinger's Body Concept Scales, diabetics described their bodies as being less coordinated, less athletic, heavier, weaker, less tough, yet stiffer and tenser. In particular, male diabetic adolescents perceived their bodies in these ways more than healthy males did.

Based on the information obtained in the interviews and in the questionnaires, we were also able to confirm the finding that healthy adolescent girls' body images were more negative than those of healthy boys. Adolescent girls did not accept their bodies as much as boys did; they perceived more failings and flaws in their own bodies, and they more often wished to change parts of their bodies. They thought they were less attractive than other girls, did not like looking in the mirror as much as adolescent boys did, and were more concerned when their appearances deviated from their normative ideas. This gender difference did not, however, apply to the sample of diabetic adolescents. In this group, boys and girls did not differ in the perceived low attractiveness of their bodies. This suggests that the psychological effects of being afflicted with a chronic illness may be such that the gender differences consistently found in healthy adolescents are suppressed.

Our results thus lend substantial support to the findings that diabetic adolescents have a negative body image. In summary, diabetic adolescents have problems in accepting their bodies; they believe that their bodies are less sensitive to change, less developed, less attractive, less competent, and more boring. Given this fundamental difference between healthy and ill adolescents, we were interested in learning whether the body image of diabetic adolescents was influenced by medical parameters, such as illness duration and metabolic control. On the whole, adolescents who had been recently diagnosed with diabetes, those who had been ill for 1 to 2 years, and those who had been ill for over 3 or over 5 years did not differ in showing a more negative body image. Differences emerged, however, with respect to metabolic control. Adolescents with poor metabolic control (high HbA_1 or HbA_1c values) defined their bodies as being uglier ($r = .33$), weaker ($r = .25$), plumper ($r = .34$), more unkempt ($r = .34$), more childlike ($r = .62$), and more rigid ($r = .42$) as compared with diabetic adolescents with good metabolic control. Thus, poor metabolic control is strongly associated with an even more negative perception of the body (see Figure 4.2). Taken together, our findings point to an important, yet insufficiently studied area in diabetes research. More research is needed to establish whether a more negative body image can directly influence metabolic control or if it can affect adherence behavior, thereby having an indirect impact on metabolic control.

Changes in the Body Image over the Course of Several Years

As a result of the illness, diabetic adolescents have trouble accepting physical changes in their own bodies. How does this perspective develop over time? Are diabetic adolescents able to acquire a more positive view of their bodies – above all, one that integrates the appropriate physical maturity? Or do the body images of ill and healthy adolescents diverge more and more as they grow older? Results from the four annual surveys conducted in our study revealed that in the more advanced stage of adolescence, the ill adolescents differed from healthy controls only in a few dimensions of the BES. Compared with healthy adolescents, the diabetic adolescents consistently evaluated their bodies as being sicker and more boring. In the third survey, when the adolescents were on average 15.9 years old, both male and female diabetic adolescents still perceived their bodies as being less adult in comparison with those of healthy adolescents, and the diabetic girls described themselves as being less curvaceous. However, by the time of the last survey, the mean values for these features had increased dramatically. This was also true for the evaluations of physical maturity. By the age of about 16.9 years, diabetic adolescents described their bodies as being less childlike and more adult. The diabetic girls' mean values even surpassed those of healthy girls' for the attributes "changeable" and "strong." It appears that the diabetic adolescents perceived the changes to their bodies much later than did healthy adolescents (with a delay of approximately 2 to 3 years), at a point when the healthy adolescents no longer described their bodies as recently and notably altered. In summary, diabetic adolescents were indeed able to adequately perceive and integrate their physical changes into their body image, albeit with a delay of several years.

One aspect of body perception showed a gender-specific development over time. Even after 3 years, diabetic adolescent girls viewed their bodies as more "regular," a feature that decreased over time in the healthy girls. This rigidity perceived by diabetic females, which we linked to the strict therapeutic regimen, is surprising. Although metabolic control did worsen somewhat across the years, most of our sample regained satisfactory metabolic control by the time of our last survey, that is, when the mean age of the adolescents was 16.9 years. We had expected that this positive development would lead to relaxation and a decrease in physical rigidity; however, this did not appear to be the case. Thus, while the diabetic adolescents were able to make up for much of their developmental delays in body perception, they continued to incorporate perceptions of their bodies as rigid in their body images and remained irritable with respect to their attitudes toward their bodies. Furthermore, whereas the older healthy adolescents tended to find their bodies as more interesting, the older diabetic adolescents continued to assess their bodies as boring. This illustrates how difficult it is for chronically ill adolescents to feel comfortable with their bodies.

"One Body for Two": Diabetic Adolescents and Their Mothers

Psychological and psychoanalytic theories differ in the extent to which sexuality is integrated into the body image. According to psychoanalytic theory, the integration of the physically mature genitals into the body image is crucial. As Laufer and Laufer (1984) have suggested, failing to accept one's physical maturity may result in a developmental breakdown. A delay in integrating physical maturity into the body image was found in most of the diabetic adolescents we studied; they experienced their bodies as being more unattractive and gender-neutral, and they were much more hesitant about beginning to have romantic relationships. As detailed above, the majority of diabetic adolescents developed a mature body concept after a delay of 2 to 3 years. There were, however, some cases in which it appeared that there had been more difficulties in integrating physical maturity into the body image and furthermore, in which the boundaries between the child's and mother's bodies were missing. In the following case study, aspects of the psychoanalytic object relationship theory, in particular Joyce McDougall's concept of "one body for two," will be analyzed more deeply with respect to some of the families caring for a diabetic adolescent. McDougall (1989), who based her studies on patients with psychosomatic illnesses, described the fantasy of the "inseparability of mother and child" (p. 269). She observed how mothers' inabilities to encourage their children's needs for autonomy or to emphasize individual physical boundaries had led to fixation of the fantasy of mother and child being fused together in a single body. According to McDougall, the small child can only develop an image of his or her body when the mother's unconscious does not hinder this step. Not only must a mother be able to sufficiently separate her body from her child's, she must meet the child's needs for physical contact as well as physical autonomy in a balanced manner. Also, if the mother is not able "to perceive her child's desires for merging, differentiation, and individuation, she runs the risk of exposing her child to conditions that can lead to psychosis or psychosomatic illness" (McDougall, 1987, p. 270). McDougall demonstrated quite convincingly that some of her psychosomatic patients were unclear about to whom their bodies belonged. Frequently the mothers knew "better" about their child's physical needs than the children did themselves, that is, the mothers were acutely aware of when their children were thirsty, hungry, or had to relieve themselves.

The following case study illustrates how a pathologically prolonged mother–child dyad renders the development of a physical separation of the body impossible. The onset of a severe physical illness can accelerate such a pathological process and/or concomitantly revive a former relationship pattern. Although the phenomenon of one body for two was not observed very frequently in our study (see Seiffge-Krenke, 1997a), it offers insight into the difficulty of establishing a separate identity and a separate body image under conditions of illness. This important aspect of dealing with the body was only observed in the diabetic adolescents, as was the existence of an extremely close physical relationship, usually between mother and adolescent. The nature of these relationships showed a marked similarity to the phenomenon of one body for two described by McDougall. In the case study presented here, this phenomenon is described as it was observed over the course of our study, during four annual interviews at home.

Tanya

In our first investigation in 1991, we interviewed Tanya, a 15-year-old girl who had been afflicted with diabetes for 6 years. Her brother was 20 years old. Her father, a long-haul truck driver, was only home irregularly and in the following years of the investigation, never participated in the interview sessions. Tanya was a plump girl with bleached, permanently waved hair, which was pinned back in a bun. She appeared rather bored and sullen; one had the impression that she was doing a favor for her mother by participating in our study. In conversation she was not very reflective and was very awkward in expressing herself. She either did not know how to begin to answer several of the questions posed to her or responded by indicating she had not thought about the issue. She was hardly able to talk about her feelings. The striking deficit in ability to articulate her feelings was certainly related in part to her socioeconomic background. According to Tanya's assessment, diabetes was fully integrated into her day-to-day life. The only occasion during the entire study in which the young girl demonstrated any kind of emotional reaction occurred when she reported that her boyfriend sometimes gave her injections–she thought this was "great."

In contrast to this stout, physically shapeless, and phlegmatic girl, her mother, Mrs. A., was extremely thin, fidgety, and very talkative. She appeared very worn-out and run-down. Mrs. A. worked as a house cleaner. She, too, had difficulties in expressing herself but was much more articulate than her daughter. Whereas the interviewer had to extract nearly every word from Tanya, her mother was spontaneously loquacious. It was clear that Tanya's illness caused her mother great distress. Yet, it almost appeared that Mrs. A. suffered vicariously, as if she had diabetes herself. After Tanya had been diagnosed as diabetic, Mrs. A. had sobbing spells for weeks, for which she received medication. Even 6 years later, she was still unable to cope with the diabetes at all; in fact, she sometimes felt that her situation was getting worse and that she was becoming more nervous and restless. In contrast, Tanya reported that being diagnosed as diabetic had not bothered her very much. She simply regarded it as a blow of fate, which she had accepted. At the time, her mother had taken care of everything, including injecting her with insulin, a task that she still continued to perform.

The topic of shame at having a sick child was an important one for Tanya's mother. She repeatedly stated at great length that parents should not be ashamed of having a sick child or hide themselves behind this fact but should face up to it. Yet, she appeared only partially capable of doing this herself. Again and again, Mrs. A. emphasized that if she could, she would gladly relieve her daughter of diabetes, even if it meant having the illness herself. In this regard it is noteworthy to mention that in the beginning, while Tanya still refused to inject herself with insulin, her mother even injected herself (without insulin), "so that I could understand my daughter's situation better."

By the time of the second interview in 1992, Tanya was much more eager to talk and less sulky than the previous year. She now shared an apartment with her boyfriend in the same building her parents resided in. Also, she had started her vocational training in a day-care center for preschool children, with which she was very satisfied. Because she ate so many sweets, her HbA₁ values were still poor. She was unable to follow the urgently prescribed diets. Her mother reported that very little had changed in the past year in either negative or positive aspects. The mother and daughter still maintained a close relationship. Although Tanya now had her own apartment, after work in the evening she first stopped in at her mother's to talk about the day's events. Also, if Tanya came home from a party late at night, she first went into her parents' apartment, entered their bedroom, woke her mother, and asked her to give her an injection or measure her blood sugar. In describing these incidents the mother vacillated between feelings of indignation and pity for her daughter. Her husband complained about her being overly concerned, but she herself appeared to be tormented by intense guilt.

Mrs. A. appeared for the third interview in 1993 looking very stressed, even thinner and more harried than before, and for the first time, thoroughly angry with Tanya. She described her 17-year-old daughter as being completely spoiled, inconsiderate, self-centered, and lacking in self-reliance. Although she lived with her boyfriend in their own apartment, the two of them showed up daily at her apartment for the evening meal but never helped with clearing off the table or any other task. The two of them behaved as if it were perfectly natural for Mrs. A. to serve them. In her judgment, both of them were too lazy to take care of their own household tasks and thus preferred to move in

*with her. Mrs. A.'s intense anger had already resulted in physical prob-
lems. She developed an intestinal infection, which her physician had
diagnosed as being of psychosomatic origin. Apparently, Mrs. A. had
reported to her physician the troubles she was having with her daughter. For the first time it appeared that the symbiotic mother–daughter
relationship was swinging into a negative phase. On the other hand,
although Mrs. A. voiced her irritation with her daughter, during the
conversation she also spoke of her guilt and great worry about Tanya,
which made it easy for her to be exploited.*

*To an outsider, the relationship between Mrs. A. and Tanya
appeared to be that of a mother and a prepubertal, sick child, and not
a nearly adult daughter, who was already working and living with her
boyfriend. There was a major discrepancy between the anxious
mother and Tanya, who appeared this time in her typical calm, phlegmatic manner, reporting about her "completely care-free life." She
enjoyed her occupational training very much. She reported that she
had recently received an insulin pump, which she found very pleasant
and with which she managed quite well. However, this development
meant that Tanya had reassigned the responsibility for self-management to the pump, which measured blood sugar levels and delivered
the appropriate insulin dosages automatically, thus relieving her
totally of having to deal with her body or the illness. She not only
accepted the pump positively but obviously also regarded it as a sub-
stitute for her controlling mother. At the same time, however, this
deferment and new delegation of control hindered her in assuming
possession of her own body. Indeed, for Tanya this was so pronounced that she even disregarded the inconveniences of the pump
(e.g., removal before showering or athletic activity), which many of
the other adolescents in our study complained about. Furthermore,
she seemed not to notice the major changes in her blood sugar levels
reported by her mother. According to Tanya, her only problem was
being so plump and unable to lose weight. Tanya's bloated body was
striking in comparison with her mother's haggard, emaciated appearance; it was easy to think of Tanya as a fat, hungry baby who suckled
her mother dry. Tanya's account of stuffing herself indiscriminately
with food from her mother's refrigerator (she reported that after work
she usually stopped by at her mother's apartment to look for and
devour sweets, despite her mother's protests), without being able to feel
full, confirms this impression and again indicates the lack of connection to her own body.*

For the fourth interview in 1994, the mother arrived home looking worn-out and stressed as usual. She immediately blurted out the most important news, namely, that Tanya was planning to get married in 3 weeks. Tanya had sprung this date on her mother without having given a thought to the matter; she had not informed herself about the necessary formalities (e.g., the availability of calendar openings for ceremonies at the city hall or the church), nor had she selected a restaurant for the reception. She had not even considered what she and her husband should wear to the civil ceremony and the wedding. Her fiancé was in southern Germany completing his military service and could not help with the preparations in any way, so Tanya had simply delegated all the responsibility to her mother. Just as Mrs. A. had been made responsible for managing her daughter's diabetes, she was now being made responsible for organizing and financing Tanya's marriage. As a matter of course, without recognizing her own behavior and the necessity of stepping back, she took on these tasks, which Tanya should have taken care of herself. Again, the close mother–daughter relationship was clear, as well as the mother's inability to firmly dissociate herself from her daughter's demands. Excited and flushed, the mother continued to relate her thoughts almost as if she were preparing for her own wedding. Instead of referring to Tanya in the third person, the mother almost invariably used "we" or made several slips of the tongue by saying "I" instead of "she." This strong fusion, or rather identification, with Tanya calls to mind the inseparability of a mother and her newborn child. Mrs. A. was hardly able to understand our suggestion that Tanya should take responsibility for her own life, even if it meant a poorly organized wedding.

To this end, it would first be necessary for Mrs. A. to offer Tanya the possibility of distancing herself by allowing her to take possession of her own body. At her age, for example, it would be perfectly appropriate to let Tanya completely and independently manage the diabetes therapy herself. Only then could a psychological separation process slowly begin. Mrs. A. appeared completely indifferent about allowing her daughter to lead her own life, despite the great demands Tanya placed on her. So, for example, Tanya was not interested in obtaining her driver's license, because it meant her having to submit various medical statements to the motor vehicle bureau. She was too apathetic, and she avoided having to deal with authorities. It was quite likely that she was also afraid of failing to receive her license because of her poor diabetes control. The result of this situation was that every morning her mother drove across town through rush-hour traffic to take Tanya to work, and again in the evening to pick her up. Mrs. A. resented having to perform this task and felt completely overburdened; nevertheless, she was unable to withdraw from this routine.

At the time of the fourth interview, Tanya was participating in a hospital course in order to improve her poor blood sugar control. As usual, she was indifferent, too lazy to speak or think, and was simply prepared to let others, in this case the interviewer, "do the hard work." She passively described her wedding plans, adding that she did not really have any concrete ideas about how it should proceed because her mother was going to take care of everything anyway. We had the impression that she experienced the relationship with her future husband on a very childish level and that she was handing over her body to him.

This case study clearly demonstrates how a severe physical illness can regressively reactivate an earlier dyadic, unseparated mother–child relationship, in which the child has become fixed in the position of the "screaming giant baby." This was particularly evident in Tanya's case. Although engaged in her work and living in her own apartment, she continued to allow her mother to care for her needs in every respect, especially orally. The image of a giant baby was a compelling one for some of the other diabetic adolescents in the sample. One mother, for example, reported that when her 15-year-old son, who towered above her, was frustrated he would climb onto her lap to suck and cuddle with the security blanket he had used in early childhood.

Above all, a failed individuation was revealed quite dramatically in a few families through the lack of physical separation between mother and ill adolescent. Thus, the mothers (not the adolescents, although they had nearly reached legal age) were the experts on the diabetes regimen, and by supervising the special dietary regulations this illness calls for, they had assumed an oral caretaking and controlling function. It became clear again and again that these mothers were not only considerably more informed about their children's illness-specific needs but also more in tune with their children's body feelings than the children were themselves. Even before the adolescent perceived a physical uneasiness, a slight dizziness, or other signs of an impending metabolic imbalance, the mother, already having anticipated the condition, fetched the syringe case or glucose candies. One mother, for example, reported how she was able to recognize an approaching hypoglycemic episode by observing her 16-year-old son's pupils. By urging him to eat a sugar drop, she avoided an impending crisis without her son being aware of it himself. The adolescent thus never experienced the feelings of an approaching metabolic imbalance and could not develop a sensitivity to changes in his own physical state.

This lack of physical separation was also evident in the mothers' repeatedly articulated wishes to assume the illness on behalf of their children. Some of the mothers we interviewed were so unable to physically separate themselves from their children's bodies that they did not even refer to their children in the third person. When speaking about the processes affecting their child's body alone, they employed the pronoun "we."

In summary, a delay in integrating physical maturity into the body image was found in most of the diabetic adolescents whom we studied; they experienced their bodies as being more unattractive and gender-neutral, and they were much more hesitant about beginning to have romantic relationships. As detailed above, however, the majority of diabetic adolescents developed a mature body concept after a delay of 2 to 3 years. The case study material presented here represents particularly pathological mother-child relationships. For the majority of the adolescents we studied, individuation occurred during the course of our study.

6

Adolescent, Parental, and Family Coping with Stressors

In this chapter the constructs of stress and coping will be discussed in greater depth, especially as they relate to the special circumstances of the adolescent suffering from chronic illness. Few concepts in health research have been as important, yet as difficult to define, as stress and coping. Lazarus et al. (1974), who have made substantial contributions to the field of coping research in adults, defined coping as

> ...problem-solving efforts made by an individual when the demands he/she faces are highly relevant ... and tax his/her adaptive resources. (p. 249)

Inherent in this definition is the close association between stressors and coping skills.

Whereas early research initially concentrated on determining which features make an event stressful, the emphasis has shifted in recent times. Stressors are now seen as ubiquitous, and many researchers have come to believe that an individual's coping skills have a greater bearing on outcome, that is, adaptation or maladaptation, than the features of a stressor per se.

In the following, the kinds of stressors with which chronically ill adolescents are confronted will be described. In addition, the questions of how such stressors may accumulate is discussed. Finally, findings related to how adolescents and their families cope with these stressors during each phase of the illness are examined. As in the other chapters of this book, data obtained in our longitudinal study through questionnaires and interviews conducted with adolescents and their parents will be referred to.

Parents' and Adolescents' Perceptions of Stress

Most models of health psychology take into account the role of stress in the etiology and course of chronic illness. As such, stressors are depicted as factors that are likely to increase the risk of poor health as well as to exacerbate existing illness (for summary, see Seiffge-Krenke, 1998a). According to Rice, Herman, and Petersen (1993), it is important to distinguish between types of stressors, whose impact on health or the course of an illness may vary. In the context of chronic illness, it is especially necessary to differentiate between everyday stressors and illness-specific stressors. In addition, stressors may vary with respect to their frequency and duration of occurrence, that is, their chronicity. Finally, an additional parameter is the accumulation of stressors.

Types of Stressors, Timing, and Synchronism of Stressors

Research on how adolescents cope with stress has generally preferred to classify stressors as either normative or nonnormative (Hauser & Bowlds, 1990). Stressors have also been categorized by Compas, Davis, Forsythe, and Wagner (1987) as minor and major events, largely paralleling the distinction made by Lazarus and Folkman (1984) between everyday hassles and critical life events. In any case, the distinction between normative and nonnormative stressors has asserted itself, most likely because it has been best able to distinguish stressors according to the variables of frequency, predictability, control, negative impact, and appropriate coping options.

Normative stressors in adolescence include all stressors that are typically observed in this period of development. Among these are physical changes brought about by adolescence, changes in family dynamics and friendships over the course of adolescence, and the transition to new, higher-level schools. According to recent findings, early adolescence is particularly stressful for girls. Because the onset of puberty generally occurs quite early in girls, they are more likely to experience the most dramatic physical changes during the period of transition from primary to secondary school. Simmons and Blyth (1987) have demonstrated conflicting demands between aspirations for popularity in girls, which is linked to physical maturity, and their scholastic achievement. In contrast, boys' slower rate of physical development in puberty usually allows them more time to cope with these two potential stressors. In early adolescence, an additional stressor may arise because of a delayed or premature onset of developments expected for puberty, that is, being "off time." In midadolescence, normative stressors are largely related to friendships and family relationships. During this period, adolescents spend more and more time with friends and have more disagreements with parents about such issues as clothing, driving, personal space, and curfews. In mid- and late adolescence, most adolescents begin to date and have intimate heterosexual relationships for the first time. Fear of rejection and feelings of incompetence can be concerns that cause the adolescent much stress. In summary, normative stressors are frequent, mildly stressful events, which are typically experienced at about the same point of development for most individuals in the age group. As a rule, most adolescents cope with these normative stressors quite competently (for a summary, see Seiffge-Krenke, 1995).

In contrast, nonnormative stressors, such as critical life events, occur rarely but are extremely stressful and can increase the risk of maladaptation. One particular nonnormative stressor that has received much attention is that related to family stress (Hill & Holmbeck, 1986). If the family situation is unstable and the parents quarrel excessively, adolescents are at risk for developing psychopathology. In the extreme case, marital discord may result in divorce, a phenomenon that is on the rise in all industrialized Western societies. Divorce and the divorce-related changes in family structure, such as stepparents (see Visher & Visher, 1988) were comparatively rare a few decades ago but are now quite common (Seiffge-Krenke, 1998a). A most disabling aspect of this family-related stressor is that its effects may persist for a long time. It is rare that parents separate or divorce from one day to the next. Rather, the quarreling, tension, and animosity between the parents as well as the overt signs of their unhappiness are usually present long before a separation occurs and may continue to affect the adolescent long afterward. Other family stressors include the death of a relative, parental abuse, parental unemployment, psychological disorders in the parents, and chronic illness in the family (Hauser & Bowlds, 1990). The onset of a chronic illness in adolescents is also a critical life event; it afflicts only a small percentage of the age group, it is hard to predict, difficult to control, and extremely stressful. Because of these characteristics, it is obvious that such a nonnormative stressor places extraordinary demands on the individual's coping skills.

Normative and nonnormative stressors do not necessarily occur or exert their effects independently of one another. Several studies have shown that different types of stressors occurring within a given period of development may interact and thus intensify the aversive effects. In a study on adults, Lazarus and Folkman (1984) found a correlation of $r = .30$ between critical life events and daily problems. Studies on adolescent samples have revealed similarly high correlations (Seiffge-Krenke, 1995). Such findings warrant the use of models of stress that take into account the interaction of different stressors within a certain time period (e.g., see Wagner, Compas, & Howell, 1988).

In adolescent research, there is much concern about the accumulation of stressors in certain subgroups. Simmons, Burgeson, and Carlton-Ford (1987) have pointed out that the number of changes is much greater in adolescence than in other developmental phases. Although the onset of a chronic illness is a statistically rare event, the individual adolescent's coping capacity may be overtaxed when it occurs in combination with the normative stressors that are present in any case. Several authors consider early maturing girls to be a risk group for development of psychological and somatic symptoms (Petersen & Ebata, 1987; Brooks-Gunn & Petersen, 1991; Seiffge-Krenke, 1998a). The onset of a chronic illness in early adolescence could, therefore, lead to particular complications in early maturing girls. However, few studies to date have examined how chronically ill adolescents react to normative stressors (Boyce, 1998; DiGirolamo, Quittner, Ackerman, & Stevens, 1997).

Several studies emphasize the additive effects of multiple stressful life events. Rutter, Tizard, Yule, Graham, and Whitmore (1977), in their study on the Isle of Wight and in urban London, found that the risk of a poor outcome rises exponentially with the number of major stressors that an adolescent experiences. Although there was no rise in psychiatric risk as long as adolescents had to deal only with a single nonnormative stressor, if two stressors occurred simultaneously, the risk of maladaptation was quadrupled. In other words, stressors potentiate each other's effects. This empirical finding is particularly relevant to chronically ill adolescents.

Taken together, the confrontation with a series of stressors belongs to adolescent development. As Riegel (1976) has argued, the function of stress may indeed be to stimulate development. For this reason, an integrative approach toward understanding stress was used for our longitudinal investigation. Thus, we examined how our participants reacted to everyday stressors as well as to critical life events. Half of the participants in the sample were faced with the critical life event of being afflicted with diabetes, a nonnormative stressor of a chronic nature. As discussed above, such a stressor is qualitatively different from the normative stressors because it has a discrete onset, affects only a small percentage of adolescents, and often leads to quite radical changes in the life-style of the adolescent and his or her family. Finally, the chronicity of the stressor has a major impact on the adolescent's ongoing life and future and in part, those of the family as well. This impact on the family system (Hauser, 1991), as well as the often subtle restructuring of family roles and relationships, suggests that the level of stress caused by the illness should be assessed not only from the adolescent's perspective but also from that of the parents. Consequently, in our longitudinal study, everyday stressors and critical life events were examined from the perspectives of ill adolescents and their parents, and these results were compared with the evaluations of adolescents in the healthy control group and their parents.

Are Critical Life Events Responsible for the Onset of Diabetes?

Some investigators have attempted to demonstrate that an increase in critical life events is responsible for the etiology and pathogenesis of insulin-dependent diabetes mellitus (IDDM) (Hinkle & Wolf, 1952; Robinson & Fuller, 1985). Early reports from Stein and Charles (1975) suggested that the onset of type I diabetes may be triggered by psychological stress in a physiologically susceptible individual. Since psychological stress can alter activity in the sympathoadrenalmedullary system, elevate plasma cortisol levels, and possibly enhance the secretion of glucagon and growth hormones, it is possible that psychosocial stress could elicit clinical manifestations of diabetes in patients with partly destroyed pancreatic beta cells. Furthermore, research examining the effects of psychosocial stress on immunological functioning (Kiecolt-Glaser et al., 1987) has suggested a possible pathway for explaining how stress influences the initiation or continuation of autoimmune beta cell functioning. More research is needed to address this underexamined area.

Although the causal relation between critical life events and the onset of IDDM is not fully clear, several studies have substantiated the significance of stressful events for the metabolic control and course of diabetes (Barglow et al., 1983; Brand et al., 1986; Chase & Jackson, 1981; Hanson et al., 1987). Further differentiation is required regarding the number, degree of stress, and controllability of events. Brand et al. (1986), for example, referred to the relationship between life stress and measures of diabetic control for negative but not for positive life changes. Delamater et al. (1987), in contrast, found no correlation between daily problems and metabolic control. Similarly, short-term psychological stress, as induced by challenging mental arithmetic tasks and public speaking experiences, did not result in increases in blood glucose in diabetic patients (for a summary, see Hauser et al., 1997). Stabler et al. (1987) suggested that stressors may have direct physiological effects, since increased anxiety raises blood sugar levels. Stressors can also alter the self-management of diabetes by influencing diet, athletic activity, or health-related behaviors, which in turn affect adjustment to diabetes. It would seem plausible that in at least some diabetic patients, acute psychological distress can cause changes in blood sugar levels, raise the concentration of free fatty acids, and even lead to long-term damage in the form of coronary illness (Delamater et al., 1987). Yet, all in all, owing to the poor differentiation between types of stressors, the existing findings are too heterogeneous to allow unequivocal interpretation.

In an attempt to evaluate the effects of critical life events (such as divorce, death of a relative, relocation of the family to a new home, unemployment, or emigration) on the onset of diabetes, the mean number of life changes were assessed by use of the Life Event Scale (LES) (Sarason, Johnson, and Siegel, 1978), based on the parents' reports. The mean number of life changes that had occurred during the previous 12 months was $M = 2.27, SD = 0.78$ in families with an ill adolescent and $M = 2.18, SD = 0.81$ in the families with a healthy control subject. Thus, apart from the onset of the illness, families with a diabetic adolescent experienced no more critical life events than families with a healthy adolescent during the previous year. This result corresponded to the findings obtained in the interviews with parents. Diabetic adolescents' parents reported very few critical life events, and these did not differ qualitatively from those listed by parents of healthy adolescents for the same period of time. In both groups, the most common critical life event was a chronic illness in another member of the family (12%), followed by divorce or a parent's remarriage (4%), moving into a new home (4%), and the mother or father becoming unemployed (1%). Few of these stressors had occurred immediately before the illness began; most dated further back.

Thus, this analysis does not suggest that critical life events were important etiological factors in the outbreak of diabetes in our sample. However, in some families, an accumulation of major stressors was found around the onset of the illness, which indeed augmented the stress resulting from the illness. The following case study report is an example of how this interaction might occur.

Martin

Martin, 14 years old, was diagnosed with diabetes 2 months after the family of four relocated from East to West Germany. The mother herself had had diabetes for 9 years and was already suffering from long-term ophthalmological complications. The family's living space was confined to two rooms in an immigrant housing complex. After a short period of unemployment, the father had just found a job, although not in the occupation for which he had been trained. The family's financial situation was poor. In view of the many problems to be solved and the limited amount of material resources, the family's mood was troubled and depressed.

It should be noted that few families in our sample (only 4%) reported such an accumulation of critical life events or severe stressors around the time of onset of diabetes. In these cases, we recommended urgent intervention and assisted the families in their efforts to obtain concrete assistance (see chapters 10 and 11).

We also examined whether families with poorly adjusted and those with well adjusted adolescents differed in the accumulation of critical life events around the time of the onset of diabetes and whether the number of non-normative stressors changed in either group over time. At the beginning of the study, the numbers of critical life events as well as the general circumstances of the families in both groups were very much the same. On the basis of both parents' responses in the LES and in the interviews, there was no indication that families of adolescents with poor metabolic control generally experienced a higher number of nonnormative stressors than families of adolescents with good metabolic control. Over the years, however, families of adolescents with poor metabolic control reported severe stressors and critical life events slightly more often than did families of adolescents with good metabolic control. Among adolescents with poor metabolic control, there was a subgroup whose parents consistently reported massive and even increasing numbers of stressors over the course of the study (see also chapter 10).

Discrepancies Between Adolescents' and Parents' Perceptions of Stress

The results presented so far suggest that in general, diabetic adolescents were not confronted with more critical life events than were healthy adolescents in the year before our study began. Furthermore, the number of critical life events over the course of the 4-year longitudinal study was remarkably similar in both groups. Adolescents' evaluations of the frequency of these major stressors corresponded to their parents' ratings. However, striking differences with respect to minor stressors emerged even at the first survey (mean age of adolescents 13.9 years). As compared with healthy adolescents, diabetic adolescents reported an unusually low num-

ber of everyday stressors. This finding was based on the results of the
Problem Questionnaire (Seiffge-Krenke, 1995), which measures everyday
stressors in seven different problem areas. Overall, diabetic adolescents had
a lower total score than those in the healthy group. As Figure 6.1 shows,
healthy and diabetic adolescents differed in various problem domains, particularly in concerns about the future, the self, and relationships with friends
and romantic partners.

Rather unexpectedly, illness duration had no significant influence on the
perception of everyday stressors. The quality of metabolic control was associated with differences in three domains: Adolescents with poor metabolic
control perceived higher stress in the domains of self, school, and leisure
time.

The basic difference between healthy and diabetic adolescents' perceptions of stress also emerged in the interviews. It was remarkable how few
concerns the ill adolescents spontaneously expressed – they claimed that
"everything was normal," or that there were "no problems." They put some
effort into presenting a normative façade, as if they wanted to be more normal than normal.

This finding strongly contradicted the parents' reports of the amount of
everyday stress they experienced. In the interviews, diabetic adolescents'
parents described considerable burdens and problems, such as a constant

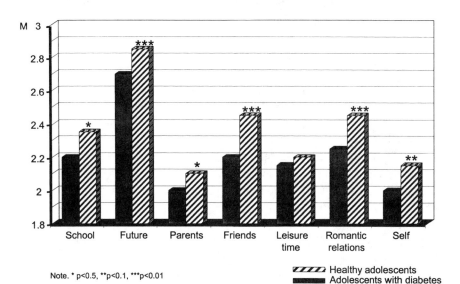

Note. * p<0.5, **p<0.1, ***p<0.01

Figure 6.1. Differences between diabetic adolescents (N = 109) and healthy adolescents (N = 119) in perceived everyday stress in various domains of life.

preoccupation with the child's illness, the feeling of being responsible for everything, the organizational overload in consulting physicians and arranging mealtimes, and supervising the child outside the home. In particular, diabetic adolescents' mothers complained about the rigid daily timetable, the influence of the diabetes on daily life, the focus on the ill adolescent, the restrictions on family activities, the general increase in negative affect (more family conflict, more problems between parents, feelings of guilt in the mother, more nervousness, and a more hectic life-style), and psychopathological symptoms (emotional lability, sleep disorders, psychosomatic disturbances, and compulsive brooding). Most of the stressors that have been described by diabetic adolescents' mothers in other studies, such as the pressure to restrict the child, the constant supervision (Hauser et al., 1993b), the feeling of isolation from the husband and of being left to deal with the problem alone (Hauser et al., 1997), chronic preoccupation with the ill child, the wish for a rest (Cole & Reiss, 1993), and fears about later damage to the child's health (Ahmed & Ahmed, 1985), were also named by the diabetic adolescents' mothers in our sample.

In conclusion, the diabetic adolescents' parents (especially the mothers) appeared exhausted and in need of psychological counseling, which they often stated they would like to receive. Their adolescent children, however, described themselves as being quite normal. They were very taciturn about identifying any particular stressors in everyday life, as if such stressors did not exist for them.

High Levels of Illness-Specific Stressors

On the basis of studies using the Coping Process Interview (Seiffge-Krenke, 1995), an interview procedure was developed for assessing coping with illness-specific stressors (Seiffge-Krenke, Moormann, Nilles, & Suckow, 1991). Nine diabetes-related problems were examined, including hospital stays, metabolic instability, drawing blood, injections, diet, and long-term damage. The adolescents were asked to indicate how stressful each problem was, what resources were available to help them cope, how they dealt with the problem, what barriers or hindrances prevented them from solving the problem, and whether these could be overcome. Figure 6.2 shows that relatively high stress values were assigned to each illness-specific problem in the first survey, when the mean age of the diabetic adolescents was 13.9 years.

Self-administered injections and metabolic instability were perceived as most stressful, followed by similarly high levels of stress associated with hospital stays, changes in therapy, and diet. Relationships with friends and

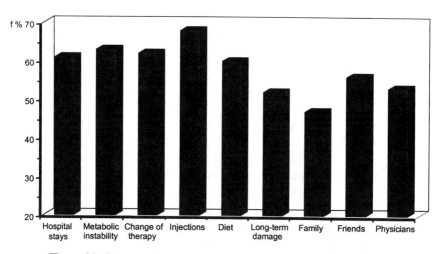

Figure 6.2. Degree of stress associated with various illness-specific stressors as perceived by 109 diabetic adolescents.

physicians were also seen as quite stressful, along with, to a lesser extent, family relationships and long-term consequences of the illness. This suggests that although the diabetic adolescents mentioned unusually few everyday stressors, they were extraordinarily burdened by illness-related stressors.

The parents were also asked about general and illness-specific stressors. The interviews with both parents made it clear that a variety of illness-specific events and measures were seen as exceedingly stressful. Parents found almost all illness management procedures to be burdensome, including injections, diet, and urine checks; in addition they feared hypo- or hyperglycemic incidents and were apprehensive about changes in therapy. The highest stress ratings were assigned to the uncontrollability of diabetes and the possibility of long-term physical damage. Altogether, the simultaneously high levels of everyday stressors and illness-specific stressors reported by diabetic adolescents' parents put them at risk for burnout.

Changes in Perceived Stress over Time

In summary, at the beginning of our study, when the adolescents were about 13.9 years old, enormous discrepancies existed between different family members' perceptions of stress. The diabetic adolescents' parents reported many everyday and illness-specific stressors. These stressors were identified in the questionnaires and openly discussed in interviews. Especially the

mothers of the diabetic adolescents appeared quite desperate, often mentioning that they would like professional help to deal with the everyday
strain and the illness-specific burdens. In contrast, the diabetic adolescents
presented themselves in the first interview as being completely normal and
untroubled by age-typical normative stressors. In addition, in the questionnaires they made even lower stress ratings than healthy adolescents.
However, they were considerably burdened by their illness. Thus, while the
parents of adolescent diabetics barely distinguished between the stressors
of everyday life and stressors stemming from the child's illness, their children differentiated strongly between the two areas.

How did the perception of stress change over time? The initially large
discrepancies in perceived everyday stress found between diabetic and
healthy adolescents at a mean age of 13.9 years continued into the following years, with one exception. Both healthy and ill adolescents showed
equally strong increases in school-related stressors from the mean age of
14.9 years onwards (see chapter 8), which suggests that the pressure to perform well in school began to increase from mid-adolescence onwards. An
analysis of the interview data in the following years revealed that diabetic
adolescents remained much more cautious in their expression of worries
and problems than healthy adolescents. Although the ill adolescents grew
more relaxed as relationships with the interviewer became closer, it
seemed as if they still needed to assert that everything was normal. Only
the diabetic adolescents with poor metabolic control were able to express
problems and concerns more openly, in particular, those having to do with
relationships and personal identity. In the interviews, they were more
likely to be open and more precise about how stressful their lives were. The
questionnaire results from adolescents with poor metabolic control similarly indicated a larger number of both everyday problems and illness-specific stressors. The high amount of stress in nine illness-specific stressors,
perceived by all diabetic adolescents at the beginning of our study,
remained constant from age 13.9 to age 16.9 years. This suggests that the
illness-specific burdens did not change much over time for the majority of
diabetic adolescents.

The perceptions of parents with diabetic adolescents showed an interesting course. In some areas, the stress abated. For example, in 1994, the parents
no longer considered routine procedures related to illness management and
everyday problems to be as demanding as they had been at the beginning of
the study in 1991, when their children were about 13.9 years old.
Nevertheless, although some stressors had become less taxing, other concerns appeared to have taken their place. Many parents complained in 1992

and 1993 that supervising their children had become much more difficult or even impossible because the adolescents spent so much time away from home. In 1993 and 1994, diabetic adolescents' parents expressed more worry about their children's private and professional futures. When the diabetic adolescents reached the age of about 16 years, their parents became more concerned about their children's difficulties in selecting an appropriate occupation or profession, in dating and developing romantic relationships, and about the possibility of the adolescent having children someday (for more detail, see the last section of this chapter). Some parents also worried about their children's increasing tendency to engage in risky activities and their decreasing compliance. This raised the question of how parents and adolescents actually coped with the stressors that they viewed so differently. This question is addressed in the following section.

Individual and Family Coping Processes

One important goal of this section is to integrate the findings generated from two divergent research trends in dealing with a chronic illness in adolescence, namely, individual and family coping. Whereas considerable attention has been paid to the study of family coping processes in cases of chronic illness in childhood, illness in adolescence has been largely neglected. This deficit is noteworthy because, as in childhood, the family continues to represent the main context for the ill adolescent's coping processes. In addition, parents' coping styles may serve as models for adolescents' coping with the illness. Because the illness represents only one, albeit a major, demand among the many others that a family must cope with in adolescence, the adolescent's and the family's coping skills in dealing with normative stressors will also be discussed.

Family Coping: A Forgotten Contribution to Adolescents' Coping with Illness?

Two consecutive meta-analyses of 334 studies on coping with chronic illness, conducted from 1970 to 1995 (Hanl, 1995; Seiffge-Krenke & Brath, 1990), showed that research methods used to assess coping varied with the age of the afflicted child. However, family coping was studied almost exclusively in cases of chronically ill children; this aspect received less attention in research on adolescent patients. Only 4% of all studies on coping with chronic illness in adolescent patients investigated family coping. Researchers concentrated on how individual adolescents themselves dealt with the illness (80% of all studies), or, at best, how they did so in combination with the family (16% of all studies). This parallels the changes in illness management from parental care in childhood to autonomous management in adolescence and may reflect the researchers' acknowledgment that the adolescents develop more autonomy in their own coping efforts. However, research on parent–adolescent agreement has revealed discrepancies between mothers', fathers', and adolescents' perceptions of adolescents' problem behaviors (Achenbach, McConaughy, & Howell, 1987; Seiffge-Krenke & Kollmar, 1998), suggesting that it might be useful to assess the individual perspectives of all persons concerned. Therefore, in studying coping with illness, we examined and compared individual and family coping.

The bulk of research on adult and adolescent sample populations has examined most coping processes on an individual level (Lazarus & Folkman, 1984; Spirito, Stark, Gil, & Tyc, 1995; Stone & Neale, 1984; Seiffge-Krenke, 1995). As a rule, coping strategies have been analyzed individually in relation to various stressors and grouped along conceptually distinct dimensions. Lazarus's distinction between emotion-focused and problem-focused coping (Lazarus et al., 1974) has become well known, as has, in adolescent samples, the distinction among active coping, internal coping, and withdrawal (Seiffge-Krenke, 1993a; 1995) or more recently, between approach-oriented and avoidant coping (Herman-Stahl, Stemmler, & Petersen, 1995; Seiffge-Krenke & Klessinger, 2000).

In chapter 2, previous research on coping with illness in adolescence was discussed, with emphasis on the various factors that influence the way the illness is dealt with. The research presented there was based almost exclusively on the individual coping strategies of the afflicted adolescent. Many coping strategies were found to be common among chronically ill adolescents, with cognitive and emotional strategies being the most frequent forms of coping (for a summary, see Hanl, 1995). Similarly, defense mechanisms (above all, denial and repression) were found quite consistently among adolescents suffering from various chronic illnesses (see Goertzel & Goertzel, 1991; Greenberg et al., 1989). In addition to those coping and defense processes commonly observed in adolescents suffering from a variety of illnesses, very specific forms of coping with particular illnesses have also been reported.

Compared with research on children afflicted with chronic illnesses, parents' perspectives have largely been neglected in research on adolescents. More recently, this trend has changed, so that more investigators have chosen also to examine the processes of the family's coping with illness. This change was certainly warranted, especially considering the fact that much evidence has accumulated showing that family variables affect the beginning, course, and treatment of an illness (Campbell, 1986). The development of the family system theory (Reiss & Oliveri, 1980) and family stress research (Hill, 1987; McCubbin & Patterson, 1982) have further contributed to this approach. Accordingly, recent work on family coping processes has generally been based on a paradigm that differs from that used for individual coping. In the analysis of family coping processes, the family is perceived as a unit, indicating that the family is more than the sum of its individual members (Hauser et al., 1993a; Hauser et al., 1993b; Minuchin, 1985; Olson, Russell, & Sprenkle, 1983b).

In our approach, we decided to incorporate both individual coping and family coping. It became clear that these processes do not exist independently of one another. For example, as described in chapter 4, illness management places a considerable burden on adolescents. Above all, this is because diabetic adolescents are generally encouraged to learn how to manage the illness successfully on their own. The procedures involving self-administration of insulin and the threat of metabolic instability are among the most stressful illness-specific events that the adolescent must cope with. Yet, these are not necessarily matters that concern the adolescent alone. Whereas it is largely up to the diabetic adolescents to carry out the procedures belonging to the treatment regimen and to closely monitor their metabolic status, the parents still need to monitor their adolescents on a continual basis. In addition, numerous family activities are interrupted or impaired by diabetes management, including mealtimes and leisure time activities (see chapter 7). The previous section showed that parents of diabetic adolescents find these changes in and restrictions on family activities very stressful, even when the adolescents assume almost all of the responsibility for the management of their illness. In addition, not only are parents obliged to accept the everyday changes to their routines, but they must also come to terms with the long-term consequences of the chronic illness for their child. Indeed, most parents of diabetic adolescents in our study (68%) found the latter to be much more stressful than their children (41%) did. In any case, it is clear that the illness affects the adolescent, the parents, and the family as a whole, whereby some aspects of living with and managing the illness may be perceived by the different parties involved as requiring more coping efforts than others.

In the following, the findings on adolescent, parental, and family coping from our study are presented, with comparison of the perspectives of the adolescents, their parents, and the adolescent and parents as a unit. As in many other aspects of our study, these perspectives were obtained through semistructured interviews with the adolescents and their parents and by using questionnaires (see chapter 3). As previously mentioned, most research on coping with chronic illness in adolescence had often neglected to examine the processes of coping with everyday stressors. This appeared to be a major shortcoming, since the illness may influence many aspects of everyday life. Thus, in gathering these perspectives we were not solely concerned with learning how the individual adolescent, the parents, and the family unit dealt with illness-related stressors. More importantly, we were interested in determining whether competence in dealing with everyday stressors, including family problems, might be helpful in dealing with a major stressor, such as a chronic illness. Furthermore, because several studies (Baumrind, 1991; Seiffge-Krenke, 1995) have demonstrated the function of the parents as models for the adolescent in coping with everyday stressors, we were interested in learning more about how the parents' coping behavior might serve as a model for coping by the adolescents, not only in illness-specific matters but in other matters as well.

Adolescents' Coping with Everyday Stressors and Illness-Specific Stressors

Adolescents' coping with everyday stressors were assessed using the Coping Across Situations Questionnaire (CASQ) (Seiffge-Krenke, 1995), which analyzes adolescents' coping in several problem domains (e.g., the future, self, school, teacher, family, friends, romantic relationships, and leisure time). The perceived stressfulness of these problems in diabetic as compared with healthy adolescents has been detailed in a previous section (see Figure 6.1). The CASQ measures 20 coping strategies, which can be collapsed into three styles of coping across problem domains: (1) active coping (e.g., mobilizing social resources in order to solve the problem); (2) internal coping (e.g., reflecting about the problem); and (3) withdrawal (e.g., avoiding the problem). Although diabetic adolescents differed from the healthy controls in the first survey in that they were less active in using social resources and contemplated their problems significantly less, withdrawal was not significantly greater. This profile – low active coping and low internal coping – was found quite uniformly across most of the eight problem domains. Taken together, at the beginning of our study, when the mean age of the adolescents was 13.9 years, diabetic adolescents were characterized by low levels of perceived everyday stress and a low level of functional coping efforts in solving these everyday problems as compared with healthy peers.

Illness duration was unrelated to the diabetic adolescents' scores on coping with everyday stressors. However, poor metabolic control was associated with higher perceived stress in several problem domains and a less active coping style. In particular, self-related problems were highly correlated with poor metabolic control ($r = .45, p = .02$). In addition, active coping ($r = -.36; p = .04$) as well as internal coping ($r = -.25, p = .05$) showed significant negative correlations with metabolic control. These results suggest that poor adjustment to the illness is associated with poorer coping skills, that is, with less activity and little consideration of potential solutions to problems.

Over the course of the following years, both healthy and ill adolescents showed an increase in active coping in most of the eight problem domains. Similar developmental increases in active coping and support seeking have been demonstrated in other studies in German sample populations (Seiffge-Krenke, 1993a; 1995) as well as in studies on Israeli, Scandinavian, and American adolescents (Seiffge-Krenke & Shulman, 1990; Seiffge-Krenke, 1992; Herman-Stahl et al., 1995). The diabetic adolescents' active coping increased continually, but even after some years their scores were only barely above the initial scores of healthy adolescents. The discrepancies between diabetic and healthy adolescents in active coping continued to be large in the fields of parents, friends, and romantic relationships, whereas active coping in school- and future-related problems differed little between groups after a couple of years.

Over time, diabetic adolescents' scores for internal coping also caught up to those of the healthy control subjects; after 3 years the diabetic adolescents' scores no longer differed significantly from those of healthy adolescents. A developmental increase in this dimension during adolescence has been reported elsewhere (Seiffge-Krenke, 1995; Kavsek & Seiffge-Krenke, 1996). No differences between the two groups or changes over time emerged for the third coping style, withdrawal. Overall, this analysis of general, non-illness-specific coping styles reveals that the diabetic adolescents were less active in using social support to solve everyday problems and that they devoted less time to reflecting about possible solutions. However, diabetic adolescents did make progress in developing their coping abilities. In particular, they showed more marked increases in using coping styles that required no interaction with others than in using coping styles involving negotiations of solutions with others or asking for help from others.

The coping processes in dealing with nine illness-specific problems (e.g., hospital stays, metabolic instability, taking blood samples, injecting insulin, diet, and long-term damage to health) were also explored in individual interviews with the afflicted adolescents. The Coping Process Interview was used to assess the kind and level of stress involved and the coping strategies used in dealing with each of these problems. The adolescents were also asked what kind of help they received, whether the problem was predictable, and whether any barriers prevented effective coping. Not only did the diabetic adolescents consider most illness-specific stressors to be highly stressful (see Figure 6.2), but their coping styles used for dealing with any of these stressors hardly differed. On the basis of the Coping Process Interview results, the following three main styles of coping could be identified: (1) emotions (e.g., strategy 10, "I was afraid"); (2) cognitions (e.g., strategy 4, "I didn't think about it, because I have no influence over the diabetes anyway"); and (3) actions (e.g., strategy 1, "I shared my experiences with other diabetic adolescents"). All nine illness-specific problems elicited many cognitive coping attempts, reflecting the importance of cognitive control in these patients. Independently of the problem, the most frequently mentioned cognitions were the adolescent's fear that his or her own diabetes was particularly bad, the perception of having no influence on the illness, and sarcastic humor. The adolescents' most frequently reported actions were retreat from social relationships ("I preferred to be alone"), assuming all the responsibility for illness management ("I had to deal with it myself"), and placing trust in physicians. Similar to the pattern observed in coping with everyday stressors, the diabetic adolescents were reluctant to use social resources in dealing with illness-specific stressors. Relatively few emotions were named in dealing with the nine stressors; among them, shame was mentioned often.

It is obvious that adolescent patients' coping strategies are linked with the course of their diabetes, affecting compliance, metabolic control, and overall adaptation. Research linking specific coping styles and diabetes outcome has, however, produced inconclusive results. According to Marrero et al. (1982), diabetic adolescents who undertake more problem-focused than emotion-focused coping show worse metabolic control than patients who employ both coping styles equally. Delamater et al. (1987) did not find significant differences between adolescents with good and poor metabolic control with respect to the use of problem-focused coping. Their results showed that poorly adjusted diabetic adolescents practiced wishful thinking and avoidance more often than those who were well adjusted, yet were also more active in seeking support. In the study by Hanson et al. (1989), the use of avoidant coping in diabetic adolescents was associated with poor adherence to the treatment regimen and with longer duration of the illness. In contrast, adolescents with short duration of diabetes were more likely to cope through the use of personal and interpersonal resources (e.g., self-reliance or seeking social support).

We also examined whether illness-specific coping styles were associated with illness duration and the level of metabolic control. Hardly any differences in coping styles were found to depend on illness duration. Diabetic adolescents who had been ill for less than 1 year named many emotions in dealing with the nine illness-specific stressors in the interviews, compared with adolescents with intermediate and long durations of illness. In contrast, large differences in coping styles emerged between adolescents with poor and good metabolic control in the Coping Process Interviews. Paralleling the pattern of hesitant use of social resources for coping with everyday problems, adolescents with poor metabolic control seldom relied on support from parents, friends, and physicians in order to deal with illness-specific problems, and they thought that they had to deal with these problems on their own. Accordingly, they blamed themselves when imbalances in their metabolic control occurred. In addition, adolescents with poor metabolic control were less capable of anticipating illness-specific problems. As compared with adolescents with good metabolic control, they reported that these problems were predictable significantly less often and also indicated more barriers that prevented them from coping.

The coping styles of the poorly adapted diabetics were prototypical of what we observed as a general trend among the ill adolescents: Most of them preferred to deal with their problems on their own. This basic approach did not change during the course of our study. The strong withdrawal from social relations and the difficulty in accepting help was an alarming phenomenon, common to many adolescents in stressful situations (Seiffge-Krenke, 1993a; 1998a). The analysis of coping styles in dealing with everyday stressors further demonstrated that diabetic adolescents' caution in using social resources was not illness-specific.

Parental Coping: Dealing with Family and Illness-Specific Problems

The diabetic adolescents' parents were also asked about both general and illness-specific coping styles. As a measure of parents' skills in dealing with everyday family stress, we applied the F-Copes (McCubbin, Olson, & Larsen, 1991), which was filled out separately and independently by mothers and fathers. Figure 6.3 illustrates the essential differences between parents of healthy and diabetic adolescents based on the total scores of the F-Copes. The total coping efforts made by mothers of diabetic adolescents were quite low relative to the high values for mothers of healthy adolescents. Similarly, as compared with healthy adolescents' fathers, diabetic adolescents' fathers were less active in coping with family stress.

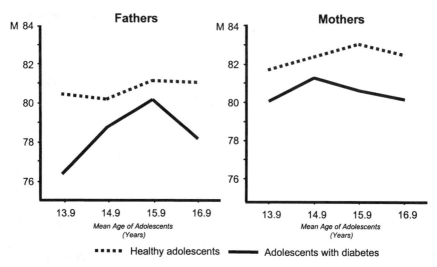

Figure 6.3. Differences in coping with family stress as seen by mothers (N = 104, 78) and fathers (N = 83, 63) of healthy and diabetic adolescents.

Noteworthy, however, were the high levels of coping efforts by mothers of diabetic adolescents as compared with those of their spouses. Healthy adolescents' mothers and fathers not only scored higher than diabetic adolescents' parents, but their coping behavior was also more stable over time. In contrast, diabetic adolescents' mothers and fathers strongly diverged in their coping behavior. Fathers showed the highest coping activity when their children were in mid-adolescence (mean age 15.9 years); before and after this time, fathers' coping activity was very low. The mothers' coping activity, despite reaching a peak at their children's mean age of 14.9 years, was more stable and on a higher level.

Interesting as well were the diabetic mothers' more ambivalent coping styles in dealing with family stress measured via subscales of the F-Copes: Mothers encompassed both active features (high in seeking and acquiring social support) and passive ones (high in passive appraisal). This ambivalence did not change across time and was largely independent of illness duration and metabolic control. Only one difference emerged: Mothers of well adjusted diabetic adolescents put more effort into motivating the family to accept help.

The parents' efforts in coping with the illness of their child (measured using the Coping Health Inventory for Parents (CHIP) (McCubbin et al., 1983) also varied at the time of the first survey, when the adolescents were about 13.9 years old. Whereas the diabetic adolescents' parents did not differ according to their child's illness duration or metabolic status, parents of girls put less effort into maintaining their children's social support, self-respect, psychological stability, and medical compliance than did parents of boys. The longitudinal analyses further revealed that both parents' coping efforts decreased over time, with fathers showing stronger decreases than mothers. This change was related neither to illness duration nor to the child's level of metabolic control but did vary with the child's gender. Fathers remained more active in coping with medical aspects of the illness if the ill child was a son. Over time, the mothers showed a decrease in family-related coping with the illness, that is, encouraging and overseeing family organization and coop-eration, and they made fewer efforts to seek medical assistance. However, over the 4 years, their activities in obtaining social support remained constant for sons but decreased for daughters. In summary, both parents showed sig-nificant decreases in coping with the illness over time, indicating that they became accustomed to the diabetes. However, they remained more actively involved in the cases of sons than in those of daughters.

Research in the past has frequently failed to assess both mothers' and fathers' perspectives. Eiser, Havermans, Kirby, Eiser, and Pancer (1993) conducted one of the few studies that have integrated fathers' perspectives on coping with a child's illness. In their cross-sectional study on 62 mothers and 45 fathers of diabetic children (mean age 11.6 years), they found that mothers and fathers differed in their child-rearing behaviors and strategies for coping. Fathers imposed stricter limits with sons than with daughters. Daughters also received more warmth and affection from their fathers than sons did. Fathers of daughters also found family coping to be more helpful than did fathers of sons. Yet, in general, fathers scored lower than mothers in all coping behaviors, including family coping, acquiring medical knowl-edge, and seeking medical support. The finding of a lower involvement of fathers in families with chronically ill children and adolescents in their study are consistent with those found in ours.

Family Coping with the Illness

Hauser and colleagues (1993b, p. 309) defined family coping as

> ...the thoughts and behaviors that the family expresses in attempting to handle or control the facts of immediate and long-term stressful situa-tions. Such responses include ways of observing, defining, acting and experiencing.

Thus, in contrast to assessments of parental coping, which take each par-ent's individual perspective into consideration, assessments of family cop-ing look at the coping style of the family as a unit.

In line with this approach, Hauser et al. (1988a) developed a standardized, semistructured interview, which elicits information on the processes involved when a family sets out to cope with a given problem or stressful event. Through these semistructured interviews, sequential phases of the family's method of dealing with a problem may be documented, for example, framing of the problem, search for relevant information, organization of the family's approach to the problem, and its emotional and overall response or solutions. We used this semistructured interview, coding the answers of families with diabetic adolescents according to the Family Coping Coding System (FCCS) (Hauser et al., 1993a). A total of 20 coping strategies used by the family as a unit were measured. Each of these strategies was assigned to one of three main categories. Appraisal-focused coping strategies were those that referred to the family's cognitive evaluation or interpretation of the stressful situation (e.g., pessimism, cognitive flexibility, blaming). Problem-focused coping strategies referred to the way the family plans the solution of a problem or takes concrete action to deal with the stressful situation (e.g., coordinating actions, seeking information, or seeking support). Emotion-focused strategies referred to the efforts of family members to monitor, accept, or regulate feelings about the problem or stressful event within and outside of the family (e.g., attempts to minimize feelings or to encourage or discourage overt expression of unhappy or negative feelings in or outside the home). The FCCS was applied from the second survey in 1992 through the fourth survey in 1994. After training the raters in the use of coding procedures described by Hauser et al. (1993a), the agreement among three raters, based on 12 randomly selected family coping interviews, was determined. Kappa values ranged from .58 to .72 for the 20 coping strategies used by the family as a unit, which can be considered as satisfactory.

Based on their studies using the FCCS, Hauser et al. (1988a; 1988b) suggested that family coping in which mastery, optimism, awareness, self-reliance, and cooperation were emphasized was related to better diabetes management. However, families that were more passive in receiving information and support from others showed a less favorable outcome. In these families, the emphasis was on routine and lack of action. Furthermore, they displayed a lack of coordination and showed signs of disjunction and functional impotence. In our study, at the time of the second survey (adolescents' mean age 14.9 years) the families experienced marked competence in coping with problems. Their appraisal was characterized by cognitive flexibility and a balanced pattern of optimistic and pessimistic perspectives. The family was perceived as a unit, but the independence of family members was also stressed. With respect to problem-focused coping, self-reliance was most important, followed by information seeking and support seeking. Coordination of activities was described frequently, but there was also a considerable mention of noncoordinated activities. Feelings were expressed directly, and family members acknowledged each other's feelings. Minimization and conscious restraint were also named.

Over time, family coping efforts in all three main dimensions decreased. As shown in Figure 6.4, coping efforts were lower in families with daughters as compared with families with sons, which confirmed our results based on the CHIP, already discussed. Overall, the families' appraisals of their situations changed. Their outlook became less pessimistic, and the illness was seen as having less of a negative impact on the family. The families' perceptions of their flexibility and mastery of the situation decreased, while at the same time it was increasingly stressed that the diabetes had to be managed by the adolescent. Problem-focused coping also decreased across time, particularly in seeking information, coordinating efforts, and alternative

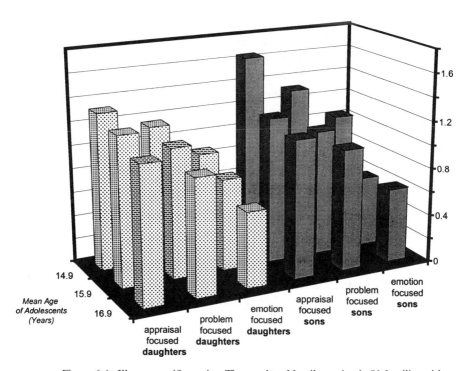

Figure 6.4. Illness-specific coping. The results of family coping in 91 families with a diabetic adolescent, broken down according to adolescent gender.

rewards. In addition, emotion-focused coping decreased. All in all, by the time of our final survey in 1994, when the diabetic adolescents were at a mean age of 16.9 years, families were much less concerned with dealing with their emotions. Ambivalent coping patterns, which were more characteristic of earlier phases, vanished. These results indicated that all families had grown accustomed to their routine. Nevertheless, families with diabetic sons continued to show a greater number of coping efforts than those with diabetic daughters.

Individual and Family Coping: An Integration

The results of our analysis of individual, parental, and family coping strategies highlight the importance of an integrative approach. Before looking at the consistency of parental and adolescent coping styles, it should be recalled that there were discrepancies in the way families with diabetic adolescents perceived stress. Parents reported consistently high levels of stress pertaining to aspects of their children's illness, such as monitoring of metabolic status and adhering to a diet plan. According to the parents, these illness-related stressors impinged on the family's everyday life, caused changes in the family climate, created family and partner problems, and eventually impaired psychological well-being. In contrast, the adolescents differentiated strongly between perceived everyday stress and illness-related stress. Although the diabetic adolescents considered illness-specific stressors to be just as much of a burden as their parents did, they believed their lives to be quite normal and free of problems. This basic discrepancy remained stable over the years.

Striking differences between healthy and ill adolescents were evident in the ways in which they coped with everyday problems in various domains (e.g., future, school, family, and friends). Diabetic adolescents differed from their healthy peers in that they were less inclined to actively exploit social resources, and they also gave significantly less thought to the problems concerning them. Altogether, it was rather surprising that the ill adolescents reported fewer everyday problems and were less active in attempting to solve these problems than were their healthy peers. These basic differences were observed throughout the study.

In general, healthy adolescents and their parents were more active in coping. Diabetic adolescents' parents were less active in coping and had children who undertook fewer active attempts to cope with everyday stressors. They were generally less prepared to use social resources, including those for illness-related problems. This phenomenon was also evident in the ill adolescents, who preferred to deal with their problems on their own. Another important finding was the greater similarity in coping styles among parents of healthy adolescents. In families with diabetic adolescents, the mothers' approaches remained ambivalent over the years: Although their coping behaviors in matters causing family stress were characteristically active, passivity, despair, and pessimism were also frequent. Over the years, however, the mothers became less and less involved in the family's coping with stress. The interest of fathers of diabetic adolescents in coping activities involving general family matters unrelated to the illness was lower than that of mothers. However, healthy adolescents' fathers were considerably more engaged overall in coping activities dealing with family stressors than were diabetic adolescents' fathers.

In general, the efforts of diabetic adolescents' parents in dealing with diabetes-related stressors decreased over time but remained higher for sons than for daughters. This finding is substantial because it emerged by using different methods of measurement. Thus, the results based on parental coping assessed with the CHIP were validated by those based on interview data assessing family coping with the FCCS. Furthermore, diabetic adolescents' mothers and fathers showed larger variations in coping depending on the type of stressor, gender of the child, and time. Altogether, these findings suggest that diabetic adolescents' parents provided their children with a less clear role model for coping.

The Influence of Gender, Illness Duration, and Metabolic Control

Finally, we need to consider differences in individual and parental coping with the illness as they relate to the adolescent's gender, illness duration, and metabolic control. According to the results of our questionnaires and interviews with the adolescents, hardly any differences in the adolescents' coping styles were found to be dependent on gender and illness duration. However, patterns of illness-specific coping and coping with everyday problems were found to differ according to the diabetic adolescent's level of metabolic control. Adolescents with poor metabolic control showed a less active coping style in dealing with illness-specific and everyday problems.

Parental coping styles reflected differences according to the child's age and gender, whereas illness duration had no impact. The strongest effect, however, resulted from the child's level of physiological adaptation to the illness. Several differences in stress perception and coping styles emerged between families of adolescents with good and poor metabolic control. As already mentioned, 4% of the families of adolescents with poor metabolic control reported somewhat more critical life events at the onset of diabetes and during the course of the illness. As compared with parents of well adjusted adolescents, parents of adolescents with poor metabolic control reacted to the diagnosis less, placed less emphasis on upholding the structure and organization of daily life, and when problems arose, overwhelmingly tried to solve them within the family. This coping style led to an increase in family conflicts.

As compared with adolescents with good metabolic control, adolescents with poor metabolic control spontaneously named more everyday problems and illness-related stressors, and simultaneously had more difficulty with requesting and accepting assistance to deal with these stressors. Given the large number of stressors with which they were confronted, it was remarkable how difficult it was for them to exploit alternative coping strategies. Our results suggest that these adolescents lacked appropriate models for coping with both everyday and illness-specific stressors. In families of adolescents with poor metabolic control, most coping efforts were characterized by reduced activity and hesitation in using social support. Moreover, the mothers of these adolescents showed ambivalent coping styles, and the parents' coping styles diverged markedly. In these families conversations revolved almost exclusively around the child's illness. This concentration on the ill child proved to be an additional disadvantage. The poorly adjusted adolescents further strengthened their excessive focus on the illness through their attitude that they had to deal with it alone, thereby exhausting their own resources. Moreover, these adolescents expressed more fears that their metabolic condition was deteriorating and were more worried about their futures.

Thus, for families of adolescents with poor metabolic control, it was possible to identify specific variables and processes that stood in the way of improving diabetic adjustment and coping with illness. By overly concentrating on the ill adolescent and confining the use of coping resources to those that existed in the family, it was quite likely that in the long run, the family became less able to devote its attention and energy toward solving each problem that arose in the family, whether illness-related or not. Moreover, as already detailed, it was difficult for the ill adolescents to find a suitable model for their coping behavior because the parents differed so much in their coping styles. This basic difficulty in all of the families with a diabetic adolescent became even more pronounced in those families with adolescents showing poor metabolic control, and it may have contributed to the child's poor coping outcome.

Stress and Coping in Different Phases of the Illness

The course of a chronic illness is characterized by several phases, related to dealing with the first diagnosis, hospitalization for initial treatment, and the corresponding curative procedures. As described in chapter 4, there is a reduction in the need for insulin replacement in the weeks immediately after the diagnosis and initial period of metabolic instability. During this remission phase, which lasts between 1 month and 2 years, a diabetic patient can achieve satisfactory physiological adjustment with only small doses of insulin. A year or two after onset of the illness, the need for insulin increases so much that the insulin must be completely replenished. Metabolic status deteriorates with the growth spurt at the beginning of puberty. Endocrinological changes, an increased and variable food intake, and the adolescent's psychological imbalance lead to large variations in blood sugar levels and an increased need for insulin. Only after puberty does a period of metabolic stability ensue, which may call for a reduction in insulin replacement. The different phases in the course of the illness are influenced by psychological variables, such as stressors, coping styles, and social support. Research has shown that social support is not equally strong in each phase of the illness. In addition, knowledge of the illness and the ability to carry out the treatment regimen increase over the course of the illness, contributing to improved adaptation.

The Initial Phase: Dealing with the Diagnosis

Several studies have demonstrated that the initial phase of the illness can be beset with crises but that families cope with the diabetes increasingly well over time (e.g., Kovacs et al., 1985). The results based on our questionnaires and the FCCS, described in the previous section, converge in showing a decrease in coping efforts over time, suggesting that the parents felt less of a need to intervene and be active. In this section, the manner in which the families in our study increasingly adapted to the adolescent's diabetes is illustrated, with the main focus on the subgroup of adolescents with recent onset of diabetes, namely, adolescents who had been ill for less than 1 year or for 1 or 2 years before the first meeting with the family.

In the first interview in 1991, the adolescents were asked about the periods before and after they had been diagnosed with diabetes. We inquired about their practical living circumstances before onset of the diabetes, when they first noticed signs of illness and how they dealt with them, and what they did when they suspected they might be ill. We also asked about the medical examinations conducted to ascertain the diagnosis, how they were informed of the diagnosis, the reactions of family and friends, and the adolescents' own attempts to cope. Both parents were also asked about the family situation at the time of onset of the illness, about their reactions to the diagnosis, and about the coping strategies they used in that initial phase.

As detailed at the beginning of this chapter, the adolescents' life situations before the onset of the illness were not unusual with respect to the number of stressors and life changes occurring at this time, compared with the life circumstances of the healthy adolescents. With respect to the first noticed signs of the illness, most adolescents mentioned polydipsia (75%) and polyuria (48%), fatigue (20%) and weight loss (13%) being less commonly cited. These symptoms caused a range of emotional responses, which included fear and worry (28%), uncertainty (19%), and repression (20%). Whereas these symptoms typically motivated the adolescents to seek explanations, they often relied on self-assurance. Some adolescents thought they might be dealing with a case of influenza (6%); others thought that they were suffering from a severe illness (8%), and a few thought they might have diabetes. Half of the adolescents did not mention their suspicions to anyone, 18% discussed them with their mothers, and 13% discussed them with both parents. Some of the adolescents did nothing, but 47% consulted a physician or went to the hospital. The parents were similarly worried about their child's poor health. All the same, the idea that their child might be severely ill came as a shock to 21% of the parents, and 14% of siblings also reported being shocked. Some of the families criticized the way in which they were informed of the diagnosis, saying that the notification of their child's illness should have been more professional (16%), that the physicians should have better prepared the family for the news (21%), or that the child should have been better looked after (17%).

Just after being informed of the diagnosis, 14% of the adolescents and their parents still hoped that the illness could be cured, and 22% hoped that medical progress would soon make a cure possible. Most (74%) of the mothers reported receiving help in coping with the diagnosis from their immediate relatives, including their partners (39%), other relatives (17%), the patients themselves (12%), or the patients' siblings (6%). The diabetic adolescents emphasized the need for family solidarity and acceptance of the illness by the family, teachers, and classmates. Almost 70% of them talked to their friends about the onset of the illness; 46% informed their closest friend first and then classmates, teachers, and relatives.

When asked about their current situation, both diabetic adolescents and their parents stressed the importance of receiving factual information from their physicians and from special diabetes training centers, as well as of sharing information with other patients. However, at the time of our first interview in 1991, 52% of the adolescents relied exclusively and 39% predominantly on their own resources for coping. Only 36% of the adolescents reported receiving emotional and instrumental assistance from their mothers and 2% from their fathers. Almost all of the adolescents and 71% of their parents believed they had a good understanding of diabetes, citing the physician (48%), a parent's acquaintance (21%), educational and training centers for diabetics (12%), scientific literature (11%), and similarly affected acquaintances (18%) as sources of information. However, 42% of the parents and 23% of the adolescents wanted more information.

In the initial phase of the illness, defense mechanisms such as denial and trivialization have been frequently found (Jacobson et al., 1986; Kovacs & Feinberg, 1982). These are related to specific conditions of the "secret" illness of diabetes. This corresponds to our own observations of the importance of denial and secrecy in the initial phase. As has been described, some of the families had trouble recognizing the symptoms of the illness; they still hoped for a cure, and one-fifth of the adolescents confessed to having "repressed" the illness. Denial and defense processes were very obvious in a few families. Three distinct patterns emerged, as illustrated by the following case study vignettes. In several families, an increase in defensive strategies by all family members made medical intervention particularly difficult, because the signs of the illness were overlooked for a long time, as in the following case. Although the patient's mother was a nurse and thus should have possessed at least basic knowledge of medical problems, this family exhibited nearly complete denial of the possibility that the daughter might be diabetic.

Orsi

The patient, a 13-year-old adolescent girl, had recently become ill. The first signs of the illness were ignored by the family for a long time. When we inquired further about the time leading up to the diagnosis, we learned that Orsi had been drinking 6 liters of mineral water per day without the family being overly concerned. No attempt to consult a physician had been made. Orsi's 18-year-old brother, who had been responsible for purchasing the family's bottled water, finally refused to transport such abnormal quantities home. He subsequently insisted on Orsi being seen by a physician.

Another family showed a dramatic increase in defensive behavior some time after diagnosis.

Edina

This 14-year-old female patient had only been ill for a few weeks when we contacted her for the first time. The family was very open, expressing fear and concern about coping with the illness. The adolescent herself was also easy to approach and agreed to participate in the study. A few months later, when a project team member called on the family to conduct an interview, he was received with suspicion. The family made it clear that they had nothing to say, that everything had already been said, and that they did not know what the interviewer still wanted from them. Edina came across as unusually reserved and withdrawn. The interviewer grew concerned that the family would cease their participation in the study.

In still another case, the parents were completely oblivious to their diabetic son's emotional strain, whereas he clearly felt helpless and troubled.

Tom

The patient was a 12-year-old adolescent boy who had recently become ill. His mother had remarried, also recently. The new family included his stepfather and a 4-year-old stepsister. The mother, an energetic and eloquent woman who dominated the family, described her son's adjustment to the illness as decidedly positive. She claimed that Tom had no problems with the illness at all and that he coped exceptionally well. She was particularly proud of his independence, which she had always very much encouraged. The mother appeared optimistic and in high spirits and was not aware of any problems whatsoever.

On careful examination, it became apparent that the boy's perspective stood in glaring contrast to his mother's. Tom was deeply depressed, lonely, and terribly anguished by fears of dying. He spent the whole day alone, because the parents had just opened a tax advisory business and his stepsister was cared for outside the home. Tom was constantly plagued by the fear of falling into a coma and dying without anyone coming to his rescue. This emotional burden was exacerbated by a difficult family situation, characterized by rivalry between Tom and his stepfather over the mother. In addition, Tom did not have a single friend, nor did he have any contact with a peer group.

This family showed a dramatic splitting in affect in the initial phase of the illness. The severity of the illness was denied so strongly by the mother that even 9 months after the illness was diagnosed, there was no physician responsible for monitoring Tom's adjustment.

For the majority of the families we interviewed, the onset of the illness was an unforeseen, highly stressful event; many families reported feelings of shock. As a consequence, defense and denial processes in this phase are to some degree understandable. As illustrated in the case studies, three different patterns of defense emerged in our study. In the first, the denial mechanisms existed before the diagnosis of diabetes, impairing perception of the symptoms and postponing treatment. A second pattern resulted in the diabetes being perceived completely differently by the adolescents and their parents. This style might have also caused a postponement of seeking or beginning to implement adequate treatment, resulting in severe medical complications. Third, some families' defensiveness increased some time after diagnosis, making cooperation with the research project difficult and signaling potential discontinuation of participation in the study. This defensiveness, often manifested in hostile and rejecting attitudes, was also a major problem for the physician.

Changes in the Years after First Manifestation of the Illness

Diabetes is not a static illness: There are times when the symptoms worsen or recede (see chapter 4). A critical time is around the start of puberty, when a dramatic increase in insulin requirements may occur. According to Struwe (1991), "satisfactory compensation for the diabetes [is] often barely possible during this time" (p. 279). The patient's metabolism does not stabilize again until after puberty, when the need for insulin, although high, remains relatively constant. It is also a period when adolescents' knowledge of the illness increases considerably (Band & Weisz, 1990; Burns, Green, & Chase, 1986), and their understanding of the illness also improves (Burbach & Peterson, 1986). For this reason, responsibility for illness management may be delegated to the patients themselves during this stage (Johnson & Rosenbloom, 1982). However, this undertaking can be difficult, because the course of the illness normally takes a turn for the worse at this time. Thus, even the most conscientious efforts to adhere to the complex treatment regimen may appear useless. Willingness to embark on and continue intensive therapy often wanes during puberty (Jacobson et al., 1986; 1990), which may, among other factors, be related to this discouragement.

The first manifestation of the illness coincided with the beginning of puberty for at least some of our sample: 10% of the adolescents (mean age

13.9 years) had become ill less than 1 year before the first interview and 22% between 1 and 2 years earlier. Yet, even for those adolescents who had already been ill for some time, the onset of puberty caused changes in the patient's health and his or her attitude toward monitoring it. How did these families respond to the situation, and how did their coping behavior change over the course of the illness? In 1992, 1993, and 1994 we asked the adolescents and their parents in separate interviews about the development of their illness during the year, about any problems related to the illness, about coping with and adjustment to the illness, and about their current relationship with their physicians. The topics of changes in social support and future worries were also explored. Finally, we asked the adolescents and their parents to consider whether a change in the course of the illness had occurred as compared with the preceding year, and if so, how they evaluated it.

In the second year of our investigation (1992), the average age of the adolescents was 14.9 years. Among the problems troubling them at the time, deteriorating metabolic control was considered to be the most important (22%), followed by problems with blood glucose levels (12%), with diet (10%), and with hospital stays (5%). The adolescents complained about the constant checking, constant food restrictions, and limitations on their spontaneous activities. They mentioned anger and fear as well as resignation. The coping strategy most frequently named was instrumental adaptation, that is, learning about and assuming responsibility for illness management procedures. The adolescents also reminded themselves that it was important to maintain discipline and not let themselves become discouraged. More emotional and instrumental support from the mother was perceived in the second year of the study (57%), although the father remained largely uninvolved (4%). The adolescents' other important coping strategies were using instrumental help and trivializing the illness. Change in the family atmosphere since the previous interview was indicated by 43% of the adolescents whereas the patient/physician relationship had remained mostly the same. By the second interview, fewer adolescents still wanted information about diabetes (16%). When asked about their perspectives on the future, 28% hoped that progress in medical research would help them; 17% hoped for a cure, and 13% strongly wished for improved metabolic control. Many adolescents (59%) were afraid of long-term damage.

In the 1992 interviews, the parents of these adolescents mentioned problems with illness management comparatively less often (injections 10%, diet 13%), yet considered the uncontrollability of the blood glucose levels to the greatest current problem (45%). Half of the families claimed that the illness had changed since the first interview a year earlier, stressing an increase in the adolescents' independence. Some of the parents said that their attitudes about the illness had also changed; 25% had come to terms with it, 14% even interpreted it positively, and 8% condemned it. When asked about the type and amount of assistance received in this year, the fathers' lack of initiative was again noteworthy (2%), whereas the help received from the ill adolescent had increased to 22%. In our second interview, the parents also mentioned relationship stressors within the family (14%) and puberty-related problems (28%). They reported changes in diabetes therapy, for example, the commencement of intensive therapy (28%), predominantly as a result of the physician's recommendation. In addition, the mothers frequently reported nervousness (37%) and irritability (13%). Nevertheless, over 70% of the parents believed that on the whole they had coped with their child's illness quite well, although their concerns about the future had grown. The parents' greatest concerns about the future were long-term physical damage (66% of the parents) and the restricted career opportunities for their children (17%). The perceived changes were more positively evaluated; 42% of the parents thought that their lives had become easier and freer, and they emphasized the adolescent's great independence in illness management.

By the third interview in 1993, when the diabetic adolescents were about 15.9 years old, a slightly larger number of parents relative to the second survey had come to terms with the illness (31%). The positive evaluation of the illness was comparatively rare (9%), and negative affect (condemning the diabetes) had become more infrequent (3%). Support for the family from the ill adolescent had further increased to 31%, whereas the father's assistance remained low (5%). As in previous years, special education centers for diabetics were considered a great help by 20% of the parents. Fewer relationship problems within the family were mentioned (13%). Although the parents reported having fewer difficulties in raising the adolescents (14%), they thought their adolescents were having more problems in school (24%). In addition, parents were concerned about their children's future career opportunities (9%), and they worried about their children's possible future problems with romantic partners or difficulties that the adolescents might have in becoming parents themselves someday (6%). Family finances had also become worries for some parents (14%). Overall, the percentage of parents who thought they had coped with their child's illness well had remained constant since the previous year, although the fear of long-term damage had risen (75%). The commencement of intensive therapy, often following the physician's suggestion, was mentioned by 22% of parents. No changes in the diabetes were reported by 50% of the parents, whereas 21% felt it had become worse and 29% recognized improvements.

In the fourth interview in 1994, the adolescents were about 16.9 years old. The parents' evaluations of how they had to come to terms with the illness were similar to those of the previous year. Fathers were slightly more involved in family matters (9%) than in earlier years. Unstable metabolic control, which had been a major issue from ages 14.9 to 15.9 years, had drastically decreased in significance. A further 11% of the adolescents had begun intensive diabetes therapy. Parents remained highly concerned about long-term damage to their children's health. They were more worried about their children's school-related problems (35%) and their children's future professions (21%). Parents reported an increase in the adolescents' leisure activities (31%) and activities involving romantic relationships (19%). The mothers' nervousness (19%) and emotional lability (8%) had significantly decreased in comparison with the beginning of our study. Overall, 67% of the parents reported no changes in the diabetes. In summary, this phase was relatively stable with respect to illness management, coping with the illness, and metabolic control.

Hardly any study to date has followed the process of coping with diabetes longitudinally by analyzing the parents' and the adolescents' reactions to the diagnosis in later phases of the illness. Kovacs et al. (1990) studied mothers of children with newly diagnosed type I diabetes and periodically assessed them over the next 6 years. Most mothers initially responded to their children's diagnosis with mild depression and emotional distress. These initial reactions subsided in about 6 to 9 months. After initial adjustment, there were slight increases in mothers' depressive symptoms over the duration of their children's illness. Overall psychological distress also increased during the course of the illness. Although symptoms increased, the stress of having a diabetic child did not pose a risk for serious maternal depression. Mothers' symptoms were unrelated to medical aspects of the diabetes and to levels of anxiety or depression reported by their children. The longer the child had the disease, the easier it became for the mothers to cope with it.

Our finding converge with those reported by Kovacs and co-workers in many respects. We also found strong family reactions, particularly in the mothers, shortly after diagnosis, yet less distress and more adaptation to the illness during its later phases. In addition, these reactions were mostly unrelated to medical aspects of diabetes. The initially high amount of family conflicts as well as the high nervousness and irritability of mothers decreased after the second year of the study. The results of the interviews further illustrate that although the overall levels of stress for the adolescents and their parents had barely diminished, there was a change in what was seen as stressful. In the first interview, when the patients were about 13.9 years old, the predominant matters of stress were related to the diagnosis, attempts to come to terms with illness management, and changes in the family. By the second interview, when the adolescents were around 14.9 years old, age-typical problems arose in the family, and the inability to control metabolic status due to hormonal changes put a great strain on the adolescents and their families. At the time of the third interview, when most adolescents were about 15.9 years old, the adolescents' increasing competence in managing the illness had allowed the parents to feel more relaxed, although metabolic control was still unstable. Concerns arose about the medical consequences of poor or unstable metabolic control (i.e., long-term damage) and the child's future occupational direction. Finally, at the time of the fourth interview, when the adolescents were about 16.9 years old, the parents' worries about long-term damage and the child's future career increased even more, along with concern about how the illness might hamper the adolescents' future partnerships and family planning. Taken together, these findings vividly illustrate the "chronic sorrow" (Hauser et al., 1993b) perceived by parents of chronically ill adolescents, as well as the complexity of concerns imposed on the family as a result of the illness (Hauser et al., 1997).

7

Chronic Illness and the Family: The Perspectives of Mothers, Fathers, and Siblings

---

The onset of a chronic illness confronts an adolescent with a situation that is highly stressful in various ways. Moreover, diagnosis and management of the illness present major long-term stressors for the parents as well (Eiser, 1985). Although some families are able to adjust to the illness by experimenting with new behaviors, other families are incapable of devising new strategies. They continue along familiar paths and rely on former methods of solving problems in order to meet the adolescent's new needs. Often one parent devotes the bulk of his or her time and energy to caring for the ill adolescent, thereby withdrawing from the other members of the family, a pattern seen most commonly in mothers of chronically ill children and adolescents (Cook, 1984). In this respect, it is important to clarify the father's role in the family's coping and whether the relationship between the ill adolescent and other children in the family is affected. Open and concealed conflicts could arise in the family, and these may undermine treatment and impair the adolescent's metabolic adjustment. A fundamental question is how the chronicity of the stressors contributes to dysfunctional behaviors in the family. The stress of an illness could, in itself, possibly be coped with well, but its chronicity might lead to a rigidity or a breakdown of coping even in a family that initially functioned well (Canning, Hanser, Shade, & Boyce, 1993; Trute & Hauch, 1988).

Conceptual Approaches for Understanding Family Dynamics in Families Dealing with Chronic Illness

The onset of a child's chronic illness is a source of stress, which spurs the family to develop coping strategies. These strategies may lead to a restructuring of family life that extends far beyond illness management and the family's coping style. The form of coping depends on the type of family and its history before the onset of the illness (Cole & Reiss, 1993). Some families develop functional coping processes that reduce the emotional stress and allow the family to deal effectively with the adolescent's needs. Other families are more preoccupied with the stress caused by the illness and its management. Although temporarily functional, the latter situation can be dysfunctional in the long term. Even in families in which functional forms of coping predominate, sustained stress can result in structural changes. Functional coping requires so much organizational control that it may eventually lead to a stifling inflexibility of interactions within the family. A rigid family style, although functional for illness management, interferes with other developmental tasks in adolescence that require flexibility.

Several conceptual approaches have been developed for understanding family dynamics in families dealing with chronic illness. According to the model proposed by Reiss and Oliveri (1980), the process of family coping involves the following three phases: (1) definition of the event and search for additional information; (2) initial reaction and preliminary solution; and (3) making the ultimate decision and final position, along with the family's obligation to it. According to Reiss and Oliveri (1980), the family's reaction when confronted with the stressor is not determined purely by the nature of the event. Over the years, each family develops its own paradigm, which provides the family with a stable orientation when it needs to cope with another stress-inducing situation. These authors propose that a family's coping abilities can be described according to three orthogonal dimensions, which they term configuration, coordination, and closure. Configuration relates to the family's ability to efficiently solve problems that face them as a group. Effective problem solving is also a sign that the family perceives the world as coherent and something they can cope with. Such families' routine actions will be orderly; they will react competently to new situations. Coordination relates to the importance the family attaches to cohesion and cooperation when confronted with a problem. In some families cohesion is the main concern: Family members are expected to act in agreement, and conflicts are avoided. In other families the individuals insist on their independence. Families with high scores on this dimension see themselves as a unit with respect to the outside world. Closure relates to the family's flexibility and openness to new information when faced with a problem. Some families seek new possibilities in adapting to actual situations, whereas others are closed to new information. Early closure in a family's attitude to the external world results in a fixed, unyielding view of the world.

According to the authors, a family that perceives the world as coherent and is in a position to operate flexibly and as a group will perceive the child's illness realistically and treat it as the concern of the whole family. In contrast, if a family considers the world to be a constant source of stress, the onset of an illness will strengthen that perspective, and the family will organize itself against the seemingly threatening environment. The family paradigm influences not merely the perception of the illness but also every further step in coping with it. Reiss and Oliveri's (1980) model thus puts coping behavior in the context of family dynamics. Families that have a fundamentally positive view of the world, whose relationships are characterized by cooperation, and that are flexible almost always develop functional forms of coping. They perceive the child's condition realistically and work together to meet the requirements of the medical therapy. For families that have difficult relationships with each other and their environment, the onset of the child's illness may become a formidable source of stress that cannot be dealt with. In some cases, these families are unable to deal with new demands, such as illness management. Owing to poor adherence to the therapeutic regimen, the child's condition can deteriorate further.

Lewis (1986) confirmed that even functional and flexible families may display increasing rigidity as the family attempts to meet the challenge of dealing with stress on a continual and long-term basis. Such a situation is certainly the case in families having to care for a chronically ill child. In any case, it is clear that structural changes occur in the family caring for an adolescent with chronic illness. Such changes may be expressed in many ways. In the case of diabetes, the family system typically becomes markedly reorganized in order to attend to and fulfill the requirements of the diabetic treatment regimen. All families must strictly follow physicians' instructions and maintain an ever watchful eye over their child's behavior for a long period of time, which as in the case of diabetes, often extends into adulthood. Injections must be given at specific times, and regular consultations with a physician are necessary. These and other requirements make it necessary for the family to observe a strict timetable of daily activities, which in turn, may make family life quite inflexible. Accordingly, interactions among family members may change radically. In his study of families with a seriously ill member, Anthony (1970) observed that the family structure changed from flexible to unyielding. Similarly, one particular member of the family might, for instance, assume a more dominant role in the family structure. This may happen when a single family member, usually the mother, becomes solely responsible for overseeing the adolescent's medical treatment, thus becoming the expert on dealing with the needs of the ill child or adolescent. Even when, as was the case in our sample, the adolescent manages the illness very efficiently and independently, the mother continues to exercise the responsibility of monitoring the day-to-day procedures involved in the management of the illness. In doing so, she may reorganize the family's daily routine so that she is able to act more efficiently. Thus, in the long run, she may assume a more active and controlling role, whereas other family members, including the father, are forced into the background. According to French (1977), such structural changes often begin gradually and are accepted with difficulty. Although in most families they initially appear in the form of organized, integrated reactions aimed at achieving efficiency and stability, an overly rigid pattern of family life may ensue. In some families, new conflicts may arise, increasing the stress already caused by the chronic illness. The family's sense of unity may suffer greatly, and coordination of family activities as well as cooperation among family members becomes stifled.

Other conceptual approaches toward describing families who must cope with a chronically ill member focus more on categorizing general family pathology. Minuchin and colleagues (Minuchin, Baker, & Rosman, 1975; Minuchin et al., 1978) described the family living with a diabetic adolescent as the prototypical "psychosomatic" family, characterized by (1) enmeshment, that is, extreme closeness and intensity in interactions, along with insufficient individuation and interpersonal differentiation; (2) oversolicitousness, that is, overprotective and restrictive parental behavior concerning the ill child; (3) stiffness and rigidity, that is, resistance to change, which may create problems in adolescence when parent–child interactions are altered; and (4) conflict avoidance. Sargent (1985, p. 220) specified that families with "psychosomatic diabetes" may be recognized by their

> ...enmeshment, overprotectiveness, rigidity, lack of effective conflict resolution, and involvement of a sick child in parental conflict.

Such family members are not adequately dissociated from one another, and attempts to achieve independence give rise to great irritation. Although enmeshment is generally an important element of the parent–child relationship, when children become adolescents they require more distance and independence. Instead, these families tend to rigidly maintain the status quo. Poor dissociation between family subsystems may be revealed by the parents' tendency to involve their children in marital conflicts. This family system theory further asserts that these psychosomatic families deal with stressors inappropriately, in that they seek solutions within the family, which leads to even more stress.

Changes in Family Climate and Family Communication

The Family's Organization Around the Illness

This chapter explores the family's perspective on living with a chronically ill family member, focusing on families with a diabetic adolescent. Based on the data of our 4-year longitudinal study, the context of the general family situation will be considered first and the different roles of mothers, fathers, and siblings in coping with the illness will then be explored. As outlined in chapter 6, the family members must deal with the illness cognitively, that is, they must understand the physiological aspects of and acquire knowledge about diabetes. All family members must cope with the emotional aspects of the illness, for example, the overt and covert expressions of sadness, despair, and anger. Diabetes management entails performing specific actions on a regular basis, including giving injections, conducting blood and urine tests, planning and keeping to a special diet, and engaging in physical exercise. The coordination of such activities forces the whole family to adopt and adjust to a new routine. Additionally, visits to physicians and hospitals can entail long stays away from home, thus compromising common family time and organization. In most cases, the adolescent is not the only child in the family; other children must also be looked after. The family's financial situation may also be put at a disadvantage. Not only do increased expenditures for special food and transportation to the physician or hospital put a strain on the family budget, but because of increased time demands or stress at home, the breadwinners of the family may not be able to live up to the responsibilities of their jobs and will thereby suffer a loss of income. In short, the family's routine is greatly determined by the adolescent's illness, on cognitive, emotional, and above all, behavioral levels (Drotar, 1998; Grey et al., 1998). Ahmed and Ahmed (1985) have described how the family's entire life-style is rearranged by caring for a diabetic child. In their study, all of the parents reported changes to the family schedule and 90% reported changes to eating habits. The amount of housework had increased for 60%, and 25% of the parents reported that their holiday arrangements had been disturbed by the illness. One-third of the parents said that their child's illness affected their employment.

It is, of course, necessary to provide details about our sample's overall home and psychosocial situations, because they represent the background against which the family's coping efforts and interaction patterns may be understood. As detailed in chapter 3, the families participating in our study were largely intact. The proportion of two-parent families was even higher in the group of diabetic adolescents (84%) than in the healthy control group (76%). The majority of diabetic adolescents were from the middle class, and most (89%) were German citizens. An average of 2.3 children was present in each family. The average ages of the fathers and mothers of ill adolescents were 45 years and 42 years, respectively. The parents had similar levels of school education: 40% of the fathers and 47% of the mothers had finished Hauptschule (a type of secondary school in Germany, encompassing grades 5 to 10); 23% of the fathers and 26% of the mothers had completed Realschule (a second type of German secondary school, encompassing grades 5 to 11); and 27% of the fathers and 24% of the mothers had completed Gymnasium (a third type of German secondary school, encompassing grades 5 to 13, successful graduation from which entitles one to pursue university studies). Most (90%) of the fathers were employed, 9% were pursuing further education or training, and 1% were unemployed. Half of the diabetic adolescents' mothers were unemployed, a relatively high proportion compared with the 37% of healthy adolescents' mothers who were unemployed. At least 5% of the fathers and 16% of the mothers indicated that their employment position had been affected by their child's illness. In particular, mothers also mentioned that they had been compelled to switch to part-time work, accept unfavorable salary conditions, or change their place of employment because of the increased demands of caring for their diabetic child.

Throughout our study, we also documented the frequency of clinic and hospital stays, the number of changes to other clinics, the distance between the clinic and the home, and the type of contact between parents and the ill child during a hospital stay. A change of clinic had been undertaken by 49% of the parents, of whom 26% changed only once and 23% changed twice or more. The trip to the physician or clinic was an average of 21 km (distances ranged from 1 to 80 km), shorter than the distances reported by other investigators for oncology patients or patients with cystic fibrosis (Petermann, 1994). The expenditures related to the illness ranged from 150 to 7,000 DM (German marks) annually, with a mean of 2,614 DM. For example, special dietary considerations and daily trips to visit the adolescents during hospital stays contributed to an increased strain on the family's budget. Of the parents in our study, 65% reported having made such trips to visit their children at clinics, which in some cases were quite far away from home. The financial burden was felt to be very substantial by 5% of parents, whereas 11% considered it to be substantial, 35% reported a noticeable strain, and only 30% did not consider the burden worth mentioning.

In summary, for most of the variables we measured (nationality, family structure, number of siblings, parents' ages, father's employment), the psychosocial situation in families with chronically ill adolescents did not differ from that in the control families. However, considerably fewer diabetic adolescents' mothers were employed, a difference that has been frequently found in research on mothers of chronically ill children and adolescents (Beresford, 1994). In addition, diabetic adolescents' parents had greater organizational concerns, experienced more changes to their employment circumstances, and had more financial worries. None of the psychosocial variables measured at the beginning of our study were associated with the adolescent's metabolic status, apart from the higher frequency of lower-class families with poorly adjusted adolescents. This trend has also been established in other studies (Ahmed & Ahmed, 1985; Silver, Bauman, Coupey, Doctors, & Boeck, 1990).

Impact on Parental Roles and Family Climate

In our sample, diabetes typically occurred at a time when the adolescents were beginning to distance themselves from the parents; yet the parents were still considerably involved in the management of the illness. Our findings demonstrate that the parents considered the increased burden of demands, responsibilities, and worries to be sizable. It is not surprising, therefore, that some studies have found adaptation problems in the patients' parents (Beresford, 1994; Canning et al., 1993; Chaney, Mullins, Frank, & Peterson, 1997; Crain, Susman, & Weil, 1986; Kovacs et al., 1990), a change in parent–adolescent relationships (Eiser & Berrenberg, 1995), and high rates of family conflict, which in turn contribute to a worsening of metabolic control in the adolescent (Koski & Kumento, 1975). In our study, the physicians emphasized that it was almost always the mother who assumed responsibility for supervising the diabetes treatment regimen, including all related medical procedures, and for accompanying the adolescent to consultations with the physician (see chapter 4). As detailed in chapter 6, mothers initially responded to their children's diagnosis with mild depression and emotional distress. During the following years, mothers described their continual supervision of the treatment regimen as a major stressor and continued to report elevated levels of psychological distress. At the time of our first survey in 1991, we found that the diabetic adolescents had already mastered a range of procedures (including blood and urine testing, giving themselves insulin injections, and observing dietary restrictions) at the relatively young average age of 13.9 years. Nevertheless, most mothers still worried about whether the adolescent was truly able to assume these responsibilities. Hauser and Bowlds (1990) have described this parental monitoring vividly. Our study further revealed that mothers received hardly any support from their spouses in everyday family duties and in responsibilities related to the illness; however, about one-third of the mothers reported that the ill adolescents supported them in dealing with the stressors associated with the illness.

Until recently, presentations in the clinical literature of a global family pathology were very prominent. As previously mentioned, Minuchin et al. (1975; 1978) and Sargent (1985) described the family living with diabetes as the prototypical psychosomatic family, characterized by enmeshment, oversolicitousness, rigidity, and conflict avoidance. The family system theories proposed by these authors assert that these psychosomatic families deal with stressors inappropriately, leading to psychopathology. Although some studies (e.g., Delbridge, 1975; Koski, 1969; White et al., 1984) have established links among pathological family relationships, an unfavorable course of the illness, and poor compliance, others have generally not confirmed the assumptions of a psychosomatic family or of psychosomatic diabetes (Coyne & Anderson, 1988; Wood, Watkins, Nogueira, Zimand, & Carrol 1989).

In evaluating the links of family relations and child psychopathology with psychopathology in families with diabetic adolescents, researchers have focused on two diabetes-specific outcomes, namely, degree of metabolic control and overall psychosocial adaptation. The achievement-oriented family climate observed by Billings and Moos (1982) demonstrates how families adjust to the management of diabetes. Families with this climate exhibited more rigid interaction styles and more control in their attempts to adjust to the management of their diabetic child's illness. Similarly, Overstreet et al. (1995) found that diabetic children showed better metabolic control in families with a high level of organization than those in less structured families. In contrast, other researchers have emphasized the importance of a positive emotional family climate (high cohesion, high expressiveness, and low conflict) in achieving good metabolic control (Hanson, De Guire, Schinkel, & Kolterman, 1995; La Greca, Siegel, Wallander, & Walker, 1992). With respect to the adolescents' developmental needs, it appears that a beneficial family climate is marked by cohesion, flexibility, and organization and is one in which personal growth is emphasized and leisure activities encouraged (Hanson et al., 1987; Hauser & Solomon, 1985; Sargent, 1985; Wolman, Resnick, Harris, & Blum, 1994). According to Wertlieb et al. (1986), active leisure activities, clear organization, and responsibility in the family are accompanied by fewer behavioral problems. A study by Hanson et al. (1992a) demonstrated that a family climate offering support as well as independence also may positively influence the illness. In this study, high levels of flexibility and illness-specific support in the family were associated with good adjustment to the illness. These findings suggest that the conditions for optimal psychosocial development in healthy and chronically ill adolescents are essentially the same. Should parents of a diabetic adolescent be able to unite flexibility in the organization and structure of family life with a positive emotional climate, one may expect to see the most beneficial effects on the adolescent's metabolic control.

Altogether, the family climate appears to be a central factor in adjusting to diabetes. The most favorable family climate is cohesive, experiences little conflict, shows well-defined structure and organization, and encourages leisure activities and an age-appropriate level of independence in the child. Our longitudinal study explored the perceived family climate from the perspectives of all family members by means of the Family Environment Scale (FES) (Moos and Moos, 1981). Ill adolescents differed in perceived family climate from healthy adolescents in several dimensions. They reported that family life was more strongly structured, organized, and controlled, and that there was greater orientation toward achievement. Although these changes are functional for coping with diabetes, they might lead to a rigid family structure, which hinders the family members' further development. Evidence of this danger was already visible in the first survey in 1991: Diabetic adolescents perceived fewer possibilities for personal growth and autonomy than their healthy peers.

The adolescents' evaluations of the family climate corresponded closely to those of their parents. However, there were also some differences, particularly with respect to expressiveness and the amount of conflict in the family. Generally, mothers of healthy adolescents indicated that conflicts were more common in their families but that feelings were more openly expressed. This view corresponds to the adolescents' perspectives. Figure 7.1 further illustrates that more mothers of healthy adolescents perceived their families as being intellectually stimulating, oriented toward leisure activities, and supportive of granting the adolescents more independence. These results concur with findings reported by Galambos and Almeida (1992), Collins and Russel (1991), and Seiffge-Krenke (1998a; 1999) for families with healthy adolescents. In these studies, adolescents' relationships with their mothers were closer and warmer but also more prone to conflict than their relationships with their fathers. In our study, no differ-

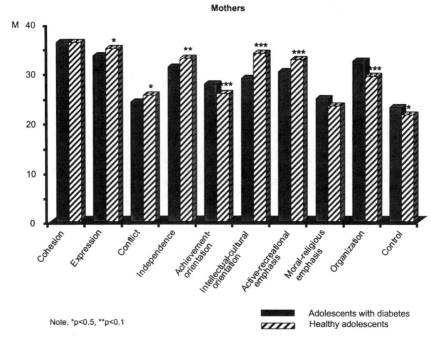

Note. *p<0.5, **p<0.1

■ Adolescents with diabetes
▨ Healthy adolescents

Figure 7.1. Differences in family climate perceived by mothers of diabetic adolescents ($N = 100$) and mothers of healthy adolescents ($N = 118$).

ences were found between fathers of healthy and diabetic adolescents in their perceptions of expressiveness and conflict in the family. However, fathers of diabetic adolescents reported more organization, control, and achievement orientation but less independence and leisure time orientation than fathers of healthy adolescents (see following section).

Altogether, families with a healthy adolescent were closer, dealt with conflicts more openly, and offered more autonomy, creating an overall atmosphere that was more beneficial to development. In contrast, families with diabetic adolescents displayed a family climate reminiscent of the achievement-oriented family type described by Billings and Moos (1982), featuring high levels of family organization, control, and goal orientation, and minimal regard for the family members' independence. In our study, this highly structured family climate was found in all families with diabetic adolescents regardless of illness duration or level of metabolic control (Seiffge-Krenke, 1998b). Families with diabetic adolescents showing good metabolic control differed from families with less well adjusted diabetic adolescents only in the better quality of their interpersonal relationships.

Similar findings were reported by Anderson, Miller, Auslander, and Santiago (1981) and Koski and Kumento (1975). Although cohesion was higher in families with well adjusted diabetic adolescents, the adolescents were not allowed more autonomy and felt subjected to more control. This highly structured family climate seems most functional for the purpose of achieving and maintaining good medical adaptation, as the majority of our sample were well or satisfactorily adjusted (see chapter 3).

Changes in Family Climate Over Time?

As detailed above, research has established links between family climate and adolescent functioning, for example, degree of metabolic control and psychosocial adaptation. The challenges posed by coping with the illness appear to be well met by increasing the levels of structure and achievement orientation in the family climate. However, the family must also deal with more comprehensive and diverse challenges related to the normal process of development in adolescence. For instance, the adolescent must achieve more autonomy (Steinberg, 1989). The distribution of authority, power, and control as well as the structure of communication in the family may be correspondingly altered. As various authors have stressed, these changes are associated with an increase in parent–adolescent and interspousal conflicts; when the new functions and roles have been established, the conflict rate decreases again (Montemayor, 1983; Hill, 1987; Seiffge-Krenke, 1999). Adolescents become more independent, while parents are increasingly relieved of their duties of care and can apply themselves to new activities.

Our longitudinal analyses revealed that the highly structured family climate observed in families with diabetic adolescents remained stable over time, showing very little potential for change. This was most clearly demonstrated in the mothers' reports; their appraisals of most of the 10 family climate dimensions that we measured remained constant. That is, as compared with the healthy adolescents' mothers, diabetic adolescents' mothers continued to characterize the family climate as being less expressive and showing less conflict but being more achievement-oriented. Little time was allocated to the pursuit of leisure or intellectual activities; family life was determined by structure and control of the individual family members and by moral principles. The mothers of the diabetic adolescents reported a decrease in organization over time, yet their scores for this aspect of family climate remained above the mean scores of those in the healthy control group. Fathers of ill adolescents made similar judgments. They perceived less open expression of emotion between family members, high levels of family organization and structure, and little interest in pursuing family external or leisure activities over time. As illustrated in Figure 7.2, this resulted in consistent discrepancies between the family climates in healthy and diabetic groups over the course of 4 years. On the average, parents of diabetic adolescents reported more structure and control in their families and portrayed a significantly worse emotional family climate than did parents of healthy adolescents. In addition, parents of diabetic adolescents perceived the family climate as being less stimulating and offering fewer possibilities for personal growth.

Because very few studies have analyzed the changes to family climate in ill and healthy adolescents longitudinally, there is little basis for a comparison with our own results. A 4-year longitudinal study conducted by Hauser and colleagues examined the links between family context and the adolescent's adjustment to diabetes. Some differences were found in the way the family context was experienced: Diabetic adolescents perceived much stronger moral-religious orientation and felt that their families placed more emphasis on organization and structuring (Wertlieb et al., 1986). Hauser et al. (1990) found that family cohesion was accompanied by good adjustment to the illness. After only 1 year, an association emerged between avoidance of conflict and poor adjustment; this remained constant over the 4 years. The parents' perceptions of high family organization correlated with good short- and long-term adjustment to the illness, but high organization as perceived by the adolescents was unrelated to metabolic control. Our results agree with Hauser et al.'s (1990) longitudinal study with respect to the importance of organization and structure in families living with diabetes. However, in contrast to their findings, we found that family conflict had only a negligible effect on poor metabolic control. Positive family dimensions, such as high cohesion and open expression of feelings, were important for maintaining the positive course of the illness in families with a well adjusted adolescent.

The Highly Structured Family Climate: Functional or Dysfunctional for Metabolic Control?

Since in our study we observed the families after the diagnosis of diabetes had been made, no conclusions can be drawn about family roles and climate before the onset of the illness. Nevertheless, we found that even in families with adolescents who were well adjusted in medical terms (that is, they had achieved optimal HbA_1 or $HbA_{1}c$ values), structure and control did not decrease over time. Over 90% of the adolescents performed their own

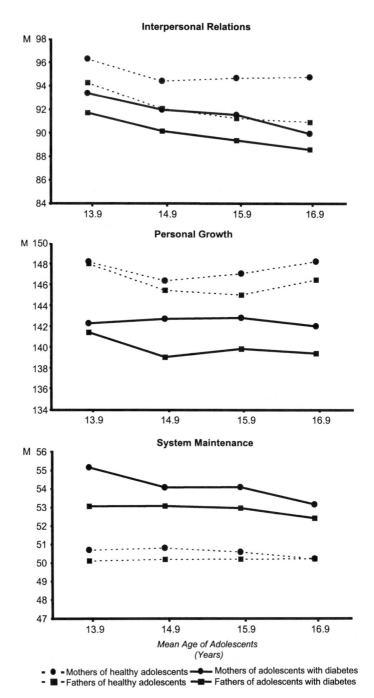

Figure 7.2. Changes in three main dimensions of family climate over time as perceived by diabetic and healthy adolescents' mothers ($N = 103, 86$) and fathers ($N = 81, 66$).

injections at the beginning of the study in 1991, when they were about 13.9 years old. In the following years, adolescents became even more independent in managing the illness, so that the mothers' – and to a much lesser extent, the fathers' – real contributions to illness management became comparatively small. Despite the adolescents' increasing independence in assuming responsibility for management of the illness, the parents, especially the mothers, remained overwhelmed with "chronic worry" (see chapter 6). Although parental supervision of the therapeutic regimen became less necessary, parental control, structure, and achievement orientation did not decrease noticeably. It appears that a high degree of control must become a central organizing principle of the family if the adolescent is to achieve satisfactory metabolic control.

As mentioned in chapter 4, the quality of metabolic control typically changes during puberty. However, we observed little flexibility in adjustment of the family climate with respect to fluctuating HbA_1 or HbA_1c values of diabetic adolescents. A change in family climate was neither apparent in periods of generally good metabolic adjustment (at about 13.9 years, and again at 16.9 years), nor in mid-adolescence, when metabolic control worsened owing to hormonal fluctuations. In addition, regression analyses revealed that neither the parents' nor the adolescents' perceptions of family climate were predictive for metabolic control over time (Seiffge-Krenke, 1998b). Also, illness duration was only associated with minor differences in family climate. As detailed in chapter 3, at the beginning of our study a recent onset of the illness could be documented for about a third of the diabetic adolescents, whereas about 46% had been ill for over 5 years. We expected levels of cohesion and control to depend on illness duration, but this was only true to a minor extent. Adolescent girls with a short to intermediate illness duration perceived a more stimulating family climate, which even increased over time, whereas girls who had already been ill for over 5 years at the beginning of our study experienced the least leisure time orientation and independence (Seiffge-Krenke, 1998b). This pattern was not precisely mirrored in diabetic adolescent boys. As with girls, boys with a short duration of illness experienced a more stimulating family climate and greater encouragement of recreational activities. However, boys who had already been ill for over 5 years at the beginning of the study reported the fewest recreational activities of all groups, and this did not vary over time. Patterson et al. (1990) have emphasized the importance of intellectual and leisure activities for coping with the illness because these activities provide opportunities of distraction from illness-specific stressors, which in turn fosters a more relaxed family atmosphere.

Whereas the families with a healthy adolescent displayed a changing pattern of relationships (decreasing cohesion, an increase in conflict, and more emphasis on the adolescent's independence), families with a diabetic adolescent were not able to offer their adolescents more autonomy. In particular, those adolescents who had been afflicted with diabetes for a long time were not offered more possibilities to achieve independence, and the emphasis on recreational activities was even less than in families of adolescents with short illness duration. Thus, it appears that individuality and independence are not nurtured in families with chronically ill adolescents. A rigid family style, although favorable for medical adaptation, interferes with developmental tasks that require flexibility in the family and are necessary for later stages of development (see chapter 9).

The question remains whether structural changes creating more control in the family are indeed functional for adjustment to diabetes. As detailed in chapter 4, two-thirds of the diabetic adolescents in our study had good to satisfactory metabolic control at the beginning of the study in 1991, when they were about 13.9 years old. During the next 2 years, HbA_1 and HbA_1c levels increased slightly with the onset of normally occurring hormonal changes and then became stable again by the time of the fourth survey in 1994, when the mean age of the adolescents was 16.9 years. The longitudinal analyses revealed that by the age of 16.9 years, 39% of the adolescents showed poor metabolic control but that the other 61% had attained satisfactory to good metabolic control. Since the majority of the adolescents showed at least adequate metabolic adjustment over the course of adolescence, one might speculate that the family climate we observed had exerted positive effects on the diabetic adolescents' physiological adjustment. However, as detailed above, neither parents' nor adolescents' perceptions of family climate were predictive for metabolic control at any time. This suggests that a highly structured family climate is not singularly instrumental in promoting physiological adjustment to diabetes. Nevertheless, this type of family climate seems to provide a context that favors the attainment of metabolic control.

Communication in Families with Diabetic Adolescents

In this section, the specific interactions within the family are analyzed. Several methods have been developed in recent years for assessing interactions and communication within the "normal" family. Such methods are valuable for those interested in learning if and how the interactions or communication patterns that a family exhibits influence the process of psychosocial development in adolescence. For our study, we selected an approach based on Grotevant and Cooper's (1986) theory of individuation. According to this theory, parent–adolescent relationships are characterized by varying degrees of connectedness and individuality, which are subject to change over time. Individuation is marked by the transformation of a unilateral, complementary parent–child relationship to one showing comradeship and mutuality. The clear advantage of this theoretical approach is that it takes into account the adolescent's need to separate from the parents emotionally without having to forfeit the existing bond based on mutual trust and understanding (see Baumrind, 1991; Youniss, 1983).

What constitutes an individuated relationship? Grotevant and Cooper (1986) operationalized individuation according to four orthogonal factors, namely mutuality and permeability, which constitute connectedness, and self-assertion and separateness, which constitute individuality. These factors are mirrored in parent–child interactions, particularly in interpersonal communicative behavior. Accordingly, a relationship featuring connectedness and individuality might be expected to display the following kind of communicative behavior: The partners are aware of their respective positions and are prepared to assume responsibility for their thoughts and feelings, which they express clearly and directly (self-assertion). They can recognize and articulate differences between the other's attitudes and their own (separateness). At the same time, they are open to the other's ideas and attitudes and allow themselves to enter into discussion about the other's position (permeability). In addition, they respect the other's ideas and wishes and are prepared to confirm and support them in their individuality (mutuality).

To assess the pattern of family communication, Condon, Cooper, and Grotevant (1984) developed the Family Interaction Task (FIT), in which the family members must solve a hypothetical problem together, namely, the family must plan a 3-week vacation, given unlimited funds. According to Grotevant and Cooper (1985; 1986) this type of task is most appropriate for studying interactions in families with adolescents. The topic allows adolescents to participate in the decision process because they are explicitly invited to contribute their competence and experience. The task is simple enough that all family members can equally participate, and power sharing processes are fostered. Indeed, these authors' central assumption is that in the optimal situation, the family members' contributions will balance individuality with connectedness. The assumptions of the model were examined by Cooper, Grotevant, and Condon (1983) in a study of 121 adolescents and their families. They confirmed the greater social maturity and personal development of adolescents who had developed an individuated relationship with their parents, as compared with adolescents whose relationships to their parents had failed to strike a balance between connectedness and individuality.

In our longitudinal study, we used the FIT twice as a tool for assessing communication in the families: in 1991, when the adolescents had a mean age of 13.9 years, and again in 1993, when they were about 15.9 years old. Following the guidelines set down in the FIT manual (Condon et al., 1984), each family was asked to plan a 3-week vacation, for which an unlimited amount of money was available. The families were asked to solve this task in the absence of the interviewer. The family's discussion was recorded on tape and subsequently transcribed. Families were allowed a maximum of 20 minutes to complete the task and were permitted to call the interviewer if they finished the task before the allotted time was over. Previous investigations using the FIT have shown that family conversations can be easily reduced to 300 chunks or fewer without losing information because most communicative behavior in the family remains relatively stable throughout the FIT (Cooper, Grotevant, & Condon, 1982). We therefore followed Cooper et al.'s (1982) suggestion to evaluate only the first 300 chunks of each family discussion. One chunk was defined as a sentence or a unit of meaning. After training the raters on the use of coding procedures outlined in the FIT manual, satisfactory agreement among three raters (ranging from 72 to 81%) was established for the four main dimensions coded in the FIT on the basis of 15 randomly selected family discussions.

It was interesting that the families with a diabetic adolescent (mean age 13.9 years) held significantly shorter discussions than families with a healthy adolescent. The mean lengths of the discussions (measured as mean number of chunks) in families with a healthy adolescent ($M = 131.19, SD = 71.60$) were much higher than in families with diabetic adolescents ($M = 86.62, SD = 38.62$); that is, families with a healthy adolescent exhibited almost twice as much communicative effort to discuss the problem as did families with diabetic adolescents. This basic difference emerged again when we used the FIT for a second time, when the mean adolescent age was 15.9 years. Although this finding might suggest that the families with diabetic adolescents were more efficient at reaching an agreement than families with a healthy adolescent, further examination of the communicative interactions was necessary to explain this finding. As compared with the healthy adolescents' mothers, the diabetic adolescents' mothers introduced more indirect suggestions and requested information or consensus from the other family members much more often. Fathers of diabetic adolescents contributed little to communication in the family, and they seldom directly and clearly rejected their spouses' suggestions. Mothers of diabetic adolescents articulated the differences between family members' positions much less often, and their interactive behavior was more uncertain and defensive. Taken together, both the fathers and the mothers in these families had very low values for the dimension of separateness, a category for which the parents of healthy adolescents scored highly. Mothers and fathers in families with a diabetic adolescent exhibited less individuality, and an atmosphere of unanimity was achieved.

The results of the FIT have not yet been analyzed with respect to the status of diabetic adolescents' metabolic control. However, an analysis with respect to adolescent gender revealed some interesting differences (Fentner & Seiffge-Krenke, 1997). The atmosphere in families with diabetic daughters was more mutual and accepting, largely because the mother–daughter interactions were characterized by many validating and confirming communicative processes. Mothers and daughters showed more openness and respect for each other's contributions overall. Daughters asked for information from their mothers, sought their agreement more often, and supported or accepted the mother's comments more often. Diabetic girls' mothers were even more accepting and interested in their daughters' needs and ideas than were the mothers of diabetic sons. Compared with the fathers of diabetic sons, fathers of diabetic daughters directly refused their child's suggestions less frequently and contradicted their wives less.

The longitudinal analysis revealed that the process of individuation as described by Grotevant and Cooper (1985) was evident in all families. Separateness and permeability decreased over the course of the survey, which suggests that in all families, the family members no longer felt compelled to assert their own respective standpoints and that less dissent about differences in attitudes took place. All families had achieved a new balance between connectedness and individuality, and communication was characterized by more comradeship and mutuality. Similar changes were observed in families with healthy adolescents and in those with diabetic adolescents. However, some differences were still noticeable when the adolescents were about 15.9 years old, which indicated that some aspects of the original pattern were maintained in families with diabetic adolescents. As mentioned, families with a diabetic adolescent required less time to find a solution for the FIT task, and they communicated less overall. Suggestions were not negotiated as much as in families with a healthy adolescent, the range of ideas expressed was narrower, and the ideas of others were less often incorporated. Instead, there was a strong need for confirmation and validation, most particularly from the mother (even more so when the ill adolescent was female). Whereas the proposals and suggestions made by the diabetic adolescents' parents were less distinct, those made by the healthy adolescents' parents were clearer and more direct. The healthy adolescents' parents also tended to show greater and more direct disagreement. In addition, healthy adolescents showed more separateness than diabetic adolescents did.

To date, few studies have examined communication in families with a diabetic adolescent. In one study, Carlson, Gesten, McIver, DeClue, and Malone (1994) analyzed communication and problem solving skills in 20 families with a diabetic child and 20 families with a healthy child (mean age, 11 years). The families participated in a simulated problem solving task (planning a weekend) while being videotaped. The investigator left the room while the family members had 10 minutes to solve the task. It was found that families with a diabetic child talked less than families with a healthy child, posed fewer questions, and gave fewer commands. In addition, families with a diabetic child generated a higher proportion of positive statements and interrupted one another less during the task. In an earlier study, Hauser et al. (1986) analyzed family communication patterns after documenting the frequency of enabling and constraining family interactions. Mothers of adolescents with recently diagnosed diabetes, in comparison with mothers of healthy adolescents, were found to be more accepting and supportive of their spouses and their diabetic children in family discussions. Diabetic adolescents' fathers, however, were found to be more judgmental and indifferent. Bobrow and Avkuskin (1985) analyzed mother–daughter relationships in 50 families with diabetic daughters, aged 12 to 17 years, using the Hill Interaction Matrix. They found differences related to the diabetic adolescents' levels of metabolic control. Female adolescents with good diabetic control (measured by HbA_1 values) had fewer diabetes-related conflicts and were more efficient at solving problems that caused conflict. The relationship between mother and daughter was warm and empathic, feelings were expressed openly, and wishes and ideas were clearly formulated. Daughters with poorer metabolic control made more negative remarks, made less of an effort to understand their mothers' viewpoints, and carried out the procedures of the medical treatment regimen on their own authority, without discussion. Their mothers accused them of showing unacceptable behavior, criticized them often, and contributed to an escalation of conflict. In summary, these findings suggest that a major stressor like diabetes may affect family communication in various ways that warrant further investigation.

Consequences of Continual Stress in Families with Diabetic Adolescents

In chapter 6, family coping processes used in dealing with the adolescent's illness were described. In this section, the questions of if and how the illness can also cause enduring changes in family organization, climate, and communication will be discussed. The results obtained in the analysis of family functioning can be explained in terms of theories of family stress and coping processes. The family pattern observed in our study did not correspond to that described by Minuchin, Rosman, and Baker (1989) in their discussion of "psychosomatic diabetics," that is, a family characterized by unclear role definitions, overprotective behavior, rigidity, avoidance of conflict, and a lack of problem solving ability. Most of the families in our study were reminiscent of families described in the framework of the family stress theory and family system models. These families put much effort into coping with illness, and they were functional with respect to illness management. Structure and organization became such central principles of family life that they became permanently embedded in their family paradigm (Reiss & Klein, 1987).

Because of the sustained levels of stress over time, increased rigidity became apparent. The temporarily functional family paradigm thus gave way to a negative outcome. During the 4 years of our study, the families did not respond flexibly to changes in metabolic control or illness duration, and they also did not take into account the increasing independence and overall good adaptation of the majority of our diabetic adolescents. This finding is disquieting, since it indicates that a family might negatively influence, that is, retard or inhibit, an adolescent's overall developmental progression regardless of metabolic control and illness duration. In addition, the family climate was less cohesive and less stimulating than in families with a healthy adolescent. Thus, in the families with diabetic adolescents, closure was comparably high, and external resources were lacking.

An analysis of the communication styles in families with a diabetic adolescent further revealed that parents and adolescents negotiated their differences less often. Diabetic adolescents' mothers and fathers displayed highly similar behavior; their suggestions for solving a task were less specific, and they communicated more indirectly. Problems were not discussed fully, and often quick, yet unsatisfactory solutions were found. Families with an ill adolescent appeared to avoid conflict, as they did not display the increased intensity of conflict observed in the control families. The many indirect and uncertain contributions to discussions indicated how difficult it was to maintain a certain position or to signal boundaries or divergent opinions. Over time, families with a diabetic adolescent achieved a new balance between connectedness and individuality, albeit a fragile one.

Overall, the families with diabetic adolescents were characterized by a mismatch between a strong family paradigm and insufficiently systematic maturation, as described by Steinglass, Bennet, Wolin, and Reiss (1987). It appears that the illness and its possible long-term consequences are so stressful to all family members that the main goal is to maintain the status quo. However, the family as a system needs to develop further in order to cope effectively with future demands, which go far beyond the illness. It would be desirable if families with a diabetic child could be relieved of some stress by assuring them that unstable metabolic control is typical for adolescence and that the course of the illness can be expected to improve over time. Perhaps some families could embrace the new developmental tasks their children are confronting if they understood that the family's influence on metabolic control is limited. Excessive organization and structuring at the peak of puberty cannot prevent a slight deterioration of HbA_1 values; in fact, it may even be counterproductive. Like so many other developmentally related (and often irritating) changes occurring in adolescence, the unstable phase of metabolic adjustment in puberty later gives way to improved control.

Fathers of Ill Adolescents: Their Roles in the Coping Process

In the previous sections, the focus of attention was on the family as a unit and in particular, the ill adolescent's mother. This section explores the father's role in family functioning and the coping process. More specifically, the questions of if and how fathers can help adolescents to achieve autonomy and independence despite their severe chronic illness are discussed. In the following it will become clear that the father's role in this process depends on the severity and duration of the adolescent's illness. If an adolescent can manage the illness independently without introducing many restrictions on the family's life-style, the father's role will be very different from his role when the illness is life-threatening, requires constant supervision, and has an uncertain prognosis. Family structure and climate may also vary with the type of illness. In other words, fathers of chronically ill adolescents must be flexible and prepared to change.

*The Distinctive Roles of Fathers in Comparison with Mothers
of Chronically Ill Adolescents*

In the meta-analyses of studies on chronically ill adolescents and their parents (Hanl 1995; Seiffge-Krenke & Brath, 1990), most of the 334 studies concentrated on the mother's reaction to the chronic illness. Responses were obtained most often from the ill adolescents themselves (58%), but the mother was also a frequent respondent (78%). Few studies included both parents (33%), and none relied solely on the father's responses. Similarly, nearly all studies dealing with terminal illnesses and coping with death and dying have relied on the mothers' perspectives. It seems that the support, help, and care a chronically ill adolescent needs can best, perhaps only, be supplied by the mother. Hardly any studies were concerned with the father's contribution to the process of dealing with illness and adolescents' development of autonomy. In contrast, numerous studies examined the worries and problems of mothers who cared for their chronically ill adolescents. This reflects a tendency to focus on registering regressive behaviors (e.g., maternal references to the ill "child"), or also to overemphasize the mothers' contribution to caring for adolescent children.

The few studies that addressed the father's perspective revealed a clear difference between the roles of fathers and mothers in coping with the illness. Since the mother usually assumed the main responsibility for the child's physical care, her intensive nursing strengthened the bond between the mother and the ill adolescent. In contrast, fathers were expected to be supportive while maintaining emotional control (Cook, 1984). Furthermore, they were expected to continue their duties as breadwinners (Gyolay, 1978). Parental reports corresponded to their roles: Mothers frequently described conflicts in the family, especially between the ill child and his or her siblings (Cain, Fast, & Erickson, 1964), whereas fathers experienced more conflicts between their occupational requirements and their desire to spend more time with the ill child (Schiff, 1972). Other studies found even more pronounced differences between the roles of mothers and fathers of ill children. In these studies, the father withdrew from the family (Binger et al., 1969) or was even excluded from family interactions (Schiefelbein, 1979).

A similar distinction between mothers' and fathers' roles has been observed in families of developmentally delayed children. Goldberg, Marcovitch, McGregor, and Lojkasek (1986) showed that fathers in these families were much less involved in family interactions than mothers. Paralleling their reduced involvement, they displayed fewer psychological symptoms, less stress, and higher self-esteem. Mothers, in contrast, were much more heavily involved and extremely stressed. Goldberg and colleagues have thus suggested that the parents of chronically ill or developmentally delayed children exhibit an extreme form of traditional family roles.

Differences between the parents' roles are especially striking in parents of terminally ill children. Cook (1984) interviewed 145 parents of children being treated for blood disorders or cancer and found that the parents reported very different problems. Mothers were most concerned with the day-to-day care of the seriously ill child; they also had to coordinate family activities around the child's care. Mothers felt responsible for keeping stressful information from the other family members. They were concerned about helping the child to overcome feelings of sadness and fear and maintaining the child's morale in adhering to treatment. Mothers frequently complained of severe emotional stress caused by the child's illness. Marital problems were reported as well. Fathers often felt neglected because of their wives' constant preoccupation with the ill child, and they often sought compensatory emotional support in relationships outside the family. Fathers felt obligated to ensure that the family's financial situation remained stable, yet the fulfillment of this responsibility was often complicated by very stressful circumstances and increased expenditures due to the chronic illness. They also felt responsible for maintaining and coordinating contact with institutions, such as insurance companies and hospitals. In some cases, fathers were shut out of the family's day-to-day activities, withdrew from their wives owing to the wives' overinvolvement with the ill child, or felt actively excluded by their wives or other family members. The fathers of ill children in Cook's study showed four typical problems, which are outlined in detail in the following.

Responsibility for Work and Family. Many of the fathers described their child's illness as a situation marked by two contradictory obligations, work and the family. Especially when the child was in the hospital, fathers had to take on additional tasks previously performed by their wives, such as looking after children who remained at home, cooking, driving, and housekeeping. These new tasks often interfered with the fathers' normal work routine, so that they often felt "pulled in different directions at the same time."

Exclusion from the Family. The fathers often reported that they felt excluded from participating in the care of their ill child, had few opportunities to be part of the child's day-to-day life, and hence, were unable to offer the child support. Because their wives usually accompanied the child to the hospital and conferred with the medical personnel, the fathers were rarely included in decisions about the child's treatment. The fathers also felt rejected by physicians and nurses. Many fathers complained about feeling almost entirely ignored, as if they were "a fifth wheel" (Cook, 1984, p. 83).

Wife's Overinvolvement with the Ill Child. Another closely related problem, and one that was described solely by fathers, was the mothers' reluctance to leave the hospital or home for any reason. Many mothers believed that their place was beside the ill child. Many fathers considered this to be overinvolvement, and they felt that they and the other children in the family were being neglected.

Desire to be with the Wife and Child. A final problem that fathers named was the conflict between their strong desire to spend more time with their wives and sick children and their inability to do so. In speaking about his ill daughter, one father lamented, "I would have liked to be with her every minute. This was constantly on my mind" (Cook, 1984, p. 84).

Although Cook's study was carried out on a very specific sample of parents of terminally ill children, its conclusions are important. More recent research has supported Cook's findings regarding mothers' and fathers' altered role requirements and responsibilities due to the illness. In a study on parents of children and adolescents suffering from cerebral palsy, spina bifida, and other physical disabilities, Sloper and Turner (1993) found that whereas fathers were very concerned with their jobs and maintaining financial resources, they were less active and competent in dealing with the ill child. In addition, there was evidence that a substantial proportion of fathers of physically disabled children and adolescents suffered from psychological distress. In the study of Eiser et al. (1993) on parents of diabetic children and adolescents, mothers and fathers differed in their reported child rearing and coping behaviors. Fathers' child rearing behaviors were dependent on the child's age and gender, whereas the mothers' were not. Furthermore, fathers found support from health care providers to be particularly helpful in coping with the illness and wanted to be present during consultations with them. Taken together, these findings suggest that both parents need to redefine their roles under illness conditions. Fathers, in particular, must learn to accept a new role in fulfilling responsibilities for taking care of children at home and assisting in the management of household affairs. It is, of course, unfortunate that most fathers must devote so much time working to provide the family with a sufficient income as well as attending to the financial and legal requirements related to the child's treatment that they have little spare time to spend with the ill child. Indeed, most fathers feel stressed by this situation and regret not being able to spend more time with their family and, more importantly, be more involved in matters pertaining to the medical treatment of their ill child. In many cases, a child's chronic illness may impose a considerable strain on the family's financial situation, so that the father's role as the main breadwinner in the family becomes even more important (Gyolay, 1978). Correspondingly, the father's inner conflict, created by having to meet income-generating responsibilities yet wanting to be with his family and more involved in the medical care of his ill child, is sharpened.

Chronically Ill Adolescents and Their Fathers

The parents' abilities to balance care and encouragement of autonomy is even more important for chronically ill adolescents than for their healthy peers. In general, any elevated level of closeness and dependence can lead to problems in a developmental phase in which achieving autonomy from parents is a central task for adolescents. Ill adolescents are dependent for a long time on their parents, particularly the mother. It is thus not surprising that they develop ambivalent and highly aggressive behaviors toward their mothers (LePontois, 1975). Adolescents with less severe illnesses are excessively mothered even in phases of relative remission (Ritchie, 1981). It is often difficult for mothers to forget the illness or disability for a while and allow the adolescent to develop autonomy, at least in a few developmental areas (Minde, 1978). As supportive and important as the family network is for the ill adolescent, unrestricted parental (especially maternal) care is a major problem for adolescents. As previously described, autonomy can be delayed, or even completely prevented. Overprotection is very common among parents, especially mothers, of chronically ill children and adolescents, and this interferes with their central developmental task of achieving autonomy. Not surprisingly, two coping strategies have been found to contribute most to chronically ill adolescents' successful adaptation: normalizing social life (maximally integrating the ill adolescent into society and the peer group) and establishing a larger social support system to share the burden of the illness (Beresford, 1994; Hauser et al., 1988b). It is interesting to note that in most families with a chronically ill child or adolescent, overprotectiveness decreases over the course of the illness, although dependence and parental control tend to increase in poorly adjusted families. These findings suggest that over the course of a chronic illness, a change from parental overinvolvement to a more individuated parent–adolescent relationship is most suitable. Unfortunately, hardly any studies have dealt with the specific contribution of fathers to adolescents' adaptation and developmental progression. In Eiser et al.'s (1993) study, indirect evidence was found to support the potential value of involving fathers in these processes. Fathers who were more involved in the consultations with health care providers had children who achieved higher efficacy scores.

In light of these findings, the fathers' perspectives were highly relevant to our longitudinal study. The different roles exercised by fathers and mothers, fathers' perceptions of family relationships, and the quality of family communication were assessed over time. Our interviews, carried out from 1991 to 1994 with 179 parents (100 mothers and 79 fathers) of diabetic adolescents, revealed clear differences in the ways mothers and fathers dealt with their chronically ill children. Obvious changes took place in family roles and duties as a result of the illness, in comparison with families with a healthy adolescent. As a rule, mothers were more involved with caring for and supervising the chronically ill adolescents. As detailed in chapter 6, only about 5% of the diabetic adolescents fathers' were actively involved in managing the illness, and this proportion hardly changed over the course of the study. In the interviews, fathers reported that their wives were overly occupied with the ill adolescent and that they felt excluded from matters concerning their child's illness. Their overall coping activities in dealing with the illness, measured by the Coping Health Inventory for Parents (CHIP), decreased over the years. Furthermore, as compared with the healthy adolescents fathers', diabetic adolescents' fathers were significantly less active in coping with non-illness-related family stress, as measured with the F-Copes (McCubbin et al., 1991).

Our analysis of family relations measured by the FES revealed that a highly structured family climate was established in all families shortly after diagnosis (Seiffge-Krenke, 1998b). As discussed in the previous section, as compared with families with healthy adolescents, diabetic adolescents and their mothers portrayed their families as possessing high organization and control, showing an emphasis on achievement orientation, allowing less opportunity for emotional exchanges, and restricting leisure activities. This perspective was mainly shared by fathers in families with diabetic adolescents. Altogether, the fathers of diabetic and healthy adolescents differed in their respective perceptions of family climate on 6 of the 10 FES scales in the first survey, when the adolescents had a mean age of 13.9 years. Fewer family activities were organized in families with a healthy adolescent at this age, more freedom to plan independent activities was granted to the adolescent, and the family atmosphere was more stimulating. Fathers of healthy adolescents also reported that leisure activities and relaxation were more important and the pressure to achieve was much less than in families with a diabetic adolescent.

Over time, mothers and fathers in all families perceived a significant decrease in family cohesion, openness, and harmony. However, despite this decrease, mothers' scores remained significantly higher than adolescents' and fathers' scores. In contrast, adolescents did not perceive much change in positive emotional family climate over time. Taken together, in families with a diabetic adolescent, adolescents and fathers shared the view of a minor change in positive emotional climate over time. Fathers of diabetic adolescents, who perceived even higher achievement orientation in family climate than mothers at the beginning of our study, perceived no change in organization and a decrease in achievement orientation as their children grew older. Furthermore, diabetic adolescents' fathers reported conflicts less often in each survey than did healthy adolescents' fathers and perceived no change over time in the frequency of conflicts. Whereas healthy adolescents' fathers reported a significant increase in independence for family members every year, diabetic adolescents' fathers only perceived this increase from the third survey onward, when the adolescents were about 15.9 years old. Compared with all other groups, the diabetic adolescents' fathers perceived the family climate to be the least positive. Their descriptions of the family climate showed the strongest lack of positive family relations and the fewest possibilities for personal growth (see Figure 7.2).

In summary, our longitudinal study confirmed that the onset of a chronic illness is accompanied by a restructuring of the family climate, in which more emphasis is placed on achievement, organization, and control. Whereas these qualities were perceived quite uniformly by the ill adolescents and both parents, there was more divergence regarding the emotional quality of family climate and the possibilities for independence. In almost all the relevant dimensions, the family climate established in families with a diabetic adolescent was retained over the years, in contrast with the more stimulating and less structured climate in families with a healthy adolescent. In the next section, some of the more specific aspects of the father's involvement in the family are treated in greater depth.

The Difficulty of Involving the Father

More recent research on father–adolescent relationships suggests that the father has a distinctive role in adolescent development and adaptation (Shulman & Seiffge-Krenke, 1997). Fathers interact differently with adolescents than do mothers, especially with respect to their focus on promoting more activity and independence. However, the majority of fathers are less involved with their children than mothers are. This difference is even more apparent in families with a chronically ill adolescent. In most of such families that we interviewed, the fathers were much more distanced than in families with a healthy adolescent. This passivity has also been described in Stuart Hauser's work on how families cope with diabetes in adolescence (Hauser et al., 1988b; 1993b). In addition, fathers have been found to be more indifferent in family communication (Hauser et al., 1986). In our study, convincing evidence was found for such a role change, particularly in the father's minimal illness-specific coping efforts (see chapter 6), as well as in the family's communicative style.

As detailed in a previous section, we used the Family Interaction Task (FIT) to evaluate communication in the family. In trying to solve this task, fathers were passive and indifferent, as compared with their wives, and they contributed very little to the discussions. The following transcript of such a family discussion demonstrates the distant, inactive attitude of one father of a diabetic son. Note how many times the son attempts to draw his father into the discussion to help solve the problem.

> *Christian:* All right then, let's go to America. How about San Diego? Hang on, that's California! Yeah! Hey, let's go to California! What do you think, Dad?
>
> *Mother:* It'd be better to take a winter holiday.
>
> *Christian:* No, no, San Diego's cool!
>
> *Mother:* A week of winter sports, all of us together...
>
> *Christian:* All right, but a week in San Diego, too.
>
> *Mother:* No!
>
> *Christian:* Oh come on, we've got enough money. Let's go to San Diego, we'll take Benny with us, too. Yeah, we can still do winter sports afterwards.
>
> *Mother:* No, we'll go to a nice hotel in the mountains where we can ski.
>
> *Christian:* But we can do that any time!
>
> *Mother:* No!

Christian: Yes!

Mother: No, I don't want to go to San Diego!

Christian: Why aren't you saying anything, Dad? You're the one who has to pay for it all!

Father: I really don't have anything to say.

Christian: Why not?

Father: Why should I be planning something?

Christian: Man, you've got no fantasy at all. You're really uncreative! I think we should go to San Diego, for one week...

Mother: No, we'll go skiing for a week, and in summer we'll go to Majorca for two weeks.

Christian: San Diego!

Mother: Just lying around in the sun and lazing at the beach...

Christian: No, no, San Diego! San Diego! I think San Diego is so cool. Come on, think about it. Make an effort! We can spend all the money we want!

Mother: No!

Christian: But of course! I think we should go to California, to San Diego. A polar expedition wouldn't be too bad either. Maybe a bit unusual, but interesting...

Mother: Now I'm sure you've gone crazy.

Christian: Yeah, or imagine a tropical rain forest, something we've never done before. So...

Mother: I don't think that's funny ... I think we should do what we've always done. We should go where there is snow for a week, right now, during the Easter holidays.

Christian: No.

Mother: A nice week in ski school...

Christian: Is my fat sister coming, too? All right, snowboarding wouldn't be too bad. Okay, but I'm really not sure. San Diego is pretty cool and unusual. I truly don't know. Say something, Dad!

Father: I really don't have anything to say. I can only say something about our last holiday.

Mother: Yes?

Christian: Last time Lisa went with us.

Father: I was on holiday with your mother, you weren't there!

Mother: Yes, we could just go without you.

Father: Actually, all our holidays have been nice.

Christian: Okay, okay. We've decided to have a winter holiday this year. We'll have a nice time. I'll snowboard; my mother and father will have a fantastic time skiing around. In short, we'll all have a lovely time (laughs). Okay?

The difficulty of getting the father involved was also apparent in a small group of diabetic adolescents who were raised by their fathers alone ($N = 5$ in our sample). Single fathers raising a diabetic adolescent displayed acquiescent, almost submissive behavior. Although they encouraged their sons and daughters to express their wishes and interests and responded to comments by confirming or accepting them, they rarely made suggestions themselves or tried to state their own interests. This behavior is very obvious in the following segment of a conversation between a father and his 15-year-old diabetic daughter. Again, this is a transcript of the family discussion based on the FIT.

> *Father:* So, would you like to spend a week with Judith [a friend]?
> *Sonja:* At least!
> *Father:* Or two weeks, or all three?
> *Sonja:* Yeah, maybe (groans).
> *Father:* Just with Nadine, or with her parents, too?
> *Sonja:* Yeah, with her parents!
> *Father:* And, hm, what about me? Should I come, too? Can I come? Do I have to come? Would you like me to come, yes or no? Hmm?
> *Sonja:* (groans) Yes, but you don't have to.
> *Father:* But I should come with you, shouldn't I? Would it bother you if I spent my holidays somewhere else, for example, if I traveled through the Eifel [a national park]?
> *Sonja:* Oh God!
> *Father:* I only meant it as an example!
> *Sonja:* (bored) If that's what makes you happy...
> *Father:* I'm only asking if you'd like me to be with you, if you'd like us to spend our holidays together.

The readiness of this father to yield to the ill adolescent's interests and needs, putting his own interests aside, was also apparent in single mothers of diabetic adolescents, although the imbalance was more pronounced with single fathers.

When the Father is Too Involved

In most of the families with a diabetic adolescent, the father was distant and passive, but there were a few cases in which the father was intensely involved. In these families, the mother had usually failed in her maternal function for one reason or another, so the fathers took on a compensatory role. In other cases, although these were rare in our sample, the father's involvement had a clearly incestuous quality, as illustrated by the following case study. This case is an example of a darker side of the way a father's involvement with the child may develop.

Janina

Janina's mother, dressed in black, greeted the interviewer stiffly at the door. The suspicion that something about her was not quite right was confirmed when the interviewer later learned that the mother had epilepsy. Her 13-year-old daughter, who had had diabetes for a year, plainly felt honored by the visit. During the discussion with the daughter, the mother intrusively interrupted several times, for example, by claiming she had to tidy up or by placing a cake directly in front of her diabetic daughter (commenting that it was intended for the interviewer, not her daughter). Janina herself reported that she got along better with her father than with her mother. The father–daughter relationship was very close: Janina virtually bloomed when her father entered but was tense in her mother's presence.

The father dominated the family interview, whereas the mother made her contributions slowly and laboriously. She was frequently interrupted by her husband and daughter. The father confirmed that when his daughter had problems, she came to him and not to his wife. He mentioned that his daughter was very interested in sex and sexuality. She talked about such topics constantly and even showed condoms to visitors. Janina's mother then told the interviewer that since the onset of the illness, her daughter slept with her father in the parents' double bed, while she herself slept in her daughter's bed.

The mother came across as weak and defeated, although her contributions to the conversation were very complex and sensitive. She often felt helpless and at the mercy of her daughter's aggressiveness. The father reported that the mother suffered from epilepsy and was often so forgetful that he had to do everything himself, just to be on the safe side. She protested, saying she was quite capable of doing things herself. The interviewer had the impression that the daughter was the "queen" of the family and that she was consciously in control of her parents.

Janina's illness obviously nurtured the further development of a quasi-incestuous relationship between father and daughter, one that had increasingly excluded the mother. The recent onset of the illness was used to legitimize the close physical contact between father and daughter. The father undoubtedly accepted his daughter's behavior and did not regard the exclusion of his wife as a problem. In fact, neither parent appeared to consider their daughter's behavior as inappropriate or unusual. In particular, the father made no attempt to justify the sleeping arrangements as supervision of the daughter, and the mother accepted the father–daughter relationship as being unalterable. In a certain way, the father and daughter were using the illness and the mother's dysfunction to fulfill their own needs.

A year later, when the interviewer returned, the relationship's incestuous quality had strengthened further. When the interviewer entered the family's home, she felt as excluded as the mother did, like a third person disturbing the close father–daughter relationship. Janina and her father remained physically close to each other throughout the interview. They continued to respond to the interviewer aggressively, and, when the interview was over, they nearly threw her out of the house.

Does Illness Solidify an Existing Pattern in the Father–Adolescent Relationship?

Clearly, both extremes – an overly distant and passive father or one who cultivates incestuous intimacy – have negative consequences for the adolescent's development. In the first example presented above, Christian's numerous unsuccessful attempts to introduce his father into the decision-making process were striking, as was his mother's dominance. Not only was she very involved in the discussion, but she knew what she wanted and that she would have her way. The son attempted to change or rearrange the problem but needed help and support from his father, who remained passive and uninvolved. In the end, Christian agreed to his mother's suggestions for vacation plans, although he really was not enthusiastic about them. In the second case, the father was very concerned about his daughter's needs but remained so distanced that he ended up excluding himself. His daughter went her own way, completely alone. In the third case, the father and daughter had already developed an overly close and intimate relationship, which was further strengthened by the onset of diabetes in the daughter. The mother was portrayed as childlike and incompetent while the father and daughter intensified their relationship. A quasi-incestuous relationship between father and daughter became increasingly established, with the mother, like the female interviewer, being forced out.

On the basis of cases such as these, it is reasonable to assume that chronic illness is likely to reinforce some preexisting patterns in the father–adolescent relationship. For example, if the father is somewhat distant, he may become even more so over time. Similarly, if he was previously very involved with his child, this involvement may increase, as seen in the last case. It is quite obvious that a reinforcement of negative patterns will impair the ill child's further development. Such relationships lack the flexibility needed for autonomous and mature development, and they fixate the adolescent in an overly childish or an adultlike position. In the last case, the adolescent became like a parent, whereas her mother was turned into the child. Such significant deviations from normal father–child interactions might even cause the illness to worsen, yet the situation can be difficult to correct simply because of the enormous gratification the adolescent derives from it. In a similar vein, preexisting interaction patterns may also be strengthened in the mother–adolescent relationship. Example of extremely close physical relationships between mothers and their diabetic children, which resulted in the phenomenon of "one body for two," were presented in chapter 5. However, because the relationships between fathers and their chronically ill children have been so little researched, it seemed particularly important to examine the nature of this dyad in the family system as it existed in our sample.

The diabetic adolescents' fathers did not support their children's autonomy and independence as much as fathers of healthy adolescents did, and their involvement with the children was low. It is difficult to explain why most of the diabetic adolescents' fathers in our study were so uninvolved. Perhaps the strict role division between husband and wife, as well as the mother's overinvolvement with the child, left the father few opportunities to develop his own initiatives. Furthermore, fathers and mothers seemed to be active in different fields. The somewhat greater efforts of diabetic adolescents' fathers in coping with non-illness-specific matters, as compared with mothers, suggest that fathers were more active in general family issues whereas mothers were more active in illness management. Although hardly involved in the practical aspects of illness management, fathers remained very concerned about the illness and its consequences.

Differences in the importance of the child's body for the father, as compared with the mother, may help to explain the passivity of diabetic adolescents' fathers. Historically, the child's healthy body was very important for fathers, particularly with respect to matters of inheritance and succession (Shulman & Seiffge-Krenke, 1997). It may be that even nowadays it is more difficult for fathers than for mothers to accept bodily distortion, disruption of normal physical functions, and loss of physical strength in their children. Research further suggests that it is harder for fathers than for mothers to deal with the maturing bodies of their children. As a rule, fathers are excluded from witnessing and acknowledging healthy adolescents' physical maturation processes (Seiffge-Krenke, 1998a), starting just prior to the first physical developments and increasing over the course of adolescence. This phenomenon, which normally has little consequence for the healthy adolescent, may handicap the chronically ill adolescent. The chronic illness is almost entirely related to the body, but because adolescents, especially daughters, do not want close physical contact with their fathers, the fathers must tread on uncertain ground. Whereas a drastic reduction in physical contact and the changed attitude about observing and exhibiting nudity are clearly marked in interactions with the mother, they are quite dramatic in those with the father. In our interviews with fathers, the value placed on a sound body and physical integrity was obvious. It is easy to understand that a child with a diseased body may represent a narcissistic insult to the father. This feeling was most strongly expressed by the fathers in our study who came from southern Europe, who lamented about their sick children's defective bodies and often complained that their sons and daughters would never have children of their own.

Finally, it should be emphasized that not only the father withdraws. The ill adolescents themselves, because of the dynamics of their development, have strong reservations about involving the father in those activities that relate to physical processes. As a result, the father's field of interaction with the adolescent is greatly restricted in comparison with the mother's. The function the father takes on with healthy children and adolescents – encouraging physical activities, such as outdoor games and sports (Shulman & Seiffge-Krenke, 1997; Siegal, 1987) – was mostly absent in the families with a diabetic adolescent that we studied, which left room only for an unfortunate fixation on achievements. This increases the diabetic adolescents' already considerable tendency to shape their world through structure and cognitive ordering (i.e., through achievement and diligence), at the expense of creative, relaxing, emotionally stimulating, and physical activities (see chapters 8 and 9).

Sibling Relationships in Healthy and Chronically Ill Adolescents

Sibling relationships are one of the most intensive kinds of interpersonal relationships. In addition, they are also among the longest-lasting, extending from birth to death of a sibling (Cicirelli, 1982). The bond between siblings endures longer than most others, even those to parents and romantic partners. This is, in part, due to the typically narrow age gap between the siblings and the early foundation of the relationship. Recently, interest in the sibling subsystem as a family variable that may influence adjustment to illness has increased. However, we still have a limited understanding about how one child's affliction with a chronic illness affects that sibling's relationship with the others. Here relevant findings from studies of chronically ill or disabled children and adolescents as well as healthy children and adolescents are presented to form the basis for a discussion of sibling relationships in families with a diabetic adolescent.

The Importance and Role of Siblings in the Family Unit

Not all children today have the experience of growing up with siblings. In 1993, 31% of German children had no siblings (Bundesminister für Familie und Senioren, 1994). The implications of this trend are yet to be fully understood. Various authors believe that sibling relationships are a fundamental experience that decisively influence personal development (Schvanefeldt & Ihinger, 1979). Indeed, growing up without siblings is seen as a psychological disadvantage, especially for the development of adolescents' and young adults' social skills (Hetherington, Reiss, & Plomin, 1994). For a long time, examinations of the effects of birth order dominated research on sibling relationships (Kammeyer, 1967; Adams, 1972), stimulated by Alfred Adler's (1926) idea of the first-born's "dethronement" as a trauma that may be the cause of sibling rivalry. Later studies focused more generally on children's perceptions of social networks and the quality of sibling relationships as compared with other close relationships. Research has also explored the functions that sibling relationships serve for the individual. Parens (1988) has named various functions that siblings can take on, such as that of an alternative attachment figure, a rival, or a target of hostility and aggression, as well as a helper in coping with the socialization processes. Negotiation with the parents and building of coalitions are additional functions. Siblings can counterbalance the parents' power as they are more likely to assert themselves as a team than individually.

Empirical research on sibling relationships has revealed age and gender differences. Rivalry and ambivalence are particularly strong when there is little age difference between the siblings and both are female. Generally, children report receiving more instrumental help from older siblings than from younger ones (Buhrmester & Furman, 1990). In addition, younger siblings mostly turn to older sisters with requests for consolation, help, and care (Whiting & Whiting, 1975), and older sisters take more care of and are friendlier toward their younger sisters than are older brothers (Abramovitch, Pepler, & Corter, 1982). Power and dependency are further dimensions of sibling interactions. The attribution of power also varies with age and gender. Older sisters and younger siblings are seen as less powerful (Sutton-Smith & Rosenberg, 1968). Gender is a factor in the dependency that younger children often establish with their older siblings: Younger girls tend to place themselves beneath their older siblings, whereas younger boys show more self-assertive behavior (Cicirelli, 1976). Overall, girls display better relationship skills with their siblings; for example, they show more care, responsibility, and assistance than boys, who strive for power and rivalry. Research on sibling relationships across the life-span has shown that these gender differences are maintained over time (Hetherington et al., 1994). A large amount of research has been devoted to describing the supervising and teaching roles that siblings take on for one another. Gender influences are evident here, too: Younger siblings are more willing to accept an older sister than an older brother as their teacher, and they learn more from a sister (Cicirelli, 1973; 1975). Thus, it appears that girls are more willing to look after their younger siblings, whereas boys are more likely to compete with them.

Sibling Relationships in Adolescence

Adolescents spend about 13% of their time with their siblings (Csikszentmihalyi & Larson, 1984), and the relationships with their siblings feature strong affective and instrumental support. For children, positive affective sibling relationships are second most important after social support from the parents (Dunn & Kendrick, 1981). In adolescence, however, siblings, particularly younger siblings, become less important and are increasingly replaced by friends of the same age. Support from siblings decreases overall, but females continue to perceive higher support from siblings than males. In addition, intimacy with siblings decreases, although early adolescents still report greater intimacy with same-sex siblings (Furman & Buhrmester, 1985). More and more, friends become the key providers of intimacy and support during adolescence, and conflicts among close friends are infrequent. In contrast, conflicts with parents and siblings increase, with conflicts occurring more frequently between siblings with smaller age differences than between those with greater age differences. Children in grades 4, 7, and 10 show the highest conflict ratings with siblings and the second highest conflict ratings with mothers and fathers (Furman &

Buhrmester, 1992). In middle and late adolescence, conflict with siblings decreases, which may reflect the developmentally normal efforts of adolescents to distance themselves from the family and devote more attention to peer relationships (Buhrmester & Furman, 1990). Finally, in late adolescence, the greater support and reduced conflict seen in sibling relationships (as well as in relationships with the parents) suggest that reconciliation in these relationships takes place as the adolescent grows older.

Such a developmental course was apparent in the study conducted by Pulakos (1989), who compared the sibling relationships of 17- to 25-year-olds with their relationships with friends. The majority of participants had an emotionally closer relationship with their friends than with their siblings. They spoke more often with friends about everyday and intimate topics, whereas conversations with siblings more commonly centered around topics related to the parents or the siblings themselves. Leisure activities were shared more often with friends, except for holidays, which were generally spent with siblings. As compared with boys, girls perceived their relationships with both friends and siblings to be closer and characterized by more reciprocity. Pulakos interpreted these findings in the context of developmental tasks, which emphasizes the adolescent's separation from the family and the increasingly intensifying relationships with friends.

The research summarized so far suggests that adolescents distance themselves from the family as a whole as they undergo the process of separation from their parents. In any case, sibling relationships generally become less intensive and more egalitarian with increasing age in adolescence. It should be noted, however, that few theories have been suggested that may explain the normal developmental course of sibling relationships. In contrast, some authors have focused their interest on understanding the influence of sibling relationships on the development of certain behaviors, for example, deviant behavior. In this regard, the temptation theory has received much attention. For example, several studies have found links between the drug use of respondents and of their older siblings. Drug use by older and younger siblings together is the most consistently reported factor in promoting the development of drug usage habits (Needle, McCubbin, Wilson, & Reineck, 1986). The role of older brothers in encouraging younger brothers' drug use was investigated by Brook, Whiteman, Gordon, and Brook (1990), who found that that older siblings, particularly brothers, had more influence on drug use than peers or parents. Other studies have examined how developmental disturbances may be related to sibling relationships. Some authors, for example, have explained symptoms of clinically referred adolescents as functional responses for balancing a problematic family system. The consistent allocation of such a function, however, makes the separation process more difficult. In an analysis of clinical cases of bulimic adolescents, Lewis (1987) identified five messages that bulimic patients wanted to communicate to their siblings:

1. *Bonding:* I want to bring us closer together through my illness.
2. *Equalization:* We are not so different after all.
3. *Distraction:* I want to protect you by taking your mind off things.
4. *Peace agreement:* I want to offer you significance and a position in the family.
5. *Dirty fight:* I want to compete with you.

As far as chronically ill adolescents and their siblings are concerned, very little empirical work has been done. Most existing studies have relied on samples showing a large age range.

Sibling Relationships of Chronically Ill Children and Adolescents

Sibling relationships in chronically ill children and adolescents have been studied comparatively rarely, although there has been extensive research analyzing the sibling relationships of disabled children and adolescents. Over one-third of published studies on sibling relationships have been carried out in families with disabled children. A change in the hierarchical status of the individual siblings represents one of the most consistent findings. A disabled child typically assumes the position of the first-born child, and the healthy sibling's privileges are curtailed. Simeonsson and McHale (1981) have identified a variety of typical situations, some of which may encourage conflict between the siblings or within the family and which emerge in families with healthy adolescents and disabled siblings. Thus, although healthy adolescents may benefit from the increased opportunity to show social maturity, they may avoid identifying with the disabled sibling, may be physically overburdened (when, for example, the healthy child must take on additional household duties), or they may show overcompensation, for example, by exceeding their parents' expectations, in an unconscious effort to make up for the disabled sibling's perceived deficiency.

In empirical studies of chronically ill children's and adolescents' sibling relationships, three main areas have been considered: (1) the influence of demographic variables; (2) the healthy child's contributions to the adaptation of the chronically ill sibling; and (3) the impairment that healthy children and adolescents may suffer by growing up with a chronically ill sibling.

Studies dealing with the effects on the healthy sibling have focused on individual variables, such as the age differences and gender of the siblings and their relevance to adjustment. In one of the most comprehensive studies, Breslau (1982) compared 237 siblings of disabled or chronically ill children and adolescents, suffering from cystic fibrosis, cerebral palsy, myelodysplasia, and various physical defects, with 248 siblings of healthy children, all aged between 3 and 18 years. Mothers assessed their children's psychosocial adjustment. Unusually high levels of aggression and psychological problems were found in the younger brothers of ill or disabled children. Breslau (1982) also observed that sisters of disabled adolescents were particularly anxious and depressive. Negative consequences resulted in boys if their ill sibling was 2 or less years older. Lavigne and Ryan (1979) also found the highest levels of psychopathology in the brothers of children with hematological illnesses. They compared the siblings of children in three illness groups (hematological illnesses, cardiac illnesses, and recovery from plastic surgery) with the siblings of healthy children, and asked their mothers to assess their social skills. According to the mothers, the siblings of ill children (especially those of surgical patients) were more socially withdrawn and irritable than the siblings of healthy children. The authors explained their findings as being the result of social stigmatization through the visibility of the illness. Surprisingly, illness severity was unrelated to the healthy siblings' psychological health. One-third of the siblings of cancer patients studied by Evans, Stevens, Cushway, and Houghton (1992) concealed the fact that their siblings were ill from those around them. This disturbingly high proportion suggests that these children suffered from severe levels of internal stress. Healthy male siblings have also been found to suffer a great deal (Lobato, Barbour, Hall, & Miller, 1987). Other investigators have reported that symptomatology in a healthy sibling generally decreases with duration of the patient's illness (Breslau, 1982; Lavigne & Ryan, 1979; Ferrari, 1984).

The findings reported so far suggest that healthy brothers are more strongly affected than sisters are, especially when younger brothers are closer in age to the ill child. These findings may lend support to the "dethronement" hypothesis set forth by Adler (1926), which maintains that the ill child assumes the position of the first-born child and absorbs the parents' attention and care, which is more difficult for a younger than for an older sibling. Older sisters' higher symptomatology may result from increased involvement and responsibility in caring for the ill child. These studies, however, were based on mothers' views and did not assess the healthy siblings' perspectives. Drotar and Crawford (1985) emphasized the mother's importance in helping healthy sibling cope with the illness. Similarly, Ferrari (1984) concluded from his own studies that a healthy sibling's psychosocial adaptation is highly dependent on individual resources and family variables, not just variables associated with the illness. It is unclear, however, how significant the sibling's independent contribution actually is or how much variance is related to other variables, such as family adaptation. This question is also relevant from the ill child's perspective. Some studies have tried to clarify the contribution of healthy siblings to ill children's and adolescents' adaptation. Sibling relationships are strongly influenced by family variables, such as cohesion, conflict, and the parents' relationship (Brody, Stoneman, & Burke, 1987). This means that the correlation between the sibling relationship and the ill child's adaptation is inflated by these variables, which makes an independent effect difficult to determine.

Basically similar findings have been obtained in families with a diabetic child or adolescent. Ferrari (1984) is one of the few to have studied sibling relationships in cases of juvenile diabetes. Ferrari spoke to 48 children and adolescents and their parents and teachers. The children were the siblings of 7- to 13-year-olds who had diabetes or severe physical handicaps or who were members of a healthy control group. The children and adolescents filled out a questionnaire on self-concept; the parents estimated their children's symptoms using the Child Behavior Checklist (CBCL) and then performed a sentence completion task to assess their children's overall psychosocial adjustment. The parents also filled out questionnaires assessing marital relationships and perceived social support. The teachers completed scales measuring the healthy siblings' self-confidence and prosocial behavior. Contrary to the hypothesis that illness visibility would make the siblings of severely handicapped children the most psychologically and socially impaired, this group was actually the most socially competent and had the lowest scores for externalizing behavior problems. No differences in self-concept were found between the groups. Healthy sisters, again, were better adjusted than brothers. Healthy siblings of the same gender as the ill child (in this study, all boys) had a poorer self-concept, inferior social competence, and less self-confidence. According to Ferrari, these results support the hypothesis of same-sex identification. Drotar and Crawford (1985) noted that adjustment is particularly poor when the healthy sibling perceives either extreme similarities with the ill brother or sister (leading to overidentification) or very few similarities (causing defense against identification, which generates fear).

Like other researchers, Ferrari (1984) found the order of birth to have an influence. Healthy younger siblings were less socially competent and had a poorer self-concept and higher externalizing scores than older healthy sib-lings. The time of diagnosis also played an important role, as did the amount of time the siblings had spent together since the diagnosis. The longer this period was, the fewer behavioral problems were seen in the healthy sibling, an effect that can be interpreted in terms of overall adaptation. Regression analyses identified the healthy sibling's self-concept as the factor most pre-dictive of his or her adjustment, followed by the social support provided by the mother and the mother's marital satisfaction. According to Ferrari, the main finding of the study was that none of the fathers' scores on any vari-ables were associated with any aspect of their children's adjustment. This result underlines the mother's importance in helping her ill child cope with illness and emphasizes her role as a mediator between siblings.

Overall, differences between illness groups were small and highly illness-specific. The siblings of diabetic children and adolescents, for example, reported more physical complaints and more often acted ill in front of the parents, for example, by imitating the sibling undergoing insulin shock. In contrast, siblings of physically disabled children and adolescents completely avoided imitating their siblings' behavior. Siblings of diabetic children dis-played the most prosocial behavior. The discovery that living with an ill child can actually be beneficial to the healthy sibling's development, for example, by fostering interpersonal skills, is most noteworthy. Several authors have emphasized the healthy sibling's learning opportunities (Gallo, Breitmayer, Knafl, & Zoeller, 1992; Simeonsson & McHale, 1981). Social development and responsibility are nurtured in the healthy siblings, and taking part in family coping strengthens their self-esteem and increases their trust in their own competence at mastering difficult situations.

In another study, the siblings of diabetic children and adolescents (Lavigne, Traisman, Marr, & Chasnoff, 1982) were compared with healthy control subjects by use of the Child Behavior Checklist completed by the mothers. No differences between groups were revealed, which corresponds to findings reported by Lobato et al. (1987), Ferrari (1984), Lavigne and Ryan (1979), and Breslau (1982), among others. Gallo et al. (1992) also found no increase in behavior disturbances among the siblings of chroni-cally ill children, a finding they explained by emphasizing the importance of family climate as a specific mediating variable. A large epidemiological study of 3,294 children and adolescents aged 4 to 16 years (Cadman, Rosenbaum, Boyle, & Offord, 1991) failed to find differences in family cli-mate between families with an ill child and control families, but the parents of ill children were slightly more nervous and irritable. Fielding et al. (1985) reported higher levels of anxiety, depression, and psychosomatic complaints in the parents of chronically ill children with final-stage renal failure, but there were no differences in behavioral problems between the siblings of these patients and of those in a healthy control group.

The studies cited above looked solely at the ill adolescent's influence on the healthy sibling's psychosocial adjustment. Hanson et al.'s (1992b) study has shed more light on the reciprocal influences in sibling relationships. This study, which lacked a control group, examined the relationship between diabetic adolescents and their siblings. The frequency of sibling conflict was the most significant predictor of problem behavior and overall adjustment in the diabetic adolescents, being even more important than the parents' marital satisfaction. However, low satisfaction with the marriage was associated with high conflict rates between the siblings, again showing that the parents represent substantial mediating factors in adjusting to illness and in the development of the sibling relationship.

Diabetic Adolescents' Stronger Bonds to Their Siblings

Unlike the studies cited so far, in our longitudinal study we acquired information about sibling relationships by directly speaking to the ill adolescents as well as to their healthy siblings. In addition, the parents' views of the sibling relationship were obtained from interviews. Using the Network of Relationship Inventory (NRI) described by Furman and Buhrmester (1985), we assessed the following 11 relevant dimensions of the sibling relationship: (1) companionship, (2) conflict, (3) instrumental help, (4) satisfaction, (5) intimacy, (6) nurturance, (7) affection, (8) punishment, (9) admiration, (10) relative power, and (11) reliable alliance. These 11 scales can be consolidated into two higher-order factors, namely, social support and negative interactions. Diabetic and healthy adolescents were asked to rate their sibling relationships on the 11 scales in each of the four surveys. Clear differences emerged between the two groups over time. In the group of diabetic adolescents, values for the dimension of social support increased over the 4 years, whereas scores for negative interactions with siblings decreased. The pattern was precisely the opposite in healthy adolescents (Figure 7.3). Over the course of adolescence, their negative interactions with siblings increased while positive aspects of the relationship, such as affection, reliable alliance, and social support decreased. In accordance with the findings of Furman and Buhrmester (1985) and Buhrmester and Furman (1990), healthy adolescents' relationships with their siblings became more distant and prone to conflict. In contrast, ill adolescents' scores tended to show the development of a closer bond with their siblings.

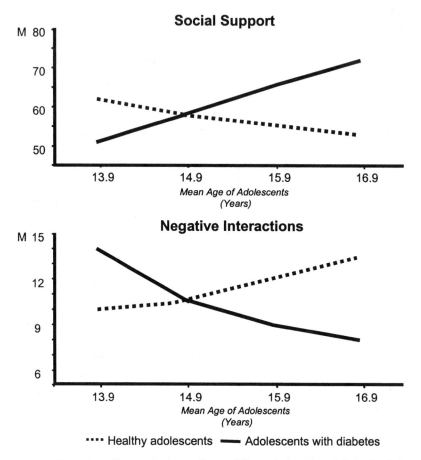

Figure 7.3. Changes in the quality of sibling relationships of diabetic adolescents (*N* = 91) and healthy adolescents (*N* = 107).

The increasingly strong bond between the diabetic adolescent and his or her siblings can be interpreted in different ways. Considering the importance of autonomy from the family in this age group, the stronger bond to the siblings may help the diabetic adolescent to develop separateness yet stay connected with the family. Siblings may compensate for imbalances in the family system, for example, for the low involvement of the father, who in families with healthy children is a model for separateness (Shulman & Seiffge-Krenke, 1997). Yet, this finding can also be interpreted as delayed development, corresponding to our other findings in diabetic adolescents of delayed separation from the parents and a slower development of close, intimate relationships with friends and romantic partners (see chapter 8).

During adolescence, not only do the parents become less important, but siblings are also pushed to the background in favor of friends. Indeed, less closeness and support but more conflict have been found in empirical studies comparing sibling relations throughout adolescence (Buhrmester & Furman, 1990). This development was evident in our healthy control group. In contrast, although the diabetic adolescents were unsuccessful in loosening their family ties, they perceived an increase in the social support provided by their siblings over time as well as a decrease in negative aspects of sibling relations, such as conflict. Whether the healthy siblings shared the diabetic adolescents' perceptions of an increasingly close relationship with their siblings was determined by the siblings' and parents' reports.

We asked the diabetic adolescents' parents to provide details about the behavior of their healthy child with respect to his or her diabetic sibling. Parents considered their healthy child's reactions to the sibling's illness to be very positive. In the first interview, parents described the healthy sibling's behavior as caring, supportive, and empathic; this perceived attentiveness increased over the next years. The diabetic adolescents' perceptions, based on the NRI results, were thus supported by their parents' observations. In addition, the healthy siblings noted nothing unusual about the relationship. Negative reactions, such as feeling disadvantaged, were named only by 2.8% of the siblings; rivalry (2.9%) and jealousy (1.9%) were also rarely named. Perceived indifference toward the sibling's illness, however, rose from 0.9% in the first interview to 6.3% in the third, a development that may simply represent the process of becoming accustomed to the illness.

As part of a general, non-diabetes-specific analysis (see chapter 3), we asked the parents of all adolescents to relate the content and frequency of quarrels between the siblings. Parents of healthy and of diabetic adolescents made very similar responses: The number of conflicts in everyday life was much the same, whether or not one sibling was chronically ill. Based on the parents' and siblings' reports, sibling relationships between an ill and a healthy adolescent did not differ from relationships between two healthy children. Healthy children were generally empathic and caring about their ill sibling, and they continued to provide support and care over time. This could well explain why diabetic adolescents cling to their siblings longer than healthy adolescents do. Rivalry and competition, which have been frequently found in other work on sibling relationships, were rarely mentioned by our families with diabetic adolescents, although in some cases they were clearly present.

Illness in a Sibling as a Family Risk Factor?

In summary, empirical research on sibling relationships in families with a chronically ill or disabled child was initially dominated by studies of the effects of single factors (e.g., age gap, birth order, and sibling gender) on the healthy sibling's adjustment. These variables have been proved to have less predictive power for explaining problem behavior than family variables, such as maternal support, marital satisfaction, and the parents' reactions to the illness. The sibling relationship can be seen as a subsystem that closely affects and is affected by family processes. As Lobato, Faust, and Spirito (1988) have pointed out, research has failed to confirm the hypothesis that siblings of chronically ill children generally exhibit more problem behavior. According to these authors, a sibling's illness can at most be considered a risk factor, whose impact is moderated by various individual and family resources. Lobato et al. (1988) cite family characteristics that can be impaired by the sibling relationship (e.g., family coping style, role differentiation) but also indicate illness-specific factors (such as cause, course, and prognosis) that can affect the family as a unit.

It has already been pointed out that a range of variables can modify the potential stress created by a chronic illness, independently of its function in stimulating the sibling's development. In some cases, though, the onset of a chronic illness presents abrupt, very stressful changes that a sibling must deal with. This is illustrated by two case studies, each detailing the reactions of an older sister to her younger brother's diabetes. In the first case, intense but temporary adjustment problems were rapidly solved by the parents' understanding and support. In the second case, the massive rivalry between the siblings was an expression of the family's inappropriate development. The daughter was excluded from the overly close mother–son relationship, and the father held a peripheral position and "escaped" to his job.

Louis

This family had four members. Louis, the patient, became ill with diabetes in 1986, when he was 9 years old. He was 14 years old at the time of the first interview, and his sister was 17. From 1984 to 1986, the mother had suffered from severe depression, which had required many stays in a psychiatric hospital. The mother described this period as being very stressful for the family. Louis's sister, who was only 9 years old at the time of her mother's first hospitalization, had served several maternal functions for her brother, which had probably required too much of her. When Louis's diabetes manifested itself, his sister initially reacted very calmly, and the parents noticed no stress in her. However, she gradually withdrew more and more. She no longer met with friends, preferring to stay in her room all afternoon, lying passively on her bed. The parents said they had not registered her behavior as being unusual, because they were so preoccupied with their son's illness and becoming familiar with the treatment regimen. For example, the mother took a special cooking course, and both parents learned how to give injections. At first, the mother especially felt overtaxed by her son's illness. She was still having considerable adjustment problems of her own after her own two-year illness, during which time she had mostly stayed in the hospital, and she was having trouble getting used to performing the many family and household duties again. She had very little time for her daughter, and most interactions with her were limited to the exchange of a few comments.

At the time of the second survey, the parents reported being completely shocked after receiving a two-page letter from their daughter in which she complained bitterly about being neglected and concluded that she saw no point in living. Only through this signal were the parents made aware of their daughter's unhappiness. As a result, they had many intense conversations with her, in which she complained further about how neglected she had felt. The parents accepted their daughter's claim and promised to improve the situation. Louis quickly learned to deal with the illness independently, so at least the greatest burden was only short-lived. Overall, the family adjusted to the illness in a relatively short time. The parents divided the work related to the illness management; for example, they shared the responsibilities of giving Louis injections at night. Thus, after his sister expressed her distress and made her parents aware of how severely depressed she had been, her mood improved rapidly. She began to take care of her brother, a behavior she had shown before he became ill.

Two years later, at the end of our study, the relationship between the siblings was completely free of stress related to the illness, and Louis's sister described it as being a normal one with the typical kinds of arguments between brother and sister. She felt that her parents now treated the two of them equally. Furthermore, she believed that something positive had resulted from his illness: She had become more health-conscious and felt that social aspects of her life had improved.

This sibling relationship went through a crisis at the onset of the illness, which developed out of the young girl's perception that she was greatly disadvantaged. Fortunately, she was able to tell her parents about her feelings, and they were able to deal with the situation constructively, so that she successfully adapted to her brother's illness. In the long term, their relationship developed positively.

Thusitha

Thusitha was 14 years old at the time of our first interview and had been ill since he was 5. His sister was 17 years old. Thusitha's illness made him the focus of his mother's life. He slept with his mother in the parent's bed, while his father slept in Thusitha's bed. This arrangement remained over the years and was still the case when we met the family for the first time. The relationship between mother and son was characterized by his complete dependence on her. It appeared that he refused to show any initiative in supervising the management of his illness regimen himself, preferring to let his mother take care of him completely. The mother knew that Thusitha would not give himself injections if she were unable to do so. This meant she could only leave the home for a few hours at a time, or that she had to excuse herself from social gatherings or activities outside of the home in order give her son an injection. Based on the conversations in the interview, it was clear that family life virtually revolved around the son. His performance in the demanding school he attended was poor, and he needed tutoring in the afternoon. He had no friends and was not interested in relationships with girls. His only hobby was fishing. Hence, the family often drove hundreds of kilometers on weekends to take him to particular rivers or lakes, then picked him up again after a few hours.

In contrast, his healthy older sister was performing well at school, was integrated into her peer group, and had a steady boyfriend. Her stable, positive development was, however, only mentioned by her mother in passing. When we interviewed the daughter alone, she explained how hurt she felt by the fact that her parents obviously neglected her. She felt lonely, poorly cared for, and could hardly wait to graduate from school so that she could leave home. She harbored a strong grudge against her brother for denying her access to her mother. According to her account, her mother had had no time for her since the onset of her brother's illness. She also had little chance to talk to her father, because he arrived home late at night, completely exhausted, and needed his rest.

Quarrels between the siblings flared up because of Thusitha's passiveness. Because he was ill, he felt he had no obligation to help in the household, and his mother did not attempt to encourage him to do so. Arguments constantly erupted between the siblings, and these became the basis for family squabbles involving the parents as well. The mother confessed to taking her son's side in the arguments, often by reminding the others that her son was ill. This embittered her daughter even more. The rivalry and bitter fighting between the two children were so central to family life that the parents remarked: "If our children didn't fight, we'd have nothing to talk about."

This last case demonstrates the problem of boundaries between chronically ill adolescents and their mothers (Seiffge-Krenke, 1997a), which leads to neglect of other family members, particularly siblings, and creates imbalance in the family system. On the other hand, the siblings' arguments may form a stabilizing factor for marital relationships and often hold the family together, a situation described to be typical for the "psychosomatic family," according to Wood et al. (1989).

8

Friendships, Romantic Relationships, School, and Career

In recent years, studies have examined the close interaction between the family system and the adolescent's external relationships (e.g., Shulman, Seiffge-Krenke, Levy-Shift, Fabian, & Rotenberg, 1995). Emphasis has been placed on the continuous nature of relationship systems involving the family, friends, and romantic partners. From the beginning of puberty onwards, adolescents spend an increasing amount of time away from their families. They seek and maintain close friendships and begin romantic relationships. Friends of the same age are very important for developing a sexual identity as well as for establishing contact with romantic partners. Friends help the adolescent in choosing and defining outward appearance and in learning age- and gender-specific behaviors. Moreover, the first romantic relationships are typically initiated with the guardianship and guidance of close friends (Furman, Brown, & Feiring, 1999; Seiffge-Krenke, 1995). Another important facet of adolescents' social environment, the transition to employment, is also moderated by peer relationships. Achievement orientation in school and the competition in and volatility of certain job markets can, however, cause relationships with peers to become a source of stress as well as social support. This issue will receive particular attention in the following analysis of the extended social worlds of chronically ill adolescents.

The Friendships of Chronically Ill Adolescents

Peer relationships and close friendships are of great importance to adolescents. One of the adolescent's central developmental tasks, highlighted in the literature on developmental psychology, is to create new, more mature relationships with peers of both genders. This task is closely related to the need to become emotionally independent from parents (Havighurst, 1972). However, studies of chronically ill adolescents have long neglected peer relationships and, above all, the important experience of close friendships. The few studies that have addressed these aspects indicate that chronically ill adolescents have difficulty with the peer group and have friendships of a poorer quality (see, for example, La Greca, 1992; Spirito, DeLawyer, & Stark, 1991). Therefore, in our study the impact of diabetes on friendships was examined.

Friendships in Adolescence: From Instrumentality to Intimacy

The adolescent's peer group fulfills special social and psychological needs and functions, which are not satisfied by the family or other interaction partners such as teachers. According to Youniss and Smollar (1985), experiences in the peer group contribute to the development of adolescent identity. Coleman (1980) stressed that friends fill the "hole" created by becoming detached from the parents and establish a forum for sharing and working out the conflicts, fears, and difficulties typical for adolescence. Nevertheless, the peer group does not replace family relationships; rather, it opens up opportunities for new interactions.

It should be pointed out that the larger group of same-aged people, that is peers, and the group of close friends, represent two relationship systems. For adolescents, these systems are closely interwoven, and even in research, clear distinctions have rarely been made between the two. However, the two relationship systems call for different social competencies and satisfy different psychological needs. Recent research has emphasized the different implications of relationships between adolescents and their peers, as compared with the dyadic relationships existing between adolescents and their close friends (Savin-Williams & Berndt, 1990). In one study examining the complexity and networking of peer relationships and close friendships in adolescence, Parker and Asher (1993) showed that the two relationship systems have different weightings and are not as closely related as one might expect. Not every high-status group member necessarily had a close friend. Of those adolescents who were highly respected by their peers, one-third were not involved in a close friendship; on the other hand, a considerable proportion of the adolescents rejected by their peer group reported having a close friend. The status in the peer group was not as important for psychological well-being as having a best friend (Parker & Asher, 1987).

Close friendships become more and more important over the course of adolescence (Furman & Buhrmester, 1992). In early adolescence, the focus is on participating in peer group activities, being accepted by the peer group, and making use of the support it offers. With increasing age, the larger group is perceived to be less supportive; conversely, friends and romantic partners become more valued. The specific nature of adolescent friendships is best understood by considering how the children's subjective concepts of friendship change as they grow older. Selman's (1980) structural approach proposes a five-stage developmental hierarchy of friendships, in which each level of friendship is built on the previous one. For younger children, the best friend is generally someone similar to them, who lives close by, and is a good partner for playing games. Children's concepts of friendship are centered on satisfying their own interests. Psychological aspects become more important in early adolescence, when reciprocity is emphasized. Thus, friendship becomes a commodity requiring care and commitment. The concept of friendship in childhood, characterized by physical proximity and instrumental motives, is thus transformed into one that includes the criteria of shared emotional closeness, support, disclosure, and trust.

The need for intimacy in the relationship with a close friend, and its realization through conversations and shared activities, increases steadily in adolescence. By mid-adolescence, the level of intimacy with close friends surpasses the level of intimacy in the relationship with parents (Hunter & Youniss, 1982). Shulman (1993) has also demonstrated a change in the nature of friendships from early to mid-adolescence. Based on observations of the interactions between adolescents in dyads of close friends as they solved a task together, two distinct types of friendship could be defined. Friends in an interdependent dyad had a great deal of mutual respect and were prepared to cooperate with one another. They balanced individuality with closeness in their interactions and thus maintained an emotional relationship even within the context of the given task. In contrast, the second type of friendship was accentuated by individuality. The two individuals worked separately, dissolving their closeness for the period of the task. The proportion of interdependent friendships increased substantially in mid-adolescence. Whereas only 39% of younger pairs of friends displayed this interaction style, 80% of 14- to 16-year-olds' friendships exhibited a balance between closeness and individuality. These changes reflect the adolescent's increasing need to experience shared intimacy with a close, trusted person. This need is fulfilled by a stable, lasting relationship that offers respect, recognition, and support.

Research has consistently generated findings on gender differences in the quality of friendships. Girls develop intimacy in close friendships at a younger age than boys (Buhrmester & Furman, 1987), and they are more intimate with their female friends than boys are with their male friends (Furman & Buhrmester, 1992; Berndt, Hawkins, & Hoyle, 1986). Furthermore, female adolescents are more interested in achieving closeness and in satisfying emotional needs through their friendships (Clark-Lempers, Lempers, & Ho, 1991; Hunter & Youniss, 1982), and they are more afraid of rejection or of a friendship breaking up (Coleman, 1980). For boys, the affective components of friendships (e.g., understanding, intimacy, and trust) are less important than the instrumental aspects (e.g., doing things together). Analyses of female adolescents' diary entries (Seiffge-Krenke, 1993b; 1995) have revealed how engaged they are in their relationships with close friends. Almost 40% of the entries described the relationship or the interactions with a close friend, whereby intimacy in conversations as well as concrete activities (such as exchanging clothes, putting on make-up, and holding hands) were mentioned most frequently. Whereas adolescent girls balance externally oriented and intimate activities, adolescent boys clearly prefer to engage in externally oriented activities with their best friends, for example, playing football (Larson & Richards, 1991; Raffaelli & Duckett, 1989). Argyle (1986) pointed out that female adolescents tend to enter into close, exclusive friendships earlier than males do. These friendships serve an important function in establishing their identity. In male adolescents, the reverse is true: Boys build their own identities first, and then initiate close friendships. Berndt (1982) has suggested that some of the gender differences could be due to girls' better abilities to talk about emotional issues. Although male adolescents do not necessarily lack the ability to show understanding for others and are not necessarily unwilling to share intimate personal details with them, they may simply be more interested in engaging in physical activity than in talking about personal issues.

Moran and Eckenrode (1991) investigated the adaptive aspects of male and female adolescents' friendships. No differences were found to exist between the males' and females' perceptions of emotional support provided by their close friends. However, compared with girls, adolescent boys gained somewhat greater benefits from their friendships in terms of social support and bore substantially fewer costs in terms of social stress. Not all studies have found gender-specific effects, but most indicate a substantial association between adolescents' friendships and psychological adjustment. For instance, Parker and Asher (1987; 1993) found that adolescents who said they had no close friend most often felt isolated and lonely, regardless of their status in the peer group. These findings have been supported by Bukowski, Hoza, and Boivin (1993), who found that close friendships protected rejected adolescents from feeling lonely and buffered the experience of negative interactions.

Several studies agree in finding that psychological adaptation depends more on the qualities than the quantities of friendships. For example, the quality of the relationship is more important for feeling secure and understood than being able to name a close friend (Frankel, 1990; Furman & Buhrmester 1992; Parker & Asher, 1987). Hartup (1993) showed that adolescents with intimate friendships displayed better psychological adjustment and social competence than adolescents who perceived their friendships as being less close. Adolescents with close friends were less aggressive, anxious, and depressive, and they had higher self-esteem. However, the connection between friendship qualities and psychosocial development and competencies may be transactional. Just as close friendships may support and promote psychosocial development, preexisting deficits in interpersonal skills and individual psychological disturbances could hinder the establishment of close relationships. This has been borne out in studies linking depression to friendships (Faust, Baum, & Forehand, 1985; Claes, 1994). Vernberg (1989) examined adolescents' experiences with peers in relation to their psychosocial adaptation at 6-month intervals and drew the following conclusion:

> These findings together paint a picture of a cycle in which poorer experiences with peers lead to increases in depressive affect, and greater depressive affect increases the likelihood of rejection by peers. (p. 195)

Which aspects of adolescent friendships, then, are conducive to adaptation and psychosocial development? The first consideration here is the friend's supportive role. For adolescents, a friend offers emotional support and comfort at a stage of confrontation with developmental tasks and role transitions. In addition, intimacy becomes increasingly important, particularly in girls' close friendships. Whereas adolescents increasingly avoid disclosing information to their parents, they confide in peers and friends more and more (Norell, 1984). This was confirmed by Kirchler, Palmonari, and Pombeni (1992) in their study of adolescents' problems and their preferred conversation partners. Three-quarters of the adolescents reported turning to others when faced with problems, and the majority chose their close friends, especially when the issues involved a romantic partner, betrayal of a secret, family problems, or feelings of emptiness and meaninglessness. Family members were called on to help with problems in school and at work. In matters of employment, parents often maintained their roles as confidants. Adolescents who felt strongly tied to their peer group were more likely to receive and more willing to accept the support and assistance provided by the individuals in this group, which gave them a better chance of coping with problems (Palmonari, Pombeni, & Kirchler, 1990). Because friendships are voluntary relationships based on reciprocity and an essentially equal sharing of power, thus distinguishing them from relationships with parents or other adults, they offer a unique domain for practicing psychosocial skills. Although conflicts between adolescent friends are frequent, they are solved differently from those conflicts that arise between the adolescent and parents or teachers (Laursen, 1993). Close friends are more willing to discuss the problem and negotiate a solution that is acceptable to both partners, so that the relationship will not be marred by the conflict (Nelson & Aboud, 1985).

Chronically Ill Adolescents' Relationships with Peers and Close Friends

Little is known about the close friendships and peer relationships of chronically ill adolescents. This is surprising, since several aspects of chronic illness may impair the adolescent's ability to develop or maintain close friendships and peer relationships. First, chronic illness is often associated with unattractive changes in physical appearance. Second, management of the chronic illness affects the adolescent's general life-style. Leisure activities may be restricted, and daily routines are often interrupted. Much of the research on adolescents with chronic illnesses has followed only a very generalized and broad approach to this topic. Most studies have suggested that chronically ill adolescents are socially less competent than same-aged peers (see, e.g., Millstein & Litt, 1990; Petermann, Bode, and Schlacker, 1990; Pless et al., 1989). Unfortunately, little empirical work has been done to assess the impact of chronic illness on the initiation, maintenance, and qualities of friendships. Moreover, illness-specific conditions, which may, of course, vary greatly according to illness type, have rarely been taken into account. It is well understood that severe, visible handicaps and a dramatic illness course may affect friendships and peer relations more strongly than a chronic, comparably stable condition that is not overtly apparent.

Attention here has been focused on diabetes, which, compared with other chronic diseases such as arthritis or cancer, places relatively few restrictions on adolescents. Most diabetic adolescents, for example, are able to participate in nearly all types of athletic and recreational activities.

Nevertheless, although the diabetic adolescent may not show overt signs of being afflicted with disease, diabetes management requires constant self-control, for example, in observing dietary restrictions, thus hindering spontaneity. Furthermore, the adolescent's activities are interrupted by daily blood sugar tests, insulin injections, and prescribed mealtimes. Meeting these demands may cause disturbances in interaction with friends. Indeed, in an earlier review of research on the psychosocial development of diabetic adolescents, Johnson (1980) concluded that of all examined characteristics, social problems with peers were most consistently associated with the course of diabetes. Since Johnson's early work, surprisingly little attention has been devoted to this issue. Instead, most of the research on peer relationships since then has examined the negative influence of peers on the ill adolescent's compliance. This is, of course, a critical component of the broader link between psychological aspects of dealing with illness and the quality of metabolic control. Failure to adhere to the therapeutic regimen can cause disturbances to health, which may sometimes be acute or enduring and in some cases, life-threatening.

From a developmental perspective, however, the effects of illness-specific stressors on the adolescent's social relationships, especially on close friendships, are equally significant. Although it is very important for adolescents to conform to their peers, diabetic adolescents may find that the disease limits their possibilities to do so. Diabetic adolescents can only participate in typical teenage activities, such as eating "junk food," experimenting with alcohol consumption, or taking vacations with friends if they accept health risks or take special precautions. The diabetic adolescent who is unable to achieve conformity may thus feel different or even isolated. Accordingly, fear of being rejected by peers was found in 35% of the diabetic adolescents studied by Sullivan (1979). In her study, which focused on compliance, diabetic adolescents often believed that they would be better liked by their friends if they were not ill. This finding converges with our results obtained with the same instrument (the Diabetic Adjustment Scale [DAS], see chapter 4), in which 12% of our diabetic adolescents felt that having diabetes hindered their friendships with healthy peers and 36% felt rejected by healthy peers. Nathan and Goetz (1984) pointed out that diabetic adolescents' relationships with friends can be adversely affected by their intensive self-centeredness. In order to achieve stable metabolism, diabetic adolescents must pay great attention to their bodies' physical processes. The intense preoccupation with the self that is necessary for the diabetic adolescent's survival can hinder his or her ability to show empathy, which is necessary to establish close, satisfying, and intimate friendships.

Aside from all the other aspects of friendships that promote development, their supportive nature is most important for diabetic adolescents. La
Greca (1992) found that the support offered by peers and friends played an
important role in helping the diabetic adolescent to deal with the illness.
Family members, as expected, contributed more supportively in everyday
management of the illness, but friends provided significant emotional support by accepting the ill adolescent, showing sensitivity to his or her needs,
and cooperating with efforts to coordinate social activities with illness-
specific requirements. La Greca (1992) stated:

> ...friends appear to be an important source of emotional support for
> diabetes. This suggests that adolescents with limited friendships or peer
> relations may be missing a significant source of support for diabetes care.
> (p. 781)

Using projective tests, Schaetz and Schaetz (1986) discovered that diabetic adolescents were often unsuccessful in creating such supportive, satisfying friendships. These adolescents were susceptible to feelings of
inferiority, loneliness, and reduced social abilities. The authors noted:

> Feeling that they are not understood, the adolescents tend to withdraw
> from their peers, which can lead to suicidal thoughts; or they try to con-
> ceal their despair by striving excessively and desperately for contact and
> a sense of belonging. (p. 188)

The difficulties that diabetic children and adolescents experience with
integration into the peer group have been discussed by Nathan and Goetz
(1984), who observed diabetic girls playing in a psychotherapeutically
arranged group. Over a period of 34 weeks, the girls failed to develop any
sense of group membership; they were more concerned with expressing
their individuality and satisfying their emotional needs through interactions
with the adult group leader.

Because of their illness-related problems, diabetic adolescents must possess better social skills than their healthy peers if they are to develop satisfactory peer relationships without having to accept extra health risks.
Petermann (1991) emphasizes how important a sense of security is to ill
adolescents in helping them to resist situations of temptation and combat
inappropriate behavior directed at them by their peers (e.g., ridicule or
pity). Equally, the adolescent must be sensitive and respectful toward others in order to be accepted in the peer group and establish friendships.
Precisely these social skills require advanced autonomy and identity. The
achievement of these central developmental tasks is considerably influ-

enced by social experiences with peers. For diabetic adolescents, social competence also affects coping with the illness, as Hanson et al. (1987) have demonstrated. They studied the link between stress and metabolic control in relation to the potential mediating variables of parental support and social competence. Stress had a direct influence on metabolic control regardless of the adolescent's adjustment to the medical regimen. This negative effect could be buffered by high social competence. Parental support did not exert such a buffer effect. The authors explained the results with reference to the adolescent's increasing tendency to deal with difficulties either alone or by talking to friends. Accordingly, high social competence enables the adolescent to maintain support from peers and cope better with stressful experiences, thus improving metabolic control.

A few studies have shown that diabetic adolescents, possibly owing to illness-related experiences, do fulfill the high demands for social competence. In comparing healthy with chronically ill adolescents suffering from diabetes or asthma, Nelms (1989) found that ill adolescents showed more empathy and a greater emotional range. Other investigators have shown that diabetic adolescents are prepared to assume responsibility for determining various aspects of daily life, including clothing, hairstyle, money, choice of friends, and leisure activities (Partridge, Garner, Thompson, Pullman, & Cherry, 1972).

Network Size and Quality of Friendships

In summary, research on friendships in chronically ill adolescents has been meager. Most of the few studies published to date have concentrated on examining integration of the chronically ill adolescent into the peer group; in contrast, close friendships have hardly been considered. In view of the special qualities of adolescent friendships described in the previous section, the peer group integration and close friendships of healthy and diabetic adolescents in our longitudinal study were explored by using semistructured interviews and the Network of Relationship Inventory (NRI) (Furman & Buhrmester, 1985). The NRI assesses 11 relationship dimensions – namely, companionship, conflict, instrumental aid, satisfaction, intimacy, nurturance, affection, punishment, admiration, relative power, and reliable alliance – which may be classified according to two general dimensions, social support and negative interactions. In addition, the adolescents took part in semistructured interviews in which we asked about the size of their peer networks as well as their current relationships with members of these groups. Concerning close friendships, the adolescents were asked whether they had a close friend and if so, how they spent their time with this friend; what was important to them in this relationship; and what kind of conflicts existed. In the following years, we also asked whether they were still close with the same friend and if not, what the reason had been for terminating the relationship, and whether they currently had another close friend.

An examination of the formal characteristics of the friendship networks (e.g., size, intactness) revealed no significant differences between healthy and diabetic adolescents. The mean number of close same-sex friends among healthy and diabetic adolescents was very similar (2.2 for healthy adolescents and 2.3 for diabetic adolescents). However, significant differences emerged between the groups with respect to the quality of friendships, both in the interviews and in the NRI. The interviews also revealed differences in the types of activities undertaken with friends.

Two questions we asked the adolescents are of special interest here: What do you especially like about your close friend? and What do the two of you do together? Even at the beginning of the study in 1991, when the adolescents' mean age was 13.9 years, healthy adolescents named intimacy as a characteristic of their friendship twice as frequently as did diabetic adolescents. Emotional support, reciprocity, and companionship in daily activities also were friendship characteristics named more frequently by healthy than by diabetic adolescents. Throughout the study, several differences in the characteristics of diabetic and healthy adolescents' friendships became more marked. In all four surveys, healthy adolescents reported a greater number and variety of leisure activities shared with their friends, along with more characteristics and attributes that they liked in their friends. However, they also mentioned more conflicts. The frequency of long talks with the close friend and the variety of topics also differed between diabetic and healthy adolescents. All in all, the healthy adolescents described their relationships with their close friends in more detail and seemed altogether more interested in discussing these relationships.

Similarly, qualitative differences between diabetic and healthy adolescents emerged in the way close friends were described in the NRI. In all four surveys, healthy adolescents' relationships with their close friends were characterized by greater intimacy, greater affection, and more companionship than were those of diabetic adolescents. For all adolescents, regardless of health status, significant time effects were found in companionship, intimacy, affection, and admiration. Although the amount of intimacy and affection in diabetic adolescents' close friendships increased over time, the level continued to be much higher for healthy adolescents. The strong increase in positive relationship dimensions from age 13.9 to 16.9 years corresponded to an increase in the general dimension of social support. As can be seen in Figure 8.1, as compared with the control group, diabetic adolescents felt much less supported by their close friends over time. No differences emerged between the two groups with respect to negative interactions. Interestingly, friends were perceived as more supportive than siblings (see Figure 7.3 in chapter 7), whereas negative interactions were not often noted as a feature of close friendships. Adolescent girls' friendships were characterized more by intimacy, affection, and conflict than were those of adolescent boys.

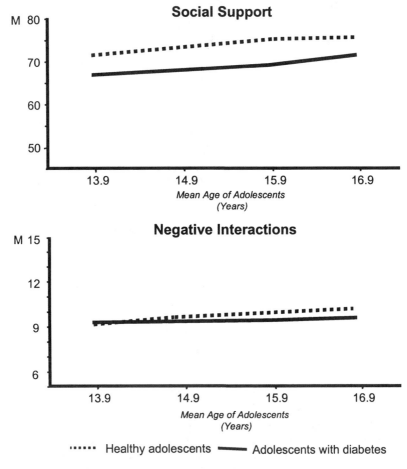

Figure 8.1. Changes in friendship qualities of diabetic adolescents ($N = 91$) and healthy adolescents ($N = 107$).

Gender differences emerged in the interviews, too. Over 4 years, female adolescents named intimacy and reflection as features of their close friendships significantly more often than did males. Adolescent girls liked to engage in conversation with their friends much more than did boys, who favored pursuing outdoor activities. Over time, the female adolescents' close friends became the most important people to whom they turned for discussing problems; such a trend was not found among the males. In the first interviews, the girls reported more conflicts with their close friends, usually revolving around rivalry. Apart from this, they provided much more precise descriptions of their friendships and their friends' personalities. When asked what they particularly valued in their friends, female adolescents were able to list more characteristics than were males. Furthermore, female adolescents were more interested in discussing the topic of peer relationships. When asked the question "What has been on your mind most over the past year?," girls spontaneously mentioned events pertaining to the realm of peer relations significantly more often than boys did.

As mentioned, healthy and ill adolescents barely differed in the number of friends they reported. This corresponds to our other findings, which demonstrated that the differences in relationships are of a qualitative nature and thus better analyzed through responses to open questions. As in other areas of the study, the ill adolescents' responses were distinguished by a strong need to portray themselves as normal, which included having one, or preferably several, close friends. However, this says nothing about the quality of the relationships, a disparity demonstrated by the following case example.

Christoph

Christoph had been diabetic since childhood. At the time of our first interview he was 14 years old. In all of the interviews he claimed that his best friend was a boy named Jürgen. He reported that they saw each other every day. Further questions revealed that Jürgen was a boy who lived on the same street. In addition, although Christoph saw Jürgen in school (they were in the same grade), they rarely met afterward or on weekends. When asked what he valued most in his best friend, Christoph said that Jürgen was very "open and friendly."

In the fourth interview, Christoph, then 17 years old, still considered Jürgen to be his best friend. At the time, however, they only saw each other on the school bus: Jürgen had to repeat a year of school and so the two were no longer in the same grade. When asked to tell more about his friendship with Jürgen, Christoph avoided the topic, claiming that he had little time for anything other than schoolwork (he was preparing for his final examinations and found this very exhausting). In addition, since his hobby was camping, he spent every weekend with his parents at a campground.

As in Christoph's case, we frequently observed the tendency of diabetic adolescents to describe peers with whom they interacted only at school as their "close friends." Also, they frequently named peers with whom they had the most contact as their close friends. Often, diabetics named interaction partners who could not seriously be considered as true disclosure or support partners because, for example, of great age differences. One diabetic 14-year-old girl named a 10-year-old mentally disabled girl, who resided in the same neighborhood, as her best (and only) friend, with whom she shared a passion for animals.

Apparently, it was very important to the diabetic adolescents simply to be able to state that they had a close friend or belonged to a clique. In the interviews, we observed that when the healthy adolescents reported having no close friends, they would focus on this topic and reflect on the reasons for this situation. The greatest differences, however, lay in the quality of friendships. Our results suggests that the friendships of diabetic adolescents at the age of 13.9 years exhibited qualities that were more characteristic for younger ages, which according to Selman's (1980) theory, included physical proximity or shared activities. Qualities related to intimacy and psychological aspects of the friendship were not as important or developed in diabetic adolescents. Although the diabetic adolescents in our study eventually began to name qualities in their friendships that could be expected for adolescents, their levels of intimacy and affection continued to be lower even at later stages of the study, when they were 15.9 and 16.9 years old on average (Seiffge-Krenke, 2000).

There are several possible explanations for this finding. It is possible that the different aims pursued by diabetic and healthy adolescents in their friendships may have led to these discrepancies. Physical closeness may have been more important for the ill adolescents than for healthy adolescents. Furthermore, the intensive self-focusing necessary for illness management may have made it difficult for the diabetic adolescents to develop intimacy and empathy in friendships. Considering the significant but small gain in intimacy in the diabetic group, it should be remembered that shared intimacy is important for adolescent friendships. Intimacy requires a certain measure of reciprocity, and it could well be that the cautious and reserved nature of the diabetic adolescents in our study was greeted with similar caution by their friends. Research on interpersonal communication has shown that the disclosure of intimate information by one communication partner typically encourages the other partner to reciprocate by disclosing intimate information as well (Cozby, 1973). Thus, because of laws of reciprocity and links between the intimacy levels of friends, the diabetic adolescents' chances of progressing in this particular relationship dimension might have been limited.

In summary, results from both the interviews and the questionnaires indicated marked differences between healthy and ill adolescents with respect to the structure and quality of their friendships. These differences continued to exist over the years, as seen in the diabetic adolescents' consistently lower scores for relationship qualities, such as intimacy and social support, dimensions that are particularly typical of close friendships in adolescence. The qualitative observations from the interviews indicate differences between healthy and diabetic adolescents in their respective definitions and understandings of close friendship. Clearly, stating only the number of friends says very little about the perceived level of support or affection in a relationship. Our results suggest that important qualities of close friendships are less developed in diabetic adolescents. This characteristic might be disadvantageous in relation to age-appropriate adaptation. Also, diabetic adolescents might thus lack adequate support from their peers in dealing with the illness emotionally (Seiffge-Krenke, 2000). Furthermore, given that friends help each other in making first romantic contacts, diabetic adolescents may lack opportunities to use the support of their friends during their first experiences with romantic love.

Developing Romantic Relationships

As the physical changes of puberty begin to emerge, adolescents begin to feel more and more like sexual beings and, under the protection of their friends, begin to initiate romantic and sexual contacts with the opposite sex. Until now, studies of chronically ill adolescents have directed little attention to their maturing bodies, and even less toward their sexual identity and experiences, as though these adolescents were believed to be incapable of sexual development. Indeed, research has been dominated by a regressive perspective (e.g., as characterized by frequent references to "the chronically ill *child*") and excessive achievement orientation (e.g., as characterized by the preponderance of analyses of illness-specific knowledge or of school performance). Whereas it must be acknowledged that school life and choosing a career are certainly important issues for chronically ill adolescents (these issues are dealt with later in this chapter), it is important to address the fact that chronically ill adolescents, in making the transition to adulthood, must also learn to develop mature romantic and sexual relationships.

Sexual Experiences and Romantic Development in Adolescence

Dating and the beginning of sexual relationships are normative and age-typical tasks for adolescents; nevertheless, not all adolescents are able to deal with these tasks with ease. There are great differences in the intensity and developmental speed with which adolescents approach such tasks (Cantor, Acker, & Cook-Flanagan, 1992). Much attention has been directed at understanding the sexual aspects of adolescent relationships; in contrast, the romantic qualities of such relationships and the links to close friendships with same-sex peers have essentially been ignored by researchers (for a summary, see Furman et al., 1999). Existing knowledge is generally of a quantitative nature, whereas the qualitative similarities and differences between both types of relationships have been overlooked.

Most notably, psychological and psychoanalytic theories place very different emphasis on adolescent sexuality as an indicator of healthy development. In psychoanalysis, sexual organization is ultimately the deciding developmental task, determining whether future development will progress normally or lead to a "developmental breakdown" (Laufer & Laufer, 1984, p. 5). Maturation processes in adolescence must incorporate the physically mature sex organs into the body image, while the body, largely passive until puberty, becomes an active translator of sexual and aggressive fantasies. When sexual organization is complete, no more changes in sexual orientation can occur. After this time, the fundamental orientation of homo- or heterosexuality is firmly established. According to this approach, rooted in the British school of psychoanalytic theory, physical maturity and sexuality are so central that a direct pathway between failure in this development and psychopathology in adolescence is postulated. Whereas psychological theories are less oriented to the "primacy of genitality" (Freud, 1905), they only highlight a few aspects of sexual development in adolescence, often excluding sexuality itself. Theories and studies of physical maturity have typically been more concerned with height, weight, and growth norms (for a summary, see Udry & Bill, 1987), whereas studies of physical attractiveness (for a summary, see Blyth et al., 1985) have rarely made reference to adolescent sexuality.

A close association between physical maturity and the onset of heterosexual contact has been reported in several studies. The appearance of visible physical changes has a direct influence on how adolescents organize their leisure time (Hendry, Shucksmith, Love, & Glendinning, 1993). Adolescents become interested in new and more complex types of leisure activities involving members of the opposite sex. For example, by the age of 13 or 14 years, adolescents show an increased interest in going to discotheques, to the movies, or to places where they can meet members of the opposite sex, and they spend a great deal of spare time in these leisure contexts, in the company of best friends (Furman, et al., 1999; Silbereisen, Noack, & von Eye, 1992). The status and timing of physical maturity play an important role in determining when the adolescent will begin to engage in such activities. The status of being "off time," that is, having begun the process of physical maturation later than normal, can have dramatic consequences for friendships and may delay the start of romantic relationships. For example, if an adolescent's physical appearance is too childlike, he or she is unlikely to be admitted to discotheques and thus cannot accompany friends. The relationship between physical maturity and dating is unequivocal (Bulcroft, 1991). A strong association also exists between physical maturity and engaging in sexual intercourse (Moore & Rosenthal, 1993). Although the age of first sexual intercourse has decreased over the last 30 years, the close association between these phenomena has not changed at all. Early-maturing adolescents begin to have sexual intercourse earlier, and late-maturing adolescents begin later, within an interval of 3 years following physical maturation (Phinney, Jensen, Olsen, & Cundick, 1990; Seiffge-Krenke, 1998a).

The processes involved in making the transition to nonvirginity have been studied almost exclusively by North American investigators (Jessor & Jessor, 1975; Strouse & Fabes, 1987). In Germany, only a handful of studies have dealt with the psychological processes and variables determining the onset of heterosexual relationships. Above all, although the studies carried out in Germany have investigated age and gender differences in the onset of heterosexual relationships, they have not considered variations in health status. In a replication of Sigusch and Schmidt's (1973) study on the heterosexual activity of adolescents, Clement, Schmidt, and Kruse (1984) found that in the early 1980s, 60% of the 18-year-old girls and 50% of the 18-year-old boys had experienced sexual intercourse. A comparison with Sigusch and Schmidt's findings from the early 1970s showed that the percentage of sexually experienced 18-year-old males had doubled, whereas the percentage of experienced girls had even quadrupled. Schmid-Tannwald and Urdze (1983) found similar distributions. They further reported that the percentage of sexually experienced adolescents increased rapidly between the ages of 14 and 18 years. One in every 30 14-year-old girls, 1-in-10 15 year olds, 1-in-4 16 year olds, and every other 17-year-old girl had engaged in sexual intercourse. These investigators also found that most adolescents had continued to have sexual intercourse regularly after losing their virginity. One year after the first sexual intercourse, every third girl and every fourth boy were still dating the partner with whom they had their first coitus. However, as a more recent replication of this study by Schmidt, Klusmann, Zeitzschel, and Lange (1994) illustrated, the trend of having intercourse at an earlier age does not seem to have persisted: The rates of heterosexual activity reported in the 1970s closely match those for the 1990s. The risk of becoming infected with HIV and developing AIDS has apparently had a marked influence on the sexual activity of adolescents, as can be seen in the trend of delaying the onset of sexual activity. This may also explain why females are more active in heterosexual situations, insofar as they take more initiative and show more control (Seiffge-Krenke, 1998a). Studies of adolescent sexual behavior in the United States also found that the age of first sexual intercourse decreased steadily until 1980, but that this trend did not continue to the 1990s (Gagnon et al., 1989).

Neubauer (1990) analyzed the motives for engaging in sexual intercourse in 14- to 18-year-old adolescents. A factor analysis revealed three categories of reasons for beginning heterosexual relationships: (1) curiosity (the adolescents wanted to know what sex was like); (2) mutual affection (the adolescents were in love and wanted to belong to each other completely); and (3) adult status (adolescents wanted to be like their friends and become an adult). So far, little is known about the characteristics of the partner in romantic relationships, except that the first sexual intercourse usually takes place with a slightly older adolescent. However, these age differences level out over time. Female adolescents ascribe a high level of commitment to their partners, and they designate affection and love as motives for engaging in sexual intercourse more often than do male adolescents, who emphasize relaxation and desire (Savin-Williams & Berndt, 1990).

Chronically Ill Adolescent's Romantic Relationships

Dating and establishing romantic relationships represent the transition to adulthood and for many adolescents are documentation of adult status. For adolescents, establishing romantic relations is a developmental step of immense importance, which decisively influences their future behavior, for example, their choice of partners (Hendry et al., 1993). As we have seen, today's adolescents begin romantic relationships at a younger age and, owing to greater social permissiveness, are granted more sexual autonomy. Nevertheless, the first sexual experience, in particular, coitus, retains a life-long significance (Furman et al., 1999; Moore & Rosenthal, 1993). It is still unknown whether adolescents whose health is chronically impaired have difficulties in establishing romantic relations and beginning sexual relations. Analyses of the literature (Seiffge-Krenke & Brath, 1990; Hanl, 1995) revealed that this topic has been neglected in studies of chronically ill adolescents. A more recent inspection of the literature confirmed that no studies dealing with this important topic were published from 1996 to 1999. Even more importantly, the qualities of romantic relationships in this special group of adolescents have not been addressed so far. In view of the fact that developing relationships with heterosexual partners is an important developmental task for this age group (Havighurst, 1972) and lays the foundation for the tasks of early adulthood, such as marriage and raising a family, this lack is all the more severe.

In our longitudinal study of diabetic adolescents (see chapter 3), an attempt was made to compensate for this deficit by investigating sexual experiences and development of romantic relationships in diabetic adolescents and their healthy peers. As in other areas we studied, two assessment methods were employed. In semistructured interviews, the adolescents were asked to talk about their romantic relationships in general and, if applicable, about their current boy- or girlfriends. We inquired about how they had met their romantic partners, how long they had been dating them, what they did together, and what they particularly liked about their partners. We asked what kinds of conflicts, if any, had occurred between their current boyfriends or girlfriends, if they had had sexual relations, and how seriously they took the relationship. Furthermore, we asked about their first experience with sexual intercourse, and whether they had had sexual relationships with other partners. In the following years, we asked whether they still dated the same partner, and if not, what the reason had been for ending the relationship, and whether they currently had a romantic partner. In addition, relationships with romantic partners were assessed by using the NRI (Furman & Buhrmester, 1985). This allowed us to make a direct comparison between diabetic and healthy subjects with respect to the qualities of relationships with romantic partners, close friends (discussed earlier in this chapter), and siblings (see chapter 7).

At the beginning of our study in 1991, the adolescents averaged about 13.9 years old; at the fourth survey in 1994, they averaged about 16.9 years old. Of course, important changes in romantic relationships could be expected to have taken place within that period. In the first year of the study, very few adolescents in the total sample had a boyfriend or girlfriend, but this number notably increased over the second, third, and fourth years. The increase was much more rapid in healthy adolescents than in chronically ill adolescents (girlfriend/boyfriend at age 13.9 years, 1% of diabetic and 4% of healthy adolescents; at age 14.9 years, 2% of diabetic and 14% of healthy adolescents; at age 15.9 years, 8% of diabetic and 22% of healthy adolescents; at age 16.9 years, 11% of diabetic and 36% of healthy adolescents). Healthy adolescents reported not only higher real involvement in romantic relations, but also more fantasies and concerns about these relationships. The interview data revealed that the mere idea of romantic relationships, even before such relationships had been experienced, was mentioned seven times more often by the healthy adolescents than by the diabetic ones. Fantasies about dating and concerns about finding a partner also increased dramatically in the healthy group between the first and second surveys, and these topics continued to preoccupy them up to the last survey. In the fourth survey, far more of the healthy adolescents considered not yet having a boyfriend or girlfriend as a deficit. These results illustrate that relationships with romantic partners – in reality or fantasy – seemed to be of minor importance to the diabetic adolescents. In contrast, real and fantasized romantic relationships were in the forefront of healthy adolescents' minds, which converges with Furman et al.'s (1999) findings.

By the fourth survey, sexually experienced adolescents reported having had an average of 2.8 sexual partners ($SD = 1.3$), with healthy adolescents reporting more sexual partners than diabetic adolescents. The majority of sexually experienced diabetic adolescents had experienced intercourse with only one partner over the 4 years. It is important to note that very few diabetic adolescents had sexual relations outside of a steady relationship. In contrast, the percentage of healthy adolescents who had sexual relations without having a steady boyfriend or girlfriend was eight times as high. It is also striking that healthy and diabetic adolescents seemed to become acquainted with their romantic partners in different social settings. Diabetic adolescents frequently met their partners during leisure activities with their parents, for example, during family vacations, or in organized leisure time settings, such as summer camps. In contrast, healthy adolescents became acquainted with their partners through their clique of friends. No differences were found between ill and healthy adolescents concerning other characteristics of romantic relationships, such as the time period of dating, common activities, frequency of dates, or seriousness of the relationship.

Differences emerged in the interview, however, with respect to the characteristics of romantic partners and their activities together (Seiffge-

Krenke, 1997b). When asked what they liked best about their boyfriends or girlfriends, healthy and ill adolescents named similar characteristics but with varying frequencies. In the fourth survey, for example, healthy adolescents named intimacy, physical attractiveness, and similar interests more often than ill adolescents. The diabetic adolescents surpassed their healthy peers in naming emotional support and instrumental aid as important characteristics of romantic relations. Other obvious differences between healthy and diabetic adolescents were found in response to the question: Generally speaking, what is important to you in romantic relationships? The results of the fourth survey showed the most differences between the two groups. On a global level, diabetic adolescents found it more important than healthy adolescents that romantic partners be good listeners, join them in carrying out everyday activities, and show understanding. In contrast, healthy adolescents stated more often than diabetic adolescents that having fun together and sharing activities were important. Whereas physical attractiveness was an important attribute of the current boyfriend or girlfriend for healthy and diabetic adolescents, it was not an important general characteristic of their romantic relationships. Healthy adolescents were generally more willing to mention sources of conflicts with their romantic partners. Rivalry, jealousy, and power relations were frequent sources of conflict in the romantic relationship of healthy adolescents. Insufficient attention was one cause of conflict named frequently by diabetic adolescents but less so by healthy adolescents.

Significant differences between groups were found with the NRI, which assesses relationship qualities on 11 scales. These scales can be collapsed into the two higher-order dimensions of social support and negative interactions. Generally, and in accordance with earlier research (e.g., Furman et al., 1999), females experienced more affection, intimacy, and nurturing in their romantic relationships than males did. In addition, the quality of romantic relationships differed depending on health status. Whereas the healthy adolescents' levels of satisfaction with the intimacy in romantic relationships were higher in all four surveys, diabetic adolescents' assessments of companionship and instrumental aid were consistently higher. In both groups, companionship, affection, intimacy, nurturing, and admiration of the romantic partner increased over time. However, the level of social support remained considerably lower in diabetic adolescents over time. In addition, negative interactions with romantic partners increased in healthy adolescents over time but did not change in diabetic adolescents. Several interactions emerged between health status and time, indicating that the developmental paths for diabetic and healthy adolescents differed.

Negative interactions as a general dimension in romantic relationships increased in healthy adolescents over time, whereas the scores decreased or remained stable in diabetic adolescents. Reliable alliance also became more important for healthy adolescents but did not change in diabetic adolescents. Over time, the diabetic adolescents perceived an increase in instrumental aid in romantic relationships, whereas healthy adolescents reported a decrease in this particular dimension. Based on the two general dimensions, healthy adolescents had higher values both in social support and in negative interactions with romantic partners. Thus, support and closeness develop over time in the relationships of healthy adolescents, but this also results in more conflict. The demands placed on the partnership grow, leading to more disagreements in the sense that "there is no fire without smoke."

Continuity and Discontinuity in Relationships with Close Friends and Romantic Partners

According to Erikson's (1968) life-span model of psychosocial development, adolescence is marked by two important life tasks: separation from the family and establishing heterosexual relationships. The formation of intimate relationships with members of the same gender may represent the missing link connecting these divergent developmental tasks. As early as 1953, Sullivan hypothesized that the intimacy and sensitivity adolescents experience with their same-sex friends is later reflected in romantic relationships. This claim has been supported by more recent studies (e.g., Miller, 1990).

In our study, we were interested in learning how changes in adolescents' close friendships were linked with the onset of their romantic relationships. Among other relationship dimensions, perceived intimacy in close friendships and romantic relationships served as a key for understanding the transition to romantic love (Furman & Wehner, 1994). We started by analyzing the formal characteristics of both types of relationships and then related them to the more qualitative characteristics. One of our most important findings concerned the marked differences between some characteristics of both relationship types in adolescents as a function of health status. Although the numbers of close friends of healthy and diabetic adolescents were basically similar, the diabetic adolescents started to have romantic relationships later and were less sexually active. The age of onset of heterosexual relationships in healthy adolescents as found in our study closely paralleled the findings reported in other studies (Anderson, Darling, Davidson, & Passarello, 1992; Furman et al., 1999; Schmidt et al., 1994).

The results reported so far show that intimacy in both same-sex friendships and romantic relationships increased over 4 years in all adolescents. However, as compared with chronically ill adolescents, healthy adolescents' intimacy scores for both relationship types were significantly higher at all four measurement points. How can the diabetic adolescent's hesitancy to begin heterosexual relationships and the specific qualities of their romantic relationships be explained? First, it must emphasized that the diabetic adolescents showed no objective deficits in physical maturity. Their levels of physical maturation corresponded to the norms for their ages; no significant differences were found between the two groups with respect to age to first menarche or semenarche (see chapter 5). Thus, differences in physical maturation did not appear to be responsible for the hesitation that diabetic adolescents demonstrated in beginning sexual relationships or for their lower rates of increase of sexual relations. However, we found differences in body image, namely, that diabetic adolescents perceived their bodies to be mature much later than did healthy adolescents. In the fourth survey, when the mean age of the participants was 16.9 years, the rate of sexual activity in healthy adolescents was three times as high than that of their chronically ill peers. Poor overall health would not account for these discrepancies, since the health status of most of the diabetic adolescents was good and their metabolic control stable. Apparently, diabetic adolescents looked for other qualities in romantic relationships, which may have caused them to become easily disappointed. Their high scores in the NRI dimensions of instrumental aid and companionship, as well as the lower scores in perceived reliability of the romantic partner, point to this possibility. Another consideration is the fact that diabetic adolescents reported taking a less active role in their romantic relationships. Diabetic adolescents had fewer arguments with their partners but also experienced less mutual support. Finally, it is worth mentioning that the diabetic adolescents were interested in having sexual intercourse only in the context of a steady relationship.

The information provided by the adolescents during the interviews sheds more light on the specific nature of these characteristics. On a global level, the diabetic adolescents felt that the romantic partner should be a good listener and be understanding. In concrete relationships, the diabetic adolescent's romantic partner had the primary function of providing security, that is, assistance and companionship in very specific daily routines. As compared with healthy adolescents, diabetic adolescents avoided situations that might result in conflict with their partner; for example, they refrained from arguing and were unwilling to date others while in a steady relationship. Thus, compared with their healthy peers, the diabetic adolescents looked for partners who could offer them more security, support, and assistance and who were more in harmony with them and more understanding.

These differences between healthy and diabetic adolescents' perceptions of romantic partners may be related to their perceptions of close friendships. Since friends help each other in preparing for romantic relationships (Seiffge-Krenke, 1993b; 1995), the quality of relationships with close friends may determine how successful adolescents are in making this important transition. Indeed, healthy adolescents perceive more affection, companionship, and intimacy in their same-sex relationships than diabetic adolescents do. Whereas intimacy has been defined in terms of disclosing personal thoughts and feelings with others (Buhrmester & Furman, 1987), it may also include such features as genuineness, trust, and emotional support. Intimate friends feel free to be spontaneous and open about themselves; their interactions are characterized by mutual trust and empathy. Achieving high intimacy in same-sex friendships is therefore a very important developmental gain in adolescence. Our findings revealed that diabetic adolescents did not achieve the levels of intimacy in friendships typical for their age. This might be indicative of a developmental delay, which could have had repercussions on establishing the first contacts with the opposite sex. The links we found between intimacy experienced in close friendship and intimacy in romantic relationships (Seiffge-Krenke, 2000) support Sullivan's (1953) hypothesis and confirm Miller's (1990) more recent finding that the intimacy and sensitivity adolescents experience with their same-sex friends is later reflected in romantic relationships.

The typical areas of conflict with romantic partners reported by healthy and diabetic adolescents also illustrate the different approaches in interactions with partners. The conflicts in the healthy adolescents' romantic relationships involved romantic partners (e.g., jealousy) and other individuals (e.g., power structure). In contrast, diabetic adolescents frequently cited lack of sufficient attention as a cause of discord. Sanderson and Cantor (1995) pointed out that adolescents differ with respect to the goals they pursue in romantic relationships. Some adolescents focus on achieving and maintaining intimacy, that is, closeness and trust, whereas for others, romantic relationships help to achieve the goal of establishing identity. However, the fusion of both goals is important. That is, an independent identity must be developed, and this identity must be merged with others in intimate relationships. Our results suggest that diabetic adolescents, possibly because of the intense self-focus that is necessary for illness management, lack empathy and intimacy with their close friends and romantic partners. They seem more concerned with the goal of establishing identity (Sanderson & Cantor, 1995). Thus, the low level of intimacy that they share with their close friends and romantic partners may then be reciprocated by equally low levels.

Nevertheless, our longitudinal analyses indicated that diabetic adolescents achieved gains in several important relationship dimensions. All in all, the results impressively show the extent to which chronically ill adolescents tried to balance out their deficits in important dimensions of close relationships with friends and romantic partners. This developmental progress was greatly dependent on the reactions of the interaction partner. Differences were still noticeable by the end of the fourth survey in 1994, when the adolescents were about 16.9 years old, but the nature and qualities of diabetic adolescents' close relationships then approached those of healthy adolescents. Future analyses carried out in late adolescence and the transition to young adulthood may reveal whether the demands on the quality of a partnership change during later years and whether they approach the levels of healthy subjects.

Chronically Ill Adolescents' School Experiences and Career Choices

Adolescents make the transition to secondary school before or around the onset of puberty. They then enter a socialization system that places increasing demands on qualifications and performance. The school environment, the type of school, and the desired qualifications exert a formative influence on the development of an adolescent's self-esteem. In light of the increasing significance of school achievement and career-related demands in adolescence, our longitudinal study of coping with diabetes in adolescence (chapter 3) also investigated whether illness-specific factors have an impact on the transition from school to the work force. According to the existing literature, there is much evidence to show that diabetics are disadvantaged in their working lives. Thus, we were interested in learning whether diabetic adolescents might be at a disadvantage with respect to their ability to meet academic standards in the schools they attend or to satisfy the prerequisites for pursuing a particular vocation.

The Constant Demand for Higher Qualifications

The amount of time that young people spend pursuing an education has steadily increased over the past decades. This is in part due to the growing awareness among young people that those individuals with higher and more specialized qualifications have a better chance of success in an increasingly competitive job market. In the German school system, there are three different kinds of secondary schools: Hauptschule (grades 5 to 10), Realschule (grades 5 to 11), and Gymnasium (grades 5 to 13), which children enter at around the age of 10 years. A recommendation for further schooling in one of the three different secondary schools is based on a pupil's previous academic performance in primary school. Entrance to university is contingent on graduation from a Gymnasium. Thus, the pressure to perform well in school may be evident at quite an early age. In any case, a clear shift in attendance percentages for the respective schools has taken place in the past 50 years. Whereas in the early 1950s, 79% of all 13-year-olds attended Hauptschule, in 1990 57% attended Gymnasium, and only 31% attended Hauptschule (Hurrelmann, 1990). Although this shift is associated with an overall improvement in educational opportunities, it also reflects the intensified pressure placed on young people to perform and compete.

It is important to recognize that longer periods of schooling prolong the time adolescents remain financially dependent on their parents. This is a critical point of reference for adolescents as they begin to make the transition from adolescence into adulthood. As such, adolescence is largely determined by the actual amount of time spent at school as well as by school-related activities and obligations, as Schulenberg, Maggs, and Hurrelmann (1997) have noted. Furthermore, the school environment and feedback about school performance influence adolescents' beliefs about their own capabilities and decidedly influence their health. Psychological stress and physical complaints are not only dependent on age and gender but also on the type of school attended. Students attending more demanding schools report, for example, a higher number of bodily complaints.

Academic stress, examination stress, and failure at school, that is, not following the normal progression of grades or not graduating, have been found to be perceived as highly stressful by adolescents in various countries, including the United States (Compas, Orosan, & Grant, 1993; Stern & Zevon, 1990; Tolor & Fehon, 1987), Australia (Frydenberg & Lewis, 1993), China (Lee, Chan, & Yik, 1992), Japan (Ogura, 1987), Great Britain (Hendry, Raymond, & Stewart, 1984), Switzerland (Plancherel, Bolognini,

& Halfon, 1998), and Germany (Seiffge-Krenke, 1995). In Germany, as in many other countries, the trend of seeking higher education is related to a marked devaluation in importance of the lowest level of high school diploma in the educational, vocational training, and job markets. In addition, adolescents today are under pressure to achieve a level of education that is higher than their parents'. Thus, the adolescent's motivation to perform well in school may indeed be influenced by parental pressure and expectations. In any case, Hurrelmann (1987) demonstrated that the gap between the parents' and an adolescent's educational levels, regardless of whether it is an upward or downward development, is often accompanied by increased stress and psychosomatic complaints. In a study by Mansel and Hurrelmann (1991), 95% of adolescents said it was very important to do well at school. In another study, Mansel and Hurrelmann (1989) compared students who were repeating a grade with those at risk of repeating one and found that the anticipation of failure in fact caused more stress than actual failure. The threat of not graduating can be very salient. Any adolescent who does not graduate from secondary school will have dramatically reduced job opportunities, possibly causing extensive, lasting stress.

The type of school and the desired qualifications guide the adolescent's career choices. In Germany, a broad range of career options is open to graduates of Gymnasium. Students in lower secondary schools are quite aware that certain career paths will be closed to them, although there is an opportunity for graduates of a Realschule to continue their schooling, obtain a higher type of diploma, and thus be eligible for admission to a university. Additionally, students in Hauptschule and Realschule must essentially choose a career relatively early in their lives, around 15 or 16 years of age, long before students in Gymnasium need to make such definite plans. The devaluation of the diplomas offered by lower-level secondary schools in Germany is closely connected to rising needs in many occupations that require specialized training, which often demands a higher level of academic preparation. In the early 1970s, 80% of all job trainees had graduated from the lowest-level secondary school (Hauptschule); today almost 50% of applicants for job training have higher diplomas (from a Realschule) or are even qualified to enter university (by having graduated from Gymnasium). Career preparation today now includes striving for the highest possible secondary school diploma and for good academic performance reports. Adolescents know very well that these are prerequisites one needs for a good start in one's working life, especially in view of the currently competitive and uncertain employment market. Indeed, German adolescents, like their peers in other European countries with high youth unemployment, are quite aware of the fact that even the most highly qualified individual is not immune from the possibility of being unemployed.

Unemployment is a macrosocial stressor affecting many adolescents today (Hammarström, 1990). About 20% of young people in Western Europe are without jobs. In Germany, about 20 to 30% of all registered jobless individuals are under 25 years old (Klink & Kieselbach, 1990; Vonderach, 1989). The rate of unemployment among adolescents in England has reached levels above the average of Western Europe. Unemployment among young people in Spain is also very high, about 48% (Kieselbach & Svensson, 1988). The effects of unemployment on health have been frequently reported (e.g., Hammarström, 1990; Hendry et al., 1993; Patton & Noller, 1984). In 1995 fear of unemployment stood alongside global fears of environmental destruction and war in adolescents' main future concerns (Seiffge-Krenke, 1995), which is perfectly understandable in light of the rising rate of youth unemployment at the time. Successful integration into the employment world and achievement of financial independence are obviously central factors in adolescents' concerns about their future. Consequently, guarding against later unemployment has been found to be an adolescent's first consideration in choosing a career (Mansel & Hurrelmann, 1991), followed by ideological orientations and the desire to have a meaningful, independent, and creative occupation.

Illness-Specific Restrictions and Discrimination in Employment

A chronic illness, including diabetes, can alter or damage work life in specific ways. Diabetic adolescents experience difficulties in the school environment and in finding a job, stemming from the need to coordinate school and work life with the demands of the diabetes therapeutic regimen. In addition, the adolescents must deal with rejection and discrimination by teachers and employers, which is often based on ignorance. Diabetes rarely causes an objective decrease in scholastic achievement. However, Ryan, Vega, and Drash (1985) found that if the illness began in children younger than 5 years old and entailed neurophysiological damage, there might be detrimental effects on intelligence, memory, speed of movement, and hand–eye coordination, all or some of which could negatively affect performance at school. Aside from the onset of a chronic illness, illness duration also appears to influence cognitive abilities. Ryan et al. (1985) found a correlation between the duration of diabetes and deficits in those cognitive functions attributed to the left brain hemisphere, such as creating verbal concepts, spelling, and forming sequences of sentences. The reason for this connection has not yet been fully explained. It may be assumed, however, that the diabetic adolescents' skills are not as much affected by an illness-related disposition as they are temporarily impaired by potentially acute complications. The most likely of these complications is hypoglycemia (blood sugar level below 50 mg/dl), which can be accompanied by sweating, shivering, and tachycardia as well as by symptoms of central nervous systems dysfunction, such as poor concentration or psychological deficits. Each of these symptoms could impair the adolescent's learning and performance abilities. In a study by Gutezeit (1987), diabetic adolescents unanimously named hypoglycemia as the most important cause of their diminished capabilities. Adolescents with poor metabolic control, including those who had had repeated severe hypoglycemic episodes, missed many days of school, which resulted in more achievement problems.

Generally, conditions of low blood glucose levels can be rectified relatively quickly and easily by consumption of carbohydrates. However, the danger of losing consciousness is particularly frightening for others, so that teachers often feel anxious about having a diabetic pupil in their classes. According to Finck (1994), diffuse fears based on ignorance and prejudice, as well as uncertainty about what to do in emergencies, give rise to teachers' unequal treatment of diabetic adolescents.

Discrimination occurs, for example, when the adolescent is excluded from school sports or not allowed to take part in school excursions or field trips. Such cases were often mentioned in our interviews. One 15-year-old boy reported that his teacher only allowed him to go on class trips if one of his parents came along. A girl explained that she had not participated in a class excursion because of her teacher's rejection. This discrimination, which can be avoided by providing teachers with adequate information about the illness, often prevents diabetic adolescents from being fully integrated into the class. As a result, they may feel that others see them as more fragile, or even as a risk. In addition, long stays at clinics, resulting in absences from school, may contribute to perceptions that diabetic adolescents need special treatment.

Education, training, employment, and success in a chosen occupation or profession take on a decisive role for diabetic adolescents, especially in the context of coping with the illness. As Petermann, Appunn, and Noeker (1987a) have shown, diabetic adolescents find themselves confronted with a major challenge when it comes to their choice of career and the associated future prospects. Although their illness-related coping strategies are dominated by acceptance of the illness and its demands, they may lack the ability to objectively evaluate and make the most of their potential. Of course, these adolescents try (as do their healthy peers) to select an occupation or profession that will accommodate their individual interests, abilities, and preferences. Also they must make their selection on the basis of the current or predicted job market trends. Yet, they also need to consider how much the chosen occupation might interfere with everyday illness-related demands. Franz and Crystal (1985) have offered suggestions to help diabetic adolescents and their career advisers in assessing career options. First, they must consider how much freedom a particular occupation leaves for dealing with the medical requirements of the disease (blood sugar checks, insulin injections, and diet). In other words, the conditions of the job cannot be such that the adolescent's health will be compromised. Furthermore, they must consider whether the illness will jeopardize the adolescent's potential to succeed in a certain occupation. If such is the case, the choice and pursuit of this occupation involves the risk of unacceptable levels of noncompliance or reduced self-esteem. Finally, adolescents should also consider whether the career is likely to involve a large amount of stress and pressure, which could undermine their attempts to maintain satisfactory metabolic control.

Other authors, however, have reported that most diabetic adolescents have little difficulty in making their choice of career, emphasizing how individual acceptance of the illness determines adolescents' capabilities just as much as metabolic adjustment does. Hasche's (1994) observations of individual cases revealed that diabetics with poor metabolic control saw themselves as highly competitive and very successful in their careers, whereas those with good metabolic control and correspondingly fewer acute complications often felt heavily restricted in their abilities. Another important aspect discussed by Gutezeit (1987) is that occupational fields involving hard physical labor can interfere with the illness and its treatment, so that qualifications for less strenuous kinds of jobs are particularly important for diabetic adolescents. Thus, even more than their healthy peers, ill adolescents are under pressure to show outstanding achievement in school in order to broaden the spectrum of careers to include those that will not necessarily endanger their health.

An important aspect in evaluating the suitability of a particular career for a diabetic adolescent involves the consideration of the type of diabetes therapy to which an adolescent has best responded. Adolescents using conventional methods of treatment are advised to seek occupations that have fixed working hours but allow for breaks. In addition, physical activities may only be carried out at particular times that are consistent with the therapy. However, an adolescent using an insulin pump is the most flexible.

Aside from the degree of personal adjustment and sense of one's own abilities, the chronically ill adolescent will inevitably feel confronted with disadvantages and restrictions in employment. These are partly the result of legal rulings and partly due to discrimination in educational institutions (Finck, 1994). Laws in Germany, for example, prohibit diabetic individuals from working in certain areas of public transportation or in the police force because of the potential risks and dangers of hypoglycemia. Although these restrictions are understandable and justified, diabetic adolescents may find it difficult to accept the limitations on their choice of occupation. This problem is illustrated in the following example case of one diabetic girl.

Carola

Carola's "dream job" was police officer. In the police department there are many fields of work that entail no increased risk to a diabetic's health. Nevertheless, her application was rejected on the grounds of her illness. This was a major problem for her, which she brought up in the fourth interview, when she was 16 years old. She perceived the rejection as an insult. Shortly after receiving this rejection, she accepted a trainee position in the administrative branch of an insurance firm, solely because of the employment prospects and the salary and not out of personal interest or inclination.

If a diabetic adolescent has not been made aware of such kinds of restrictions for certain professions until late in the process of choosing a career, as in Carola's case, the chance of making a satisfactory alternative choice may be severely hampered. It is inadvisable that adolescents be forced into making such a major decision so hastily, especially when they have been disappointed, are without proper perspectives for the future, and are confronted with a revived sense of being restricted and "different." Gutezeit (1984) found that such situations occur all too often. In this study, career advisors reported that 82% of diabetic adolescents had not known that certain occupational fields were closed to them until their first consultation. There is clearly a need for more instruction in this matter, perhaps as part of regular schooling. Apart from the restrictions that may be thought of as legitimate discrimination, Finck (1994) has pointed out a variety of illegitimate ones. Diabetic adolescents are more frequently rejected from training or employment positions, even when they are highly suitable. In Gutezeit's study, responses gathered from advisory centers and businesses showed that employers believed that potential employees with diabetes have reduced capabilities and are at a greater risk for causing or being involved in accidents. Nevertheless, companies were more willing to accept diabetic adolescents into training programs than the career advisers had estimated. Surprisingly, prior experience with diabetic adolescents in training situations did not improve the companies' willingness to employ them. According to Gutezeit, training difficulties can arise from two sources. In Germany, for example, apprenticeship or practical training for some kinds of occupations is often begun early in adolescence. Thus, this training may coincide with the onset of puberty-related metabolic instability. Moreover, some kinds of job training entail irregular hours, and so the altered daily rhythm of activity may provoke variations in metabolism. Because of the hidden nature of the illness, employers might misinterpret any short-term deterioration of abilities as a lack of motivation or decreased willingness to work.

Discrimination in the work force appears to have a large impact on the lives of employees with diabetes. In a study of adults with type I diabetes, 21% claimed that their job applications had been rejected on the grounds of their illness (Petermann et al., 1987b; Petermann, Pliske, & Seefried, 1993). However, other findings indicate that job applicants with diabetes receive equal treatment. Robinson, Busch, Protapapa, and Yateman (1989) found that only 1% of the employers they studied said they would not hire a diabetic applicant. There are two possible interpretations of these contradictory findings on illegitimate discrimination against diabetics. On the one hand, employers' responses might be influenced by factors related to social desirability. Despite a fundamentally positive attitude towards diabetic employees, employers would still prefer to take on a healthy employee, other aspects being equal. On the other hand, the subjective experience of being disadvantaged, as reported by the diabetic job applicants in the study by Petermann and colleagues, cannot be objectively verified and could be based on incorrect assessments of their own abilities and aptitudes. In summary, along with the justifiable restrictions, diabetic workers are highly aware of illegitimate discrimination (although it might only occur to a minor extent in reality). For this reason alone, diabetic adolescents may suffer uncertainty in choosing a career and finding a training vacancy.

In our longitudinal study (chapter 3), diabetic adolescents and their healthy peers were asked about stress and coping strategies related to school and to career and future-oriented plans and concerns. Semistructured interviews were used, as well as two standardized pencil-and-paper tests: the Problem Questionnaire (Seiffge-Krenke, 1995) and the Coping Across Situations Questionnaire (CASQ) (Seiffge-Krenke, 1995).

Coping with Problems at School

The results of our assessments of everyday stressors were discussed in detail in chapter 6. Whereas at the beginning of the study, the adolescents (at the time about 13.9 years old) did not consider school problems as major causes of stress, this changed over the following years. The adolescents' fears and problems related to school increased sharply with time, in both ill and healthy groups. Adolescents in both groups experienced a strong increase in school stressors over the years between the ages of 13.9 and 16.9 years. However, the groups did not differ significantly with respect to their perceived levels of stress related to academic achievement pressure, problems with teachers and other students, and other school-related concerns. The homogeneous increase in school-related problems and concerns is depicted in Figure 8.2.

These findings are consistent with those reported by other investigators, who have found that school- and achievement-related problems grow in importance in this phase of adolescence (Schulenberg et al., 1997). The adolescents' comments in the interviews confirmed the questionnaire findings. In response to the questions "What's on your mind most at the moment?" and "Do you have any concerns about the future?," all adolescents spontaneously gave more responses over the years that were associated with

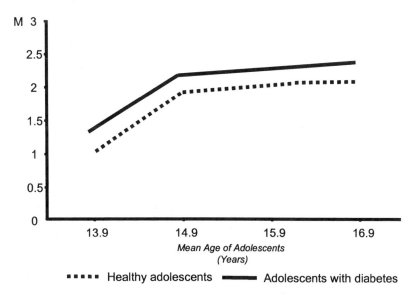

Figure 8.2. Changes over time in school-related stress, perceived by healthy adolescents (N = 107) and diabetic adolescents (N = 91).

school or achievement. However, in the open responses, unlike the answers in the Problem Questionnaire, the increase was only significant for the healthy adolescents. To qualify this finding, it should be recalled that the diabetic adolescents mentioned fewer problems than their healthy peers at all times of measurement; in fact, they were generally reluctant to name any stressors at all (see chapter 6).

It is interesting that although both groups had comparably high levels of school stress, they differed in the way they dealt with their problems. Longitudinal analysis of the CASQ, which assesses coping strategies in various fields in which adolescents typically have problems, showed that diabetic adolescents applied fewer active and internal coping strategies to school-related stressors. Healthy adolescents went to much greater effort to solve these problems by reflecting and thinking about them, actively seeking information, and/or using social resources. Withdrawal and avoidance were rare in both groups. This result corresponds to earlier findings that emphasize adolescents' high problem-solving competence and low levels of dysfunctional and avoidant coping strategies (Seiffge-Krenke, 1993a; 1995). Earlier results indicating age and gender differences in coping behavior were also confirmed. In coping with school problems, female adolescents used active strategies (such as seeking social support) more often than males did. Time and gender effects were found in both the healthy and the diabetic adolescents.

In the interviews, adolescents were asked to talk about their favorite as well as their best school subjects. Healthy adolescents indicated more subjects in which they did well, as well as a larger number of favorite subjects. As compared with the diabetic adolescents, they preferred subjects of a musical or artistic nature, along with sports. Correspondingly, they judged their performance in these favorite subjects, as well as in language-related subjects, to be "quite good" significantly more often than did the diabetic adolescents did. Healthy adolescents' interest in creative pursuits was evident not only in the school arena but also in leisure time activities: They showed significantly higher scores for musical and artistically related activities. This finding is rather surprising, since one would expect the diabetic adolescents to be more inclined to pursue less physically demanding hobbies, such as playing an instrument or engaging in creative crafts. Differences in the family climate (see chapter 7) may be responsible for this finding; families with a diabetic adolescent displayed stronger achievement orientation and rigidity, along with less emphasis on leisure activities and the external world. This could explain at least some of the ill adolescents' low involvement in creative activities.

Career Wishes and Decisions

Our results from the world of school were also paralleled in adolescents' perspectives on careers. In the first interviews, the healthy adolescents (aged 13.9 years) had much clearer ideas about their future jobs than did the diabetic adolescents. Here, too, they had artistic areas in mind, along with technical and scientific occupations. Hobbies and career wishes were closely connected in this age group. In the later years of the study, the two groups no longer differed in the number and specificity of their career ambitions, but differences in their preferences were still noticeable. Whereas healthy adolescents continued to favor careers in artistic or more unusual areas, the diabetic adolescents named preferences for occupations in administration or trade significantly more often. Thus, the ill adolescents not only reported a more limited range of interests both inside and outside of school but also a narrower variety of employment wishes than healthy adolescents did.

At each time of measurement, the adolescents in both groups were clearly realistic about their career choices with respect to their own skills or the school qualifications they expected to receive. Reality orientation even increased with the years. Surprisingly, we found no substantial evidence that the diabetic adolescents in our sample experienced the difficulties or discrimination in their choices of occupation that were reported in the studies discussed in the previous section. In fact, diabetes-related concerns were only mentioned by 4% of the diabetic adolescents in our study. It is possible that they had already eliminated those careers that could interfere with the demands of diabetes. From the third interview onward, career-related matters concerned ill adolescents significantly more than healthy adolescents.

As with school-related stressors, diabetic adolescents indicated far fewer active and internal coping problems in dealing with the domain of career choice than did healthy adolescents. This is surprising, because reflecting about possible careers and actively seeking information and advice would help the adolescent to choose an appropriate career.

Perspectives and Concerns about the Future

Growing concern about the future has become a major issue for today's adolescents. A low-grade anxiety about the future among adolescents living in different European countries and the United States has persisted for decades (McKay, 1977; Mönks, 1968; Seiffge-Krenke, 1998a). Similarly, our longitudinal study revealed that healthy adolescents were more concerned about the future than were their diabetic counterparts. This difference remained constant over the 4 years of the study. The two groups differed not only in the number of problem-related topics mentioned but also in their types of worry. In their open responses to interview questions, healthy adolescents were more concerned about world and political matters, such as environmental pollution and the threat of war. Over the course of the study, they also became more concerned about their own physical changes, finding a partner, and as already mentioned, problems relating to school and employment. Thus, the rankings of adolescents' fears about the future corresponded to the pattern that has existed for decades (Seiffge-Krenke, 1995).

The diabetic adolescents reported fewer generalized worries, but, as expected, they had many concerns regarding their illness and its course (see chapter 6). Diabetes and its possible complications seemed to be such major concerns that other topics, particularly sociopolitical or environmental issues, were overshadowed. Diabetic adolescents' anxieties about their personal futures ranked highest among their concerns about the future, including those related to society and the environment. Differences in coping were also evident with respect to the future-related problems listed in the CASQ. Overall, all adolescents increased their use of internal and active coping strategies over time. However, as was the case for problems related to school and career choices, the diabetic adolescents applied fewer functional coping strategies in coping with future-related problems than did their healthy peers.

Some conclusions can be drawn from comparing the results of the problem areas of school, career choice, and future. School and career issues are highly important in adolescence; accordingly, academic achievement and job selection represent the bulk of the adolescent's concerns and problems. Diabetic adolescents appear to have relatively few problems regarding their integration into the employment world, which is surprising in view of the illness-related difficulties they are confronted with. This was borne out in the finding that diabetic adolescents rarely mentioned any diabetes-related concerns in connection with their career choice. Although there were comparable levels of perceived problems in the two groups based on the results of the standardized questionnaires, in the interviews the diabetic adolescents mentioned fewer worries overall than the healthy adolescents did.

Altogether, the diabetic adolescents in our study did not feel confronted with any particular difficulties or stress associated with school or their proposed careers as long as they had not chosen lines of work that were closed to them by law. However, this somewhat reassuring finding must be qualified by taking into account the typical choices of career that diabetic adolescents actually made and the kinds of coping behaviors they relied on. Compared with healthy adolescents, the diabetic adolescents displayed active coping and internal coping significantly less frequently, although the rates of withdrawal and avoidance were equally low in both groups. This result means that the chronically ill adolescents did in fact use functional forms of coping but with a much lower level of activity. They did not contemplate their school- and career-related problems as much, and they sought information and social support less often. Simultaneously, they preferred to work in administrative, trade, or business fields, whereas their healthy peers favored unusual occupations more often. Overall, diabetic adolescents were less active in solving problems associated with school and employment, and their selection of "safe" careers is noteworthy.

Considering how important the choice of career is for the developing personality, the ill adolescents' minimal involvement in employment-related topics is surprising. The result may be interpreted with the aid of findings regarding the adolescents' fears about the future. Here, too, diabetic adolescents perceived themselves to be far less stressed; the classical fears, such as those related to environmental destruction or war, along with more personal concerns about finding a partner or choosing a career, were of low priority for them. Self-related topics, such as current modes of coping with the illness and the threat of later damage caused by the illness, were much more important to diabetic adolescents. In this respect, it is easy to see why the ill adolescents indicated relatively few problems with school and career. However, their different priorities and coping preferences were not necessarily alternatives without consequence. The transition to a working life may serve a significant function in stabilizing identity and supporting coping with the illness (Gutezeit, 1984). One would expect higher levels of reflection and analysis, especially as illness-specific factors must influence the choice of career.

The results presented so far did not indicate whether the diabetic adolescents' optimistic perspectives on careers, as seen in their rare mention of restrictions or discrimination due to the illness, corresponded closely to the actual situation of seeking training or a job. This is largely because only a few of the diabetic adolescents had had concrete experiences in the employment market by 1994, when they were about 16.9 years old. Most were still in the transition phase between leaving school and beginning a career. An analysis of data from follow-up surveys in 1997 and 2000, conducted in late adolescence and during the transition to young adulthood, may reveal whether the diabetic young adults have been successful in pursuing their career plans.

9

Successful Adaptation or the Development of Psychopathology?

This chapter discusses the question of whether the outbreak of a chronic illness in adolescence leads to delays in developmental progression. This question, which is undoubtedly just as relevant to younger age groups and to other illnesses, is investigated by using the paradigm of diabetic patients. Once again, the data are taken from our longitudinal study of diabetic and healthy adolescents and their families (see chapter 3). In addition, the prevalence of psychological disturbances in adolescents suffering from other chronic illnesses will also be examined. As already mentioned (chapter 2), numerous yet contradictory findings on this matter have been reported. Although some studies appear to have demonstrated that chronically ill adolescents have two or three times the risk of developing psychopathology, others have documented that most ill adolescents cope with their disease without showing any clinical symptoms. The results obtained from our longitudinal study will be analyzed further in chapter 10 with respect to the different pathways that may be involved in the development of psychopathology, and adolescents and their families that coped successfully with the illness will be compared with those that did not.

Does Chronic Illness Lead to Developmental Delays?

If individuals are particularly vulnerable during transition phases (Antonovsky, 1981), then the occurrence of a critical event, such as the onset of a chronic illness, during these times becomes especially significant. Adolescence is the epitome of a developmental transition period, in which multiple changes (such as entering new types of school, physical maturation, and separation from the parents) take place. Adolescents usually cope with these developmental stressors without manifesting any psychological symptoms. Still, the onset of a severe, incurable physical illness may represent a nonnormative stressor that exceeds their coping capacities. Aspects of coping with illness have been studied frequently (for a summary, see chapter 2); however, most research has been restricted to studying illnesses with extremely low prevalence yet high mortality rates. Only recently has attention been focused on more common, treatable illnesses. Although this trend represents a positive development, future studies of coping by the chronically ill adolescent should explicitly acknowledge the adolescent's developmental status, thereby allowing for a more complex and more appropriate representation of the context of coping. By following this approach, researchers may be more likely to examine the adolescents' own perspectives and thus learn how much importance they attach to the chronic illness, which is only one aspect of their lives. In this chapter, the adolescent's and family's perceptions of the adolescent's developmental progression in various domains will be analyzed. More specifically, the ways in which diabetic adolescents perceive their achievement of age-typical developmental tasks and the question of whether there is any indication of a developmental delay will be discussed.

Developmental Tasks in Adolescence

Traditional theories of adolescence have been based on the idea that this developmental period is one marked by crisis. Concepts such as identity crisis, generation gap, and storm and stress portrayed the adolescent as a defective social being. This perspective, which prevailed long into the 1950s, was strongly influenced by the choice of sample populations in studies. Although most studies were based on highly selective samples of adolescents with clinical disorders or were taken from families with multiple problems or in psychotherapy, the results were generalized to typical adolescent development. It was not until the 1960s and 1970s that studies of large representative samples were introduced, many of which used a longitudinal design. The results from these studies led to a revision of the inappropriate conceptualization of adolescence as a period marked by crisis and confirmed the consistent, stable nature of this phase of development. As a consequence, adolescents have come to be seen as "producers of their own development" (Lerner, 1987, p. 29), who actively tackle diverse demands and take on new tasks and roles. In the process, the value of Havighurst's (1953) early conceptualization of developmental tasks has been more full appreciated. According to Havighurst (1953, p. 2), a developmental task is one

...which arises at or about a certain period in the life of the individual, successful achievement of which leads to happiness and to success with later tasks, while failure leads to unhappiness in the individual, disapproval by the society and difficulty with later tasks.

Havighurst described eight age-specific developmental tasks for the adolescent period: adolescents must learn to accept their own body, adopt a masculine or feminine role, develop close relationships with friends, prepare for an occupation and romantic relationships, achieve emotional independence from parents, establish values and an ethical system to live by, and strive for social responsibility. Havighurst's concept of developmental tasks is unique in that it integrates challenges from three different domains: (1) physical development and bodily sensations, (2) adolescent personality and identity, and (3) society's expectations. In addition, the individual's activity in integrating these demands and linking the developmental tasks of different life phases is stressed. Accordingly, the developmental tasks of adolescence are related to tasks of early adulthood, which include, for example, choosing an occupation, establishing a relationship with a life partner, starting a family, raising children, and building a social network.

Havighurst's theoretical work was very influential in counteracting the myth that adolescent development is tumultuous and inevitably controlled by pubertal hormones (Hall, 1904), and it stimulated theory and research. Theoretical contributions from other investigators (e.g., Coleman, 1978) helped to explain the apparent contradiction between the large number of tasks to be achieved during adolescence, on the one hand, and the relatively successful adaptation of the majority of youths facing these demands, on the other. Havighurst's ideas also encouraged other investigators to acknowledge the importance of the context in which adolescents develop (Lerner & Foch, 1987) and to analyze how biological changes in adolescents interact with and stimulate changes in other domains of development (Brooks-Gunn & Reiter, 1990). As early as 1979, Neugarten's concept of a "social clock" illustrated how social expectations and subjective timing are closely connected. More recently, Galambos and Tilton-Weaver's (1996) concept of subjective age, that is, an individual's perception of being "in time" or "off time" with respect to age-specific development, emphasizes the importance of how society's expectations are interwoven with the subjective understanding of one's own competencies and physical maturity.

Nevertheless, research on adolescent development has not produced conclusive evidence to support the Havighurst theory and more recent conceptualizations. Many questions remain unanswered. Do adolescents see themselves as "producers of their own development," as Lerner (1987, p. 29) suggested? How important are certain developmental tasks for them during certain periods in adolescence? Do adolescents exercise their own competencies and pursue their own aspirations in accordance with society's expectations?

Despite the key role of developmental tasks, literature on this topic is quite limited. More importantly, these questions have not been approached from a longitudinal perspective. A review of the psychology literature conducted in 1996 generated 241 entries since 1979 that used the key words "developmental task." In most of these contributions, however, only general reference was made to the theoretical framework of developmental tasks, and only few provided cross-sectional data about these issues (for a summary, see Seiffge-Krenke, 1998c). Earlier studies focused mainly on rating the relative importance of various developmental tasks. They showed that work and career are of high subjective importance for both male and female adolescents (Dreher & Dreher, 1985; Engel & Hurrelmann, 1989). As compared with adolescent boys, girls consistently described their physical development as being more accelerated. In addition, the importance of particular tasks varies with age: Establishing romantic relationships and achieving autonomy from parents were much more important for older than for younger adolescents.

Although age influences the importance an adolescent attaches to a task as well as the sequence in which tasks are approached, culture also plays an important role (Nurmi, Poole, & Kalakowski, 1994). For example, in comparing Finnish, Australian, and Israeli adolescents, Nurmi, Poole, and Seginer (1995) found a culture-specific timing of certain developmental tasks. Australian youths expected their educational and occupational goals to be realized earlier than did Finnish and Israeli adolescents. Discrepancies between desired goals and current developmental status were found in a study comparing German and Polish adolescents (Schoenflug & Jansen, 1995). In addition, family and peer contexts have been found to influence how adolescents accomplish developmental tasks. Sessa and Steinberg (1991) have demonstrated how family structure and the parents' marital status influence the major task of autonomy development. Conflicts experienced by immigrant or bicultural adolescents in their attempts to master developmental tasks have been identified in several studies (see, for example, Gibbs & Moskowitz Sweet, 1991). In particular, problems related to adolescents' desires to avoid or delay autonomy from parents have been reported. Finally, peer group activities provide the resources that help the adolescent to master developmental tasks successfully (Kirchler, Palmonari, & Pombeni, 1993).

In summary, previous research has emphasized the subjective importance of developmental tasks for the adolescent, thereby calling attention to the diversity of adolescents' perceptions. Age-, gender-, and culture-specific differences have been noted. Cultural variation in the time span allotted for the achievement of several tasks has been addressed, as well as individual and family factors that contribute to the perceived mastery of developmental tasks. However, a neglected area of research concerns individual differences in health status. Although epidemiological studies have shown that a rather large number of adolescents are afflicted with chronic physical illnesses, such as cystic fibrosis, diabetes, arthritis, epilepsy, or cancer (Gortmaker et al., 1990), remarkably little is known about how youths with chronic health conditions complete the transition to adulthood. Are chronically ill adolescents able to cope with the various developmental tasks under illness conditions? Do they aspire to achieve the same developmental goals as their healthy peers? In addressing these and related questions, it should be considered that puberty may be the time when adolescents are most at risk for the effects of chronic illness. In particular, early adolescents are especially vulnerable owing to the cumulative effects of changes in body contour, relationship patterns, and school environment and demands.

Is Development Impaired by Chronic Illness in Adolescence?

Generally, adolescents set personal goals for their own development in terms of normative expectations. If their current developmental status deviates from the desired status, they try to prevent or eliminate the developmental pressure of the perceived discrepancy (Lerner & Foch, 1987). This process of self-regulation, by which the adolescent initiates all necessary developmental steps alone, can have a completely different course in healthy and chronically ill adolescents. The developmental status may also have different connotations for ill and healthy adolescents. Chronically ill adolescents may be severely restricted in their capacities and possibilities, so it is relevant to analyze the norms to which they aspire as well as their achievements of developmental tasks. It is particularly interesting to see how these adolescents deal with discrepancies between their current and desired developmental status. Moreover, developmental tasks are interrelated, so changes in one area can bring about changes in another. Attaining professional competence is often associated with separation from the parental household, and establishing romantic relationships occur in about the same time frame. Because of these interrelations and the sequential course of developmental tasks, cumulative deficits may occur in chronically ill adolescents.

Various authors have pointed out the strong impact of the onset of a chronic illness, speaking of interruption of the developmental course or even of "developmental breakdown" (Jamison et al., 1986, p. 616). They stress that the adolescents cannot cope appropriately with normative developmental stressors when faced with additional, illness-related stressors (Ben-Sira, 1984). There are a variety of reasons to expect increasing difficulties in successfully tackling the various developmental tasks. First, having a chronic illness may be associated with increased school absence, because of the illness itself or because of treatment and medical appointments (Weitzman, 1984). Second, academic and vocational performance may be influenced by fatigue, pain, or medication (Cowen et al., 1984). Third, a chronic illness may alter or restrict competencies and future perspectives. For example, some investigators have reported that chronically ill adolescents acquire driver's licenses less often or later than healthy adolescents (Orr et al., 1984).

Their orientation toward the future may also be altered. In a study conducted by Fröhlich (1986), ill adolescents reported career plans less frequently, and their favored occupations were in the medical field. Fourth, social interactions may be influenced. Medical treatment and physical impairments restrict participation in leisure activities, so that the adolescent is unable to become fully integrated into the peer group (Grey, Genel, & Tamborlane, 1980). Some authors have reported that chronically ill adolescents take up romantic relations later than healthy adolescents (e.g., Sinnema, 1986). Finally, there is also evidence that parents of adolescents with a chronic illness exhibit different forms of parenting. It becomes more difficult for the chronically ill adolescent to separate from the parents as role expectations and responsibilities within the family change (Becker, 1979), and the ill adolescent becomes the focus of the family's anxiety and attention. Constant parental monitoring and overprotection may hinder adolescent separation from the family. Some studies have even demonstrated that the illness may encourage the development of a "regressive pull," whereby the adolescents become more dependent and childlike (Hamlett, Pellegrini, & Katz, 1992, p. 41). Although these difficulties are common for a variety of chronic illnesses (Pless & Perrin, 1985), their incidence and the extent to which they exert an effect may depend on the type of illness and particularly on its severity and visibility.

Compared with other chronic illnesses, such as arthritis and cancer, diabetes places relatively few restrictions on adolescents; they can still participate in nearly all types of athletic and leisure time activities and are mostly able to pursue the occupations of their choice. Nevertheless, although diabetic adolescents may not show overt signs of being afflicted with the illness, diabetes management requires that they constantly exercise extreme self-control. The adolescent must live by the clock, remembering to eat and to administer insulin at predetermined times. Diabetic adolescents can only participate in typical teenage activities, such as eating so-called junk food, experimenting with alcohol consumption, or taking vacations with friends by accepting health risks or taking special precautions.

In light of the characteristics just described, that is, the mismatch between illness management and the adolescent's striving for autonomy, the nonobvious nature of the illness, and the responsibility placed on the adolescent, one may consider diabetes suitable for analyzing developmentally related as well as illness-related changes. In fact, one of the most common questions asked by the parents and physicians of diabetic adolescents in our study was whether particular behaviors were developmental or illness-specific.

Deficits in Adolescent-Specific Developmental Tasks

The results of our study presented in the previous chapters indicate that most of our diabetic adolescents coped well with the illness. The majority displayed satisfactory to good metabolic control, a high level of knowledge about the illness, good compliance, and a high level of activity in illness management (see chapters 4 and 6). An analysis of illness-specific coping strategies revealed that diabetic adolescents relied heavily on their own resources and were ambivalent toward seeking help from others. Discrepancies in the size and intactness of their social networks and the quality of their relationships were also evident. Family relationships were described as being rigid, highly structured, and controlling; in addition, there was a strong focus on achievement, leaving little room for autonomy (see chapter 7). Diabetic adolescents' relationships with close friends and romantic partners were characterized by less intimacy and more instrumental help than those of the control group. Finally, diabetic adolescents were more restricted in their school- and career-related interests (see chapter 8). Thus, an apparent discrepancy may exist: On the one hand, adolescents coped well with the illness; on the other hand, they were less developed in the area of relationships.

On the basis of Havighurst's (1953) theory of developmental tasks, we explored the adolescents' current status and future intentions in 11 devel-

opmental tasks involving peer group integration, physical maturity, autonomy from parents, occupational competence, close friendships, and romantic relationships (Seiffge-Krenke, 1998c). The adolescents were asked about
their current developmental status and what they hoped to achieve in the
future, that is, about their intended or desired developmental status. The
discrepancy between current developmental status and intended level was
termed *developmental pressure*.

It is important to note that the healthy and diabetic adolescents in our
study did not differ with respect to their *desired* developmental status in
most of the 11 developmental tasks in the first survey. A difference emerged
only with respect to sociopolitical awareness: Healthy adolescents found it
more important to achieve sociopolitical awareness than did diabetic adolescents. Close friendship, autonomy from parents, romantic relationships,
and occupational competence were developmental tasks of high importance in both groups. This confirms findings of earlier studies that established the importance of these tasks (Dreher & Dreher, 1985; Engel &
Hurrelmann, 1989). However, significant differences between diabetic and
healthy adolescents emerged in the perceptions of *achieved* developmental
status in the first survey, when the adolescents were about 13.9 years old.
Healthy adolescents perceived higher levels of achieved developmental status with respect to physical maturity, increasing autonomy from the parents,
and developing an individual life-style than did diabetic adolescents.

Figure 9.1 illustrates differences between healthy and diabetic adolescents in developmental pressure (i.e., the discrepancy between achieved
and aspired developmental status). In the first survey, the greatest developmental pressure experienced by diabetic adolescents was in the field of
developing professional competence. This developmental task was also of
the most concern to healthy adolescents. Additionally, healthy adolescents
showed a greater developmental pressure with respect to establishing close
friendships and romantic relationships than did diabetic adolescents. In
contrast, healthy adolescents experienced less developmental pressure than
diabetic adolescents regarding physical maturity. Diabetic adolescents
tended to have higher developmental pressure in achieving an independent
identity. Some gender differences emerged, too. Generally, because of their
advanced physical maturity, females experienced less developmental pressure than males in this task. In the group of diabetic adolescents, the girls
felt significantly more developmental pressure than boys regarding autonomy from parents.

The subjective perception of developmental delay was greater in poorly
adjusted than in well adjusted diabetic adolescents. Adolescents with poor

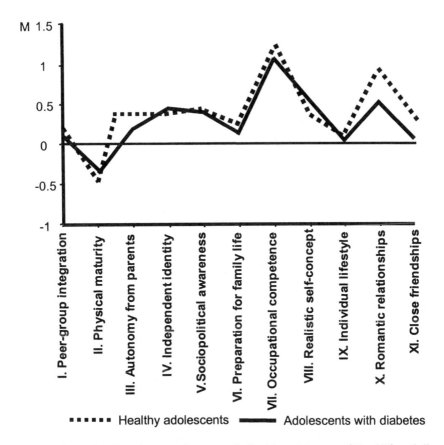

Figure 9.1. Developmental pressure in healthy adolescents (N = 107) and diabetic adolescents (N = 91).

metabolic control reported discrepancies between their current and desired developmental status in several fields. The high developmental pressure felt by poorly adapted diabetic adolescents in establishing romantic relationships is noteworthy. In addition, their scores in achieved developmental status differed significantly from those of better adjusted peers in two developmental tasks, namely, autonomy from parents and close friendships. This means that diabetic adolescents with poor metabolic control were aware of their deficits in their development of close friendships and did not feel adequately independent in their relationships with their parents. This finding was also substantiated by the pattern of correlations between developmental tasks and metabolic adjustment. Significant correlations emerged between poor metabolic control (HbA_1 > 9.5) and the developmental tasks of establishing separate identity ($r = -.37$), autonomy from parents ($r = -.47$), and close friendships ($r = -.38$), which shows that high HbA_1 values were associated with low developmental status in these tasks. The high developmental pressure in establishing romantic relations observed in the poorly adapted diabetic adolescents suggests that they greatly aspired to achieve this task, although – or perhaps precisely because – they were not appropriately developed in their relationships with parents and friends.

These results were only partially confirmed by the reports of their parents and physicians. In the interviews, the parents estimated their child's physical, social, and cognitive developmental levels as average to good. Likewise, the physicians considered a large number of the adolescents they treated as being typically developed for their age, both physically and cognitively. Parents seldom mentioned their ill adolescent's social development, whereas physicians did not discuss it at all. This indicates that diabetic adolescents perceived delays in their development that their parents and physicians did not.

Do Diabetic Adolescents Catch Up to the Developmental Level of Healthy Adolescents over the Course of Several Years?

At the beginning of our study, diabetic adolescents showed developmental delays in the field of relationships. These contrasted sharply with their age-typical development of cognitive capacities and performance and their very strong orientation toward a future career. Their career orientation was remarkable: Developing occupational competence exerted by far the greatest developmental pressure, meaning that adolescents were greatly concerned with achieving this goal. The strong focus on achievement and career applied to the entire group of diabetic adolescents but was even more pronounced among adolescents with good metabolic control.

The next question we addressed was whether the delays found in the first year of the study become even more pronounced with time or whether they approached levels found in healthy adolescents. A longitudinal analysis revealed no differences between healthy and diabetic adolescents with respect to desired developmental status. This suggests that the developmental goals aspired to were the same for both groups and did not change over time. In addition, significant time effects in current developmental status suggested enormous developmental gains in most tasks. Like their healthy peers, diabetic adolescents perceived significant developmental progression in diverse tasks, such as physical maturity, integration into the peer group, establishing a separate identity, and developing occupational competence (Seiffge-Krenke, 1998c). Thus, despite the considerable burdens of the illness, they described impressive competence in mastering the developmental tasks typical for this age group. Four years later, the diabetic adolescents in our study perceived themselves to be as developed as their healthy peers and judged their development as being in time for most of the 11 developmental tasks.

However, some differences need to be stressed. At the beginning of the study, at age 13.9 years, diabetic adolescents scored lower in the tasks of physical maturity and individual life-style. As can be seen in Figure 9.2, these differences decreased over the course of 4 years. In a third task, occupational competence, the diabetic adolescents started from the same developmental status but perceived enormous gains, surpassing those of their healthy peers. In another task, establishing romantic relationships, there was significantly more developmental progression in healthy than in diabetic adolescents.

How can the diabetics' perceived developmental delays in some tasks (e.g., those related to body image, individuality, and establishing romantic relationships) and their strong progression in others tasks (e.g., those related to job aspirations and future careers) be explained? Regarding the diabetic adolescents' perceived setbacks in physical maturity, it must be stressed that they had no objective correlates. As detailed in chapter 5, the physical development of diabetic boys and girls was normal for their ages. Thus, diabetic adolescents only perceived an increase in achieved developmental status in this task over time, which confirms earlier results reported in chapter 5 about the slow but progressive change in body image toward a more mature, adult body. Individual life-style was another task in which diabetic adolescents initially perceived a lower developmental status than their healthy peers. It is well understood that diabetes forces the adolescents to adopt a strict schedule, which leaves them little opportunity to develop individuality. In this task, too, there was developmental progression, probably related to the decrease in compliance found in our sample over time (see chapter 4). Whereas the strong gains in individual life-style can be explained by the need to reduce the gap between current developmental status and developmental goals, the latter being similar for healthy and diabetic adolescents, the situation is different with respect to occupational competence. At first, both healthy and diabetic adolescents showed the same perceived developmental status, but diabetic adolescents made much stronger gains over time. This may be related to the finding that they had already experienced the highest developmental pressure in this particular task at the beginning of the study. With respect to another develop-

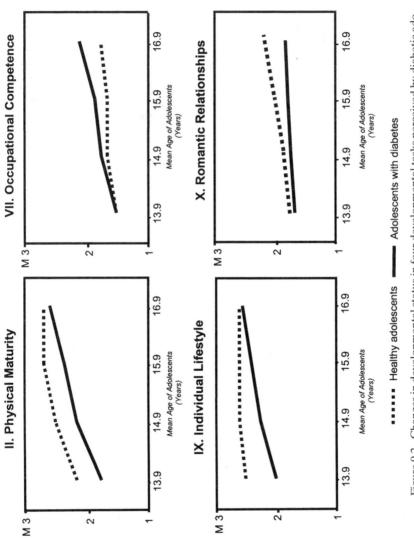

Figure 9.2. Changes in developmental status in four developmental tasks perceived by diabetic adolescents ($N = 91$) and healthy adolescents ($N = 107$).

mental task, establishing romantic relationships, the greater developmental pressure already perceived by healthy adolescents at age 13.9 years was probably responsible for the gains in developmental status in this particular task over time.

Rather unexpectedly, the duration of the illness did not influence developmental progression: Adolescents who had been ill for more than 5 years did not perceive themselves as more developmentally delayed than adolescents who had been ill for less than 1 year. In addition, metabolic control had no impact on perceived developmental progression. This lends support to the hypothesis that most diabetic adolescents share the same developmental context, with similar experiences and limitations. Thus, the impact of the illness seems to be pervasive, regardless of illness duration and adaptation to the illness.

Conditions That Contribute to or Maintain Developmental Delays

The results reported in this chapter with respect to achieved and desired developmental status in various tasks were highly consistent with the results from our interviews and other questionnaires, as reported elsewhere in this book. This uniformity was evident not only for different assessment methods but also among different respondents (adolescents, parents, and physicians). It is also striking that the diabetic adolescents caught up to their peers in some areas. These gains did not occur in all developmental tasks with the same speed or to the same extent. Before this phenomenon is discussed further, some consideration should be given to the question of how the delays in development may have come about.

Developmental psychologists have found Coleman's (1978) focal theory of development to be instrumental in explaining how adolescents cope with developmental tasks in this stage of life. According to this theory, the adolescent focuses on particular developmental tasks and works through them in succession. Thus, the ability to focus on and cope with each developmental task sequentially is the key to successful developmental progression. Coleman (1984) later described the focusing process more precisely. A promising developmental path emerges if the adolescent is successful in setting priorities and dealing with each goal in turn. Nevertheless, developmental stress may result if the adolescent's knowledge and capacities are not enough to solve a developmental task of high subjective urgency. The more that the adolescent attempts to achieve different developmental tasks simultaneously, the more likely this outcome is.

We observed that diabetic adolescents solved the problem posed by the accumulation of stressors due to the chronic illness and the need to achieve developmental tasks by considering illness management to be the single most pressing (and life-preserving) task. This was done at the expense of developmental tasks that healthy adolescents of their age would be able to achieve. Although the developmental progression of the diabetic adolescents was impressive, the selective choice of which developmental tasks they tackled requires some explanation. Among all the possible developmental tasks, occupational goals were focused on more strongly and also better achieved than were tasks involving relationships and individuality. This was consistently found throughout our study. For that reason, we analyzed what conditions contribute to selecting and focusing on certain developmental tasks at the expense of others.

The Adolescent. Much evidence in our study emerged to suggest that diabetic adolescents were hesitant in approaching relationship-based developmental tasks because of certain conditions, most importantly the ill adolescents' poor self-concept and negative body image. One consequence of having a low or depressive self-concept could possibly be a disinclination to become involved in social systems outside the family. Diabetic adolescents perceived their bodies as being more rigid, less flexible, and more childlike. As already mentioned, the perceptions of the body as being less mature were not related to objective indicators of delayed maturation processes. The perceived differences in body image may have contributed to diabetic adolescents' reserve in establishing close friendships and romantic relationships. The diabetic adolescents' body images did begin to catch up somewhat (see chapter 5), but even in the third survey at a mean age of 15.9 years, they still thought their bodies were less adult than healthy adolescents did. This may explain the continued discrepancies in developmental levels regarding romantic relationships and close friendships with peers. Another striking result was the different expectations that diabetic adolescents had of their close friends and romantic partners. Diabetic adolescents expressed a strong need for security and a desire for concrete instrumental help (see chapter 8). In these areas, healthy adolescents were more critical, open to experimentation, and independent, and they were able to fulfill their sexual needs outside of a fixed partnership. Because of their demanding, atypical expectations, diabetic adolescents were sometimes disappointed in friendships and romantic relationships, which dampened their initiative even further. They put considerable effort into personal achievements and were extremely concerned about school and their future professions. Although their developmental status in these tasks was similar to that of healthy peers at the beginning of our study, they made considerably more progress over time. This is probably related to the high developmental pressure experienced in this particular task. The results of this study further suggest that the family context might help to explain this accelerated progression.

The Family. As described in chapter 7, the family climate in families with a diabetic adolescent differed considerably from that in families with a healthy adolescent. Families with a diabetic adolescent (regardless of the diabetic's metabolic control) were more structured, organized, and controlled and more strongly oriented toward achievements. In addition, family communication was more curtailed and less elaborate, and there was less negotiation about possible solutions of family problems. Although these qualities could be considered as being functional for coping with the illness, they could have discouraged or inhibited the further development of individual family members. This danger was demonstrated in the diabetic adolescents' lower values for personal growth and autonomy, as well as in their subjectively perceived developmental delay in individual life-style. This type of family functioning persisted over 4 years (see chapter 7), although the improvement in metabolic control and generally acceptable course of the illness seen in most patients could have allowed the family climate to grow more relaxed and to take the adolescents' developmental possibilities into account. Whereas the very strict family climate supported the adolescents' efforts to show achievement, it failed in encouraging autonomy and individuality. Fathers made a strikingly negligible contribution to the diabetic adolescents' acquisition of independence, and the ill adolescents had unusually close relationships with their siblings. Because of the distinctive dynamics of the families, it is reasonable to assume that the adolescents aimed most strongly for and achieved developmental goals that conformed to the family's strong achievement orientation.

The Adolescents' Physicians. Our adolescents generally rated their relationships with their physicians as being extremely important for coping with the illness at the beginning of the study (see chapter 4). The adolescents not only discussed a variety of illness-related topics with their physicians, but they also asked them for advice on many other problems, such as those concerning parents, friends, or school. However, patient–physician relationships and compliance with the physician's instructions worsened over the course of the study, paralleling the increasingly individual life-styles of the adolescents. It is important that experts in the medical field – physicians, nurses, dietitians, and so on – be aware of their patients' developments and adopt a more complex, holistic view of the adolescent. In view of the adolescent's overall development, a more tolerant attitude to deteriorating HbA$_1$ values and metabolic instability would be desirable, at least within a range that rules out the chance of later damage. However, our data show that most physicians failed to notice any deficits in the social field or in important relationships.

How can parents and physicians help to minimize or prevent developmental delays? It should already be clear that for various reasons, diabetic adolescents are forced to proceed in their development hesitantly. The diabetic adolescent's focused attention on the most pressing issues, such as illness management and the therapeutic regimen, is not only understandable but also functional in the sense of preventing psychological overload. Only when adolescents have learned to cope reasonably well with the illness can they turn their attention to and apply themselves toward achieving age-appropriate developmental tasks.

It may take a considerable amount of time for the diabetic adolescent to learn how to cope competently with and manage the illness. However, some developmental tasks can rarely be postponed for this long. Adolescents may thus perceive the need to attend to illness management and the desire to proceed with age-typical development as being irreconcilably in conflict. Consequently, they may wish for a more lenient therapeutic regimen that allows them more freedom to develop. Tolerance and understanding from all involved parties are necessary. In the long term, excessive concentration on the adolescent's health status or unyielding parental control and restrictions may backfire (see chapter 10). In addition, encouragement of developmental progression from adults would be most valuable, because the adolescents approach some developmental tasks quite cautiously owing to their more negative self-concept, negative body image, and tendency to withdraw. However, the diabetic adolescent's achievement orientation tends to be so strong that any additional parental pressure to accomplish career plans should be avoided.

Psychopathology in Chronically Ill Adolescents

In the following section, a brief overview of adolescents' general susceptibility to psychopathology is presented, after which the question of whether a chronic illness may increase the risk for psychopathology in adolescence is addressed. Although many studies on coping with illness (see chapter 2) have focused on these topics, most of them have adopted a perspective that is more clinical than developmental. Moreover, findings in this research area have been heterogeneous, controversial, and difficult to evaluate. In order to best identify the origins of the differences and discrepancies, individual studies will be discussed in detail in the following section.

Prevalence of Psychological Symptoms and Disorders in Adolescence

Most adolescents pass through their teenage years without salient psychological problems or behavioral disorders. Large epidemiological studies on nonselective samples, such as the Ontario Child Health Study (Offord et al., 1987; Boyle et al., 1992) have shown that the overall prevalence rates of psychological disturbances during adolescence do not differ significantly from those in childhood; however, the prevalence rates of various disturbances vary with age. Disorders frequently seen in childhood, such as enuresis, hyperactivity, or conduct disorders, decrease in adolescence (Bird et al., 1988; Kashani, Carlson, & Beck, 1987). Simultaneously, adolescence is characterized by initial manifestations of depressive disorders, schizophrenia, eating disorders, drug abuse, and suicidal behavior (Hawton, 1986; Lewinsohn, Klein, & Seeley, 1995; Seiffge-Krenke, 1998a). Of these disorders, 60% develop during puberty; they are rarely seen, for example, in 10-year-old children (Rutter et al., 1977).

Offord et al. (1987) investigated the frequency of various forms of disturbances in a total of 1,869 children and adolescents aged between 4 and 16 years. They found that the 6-month prevalence rates of one or more of these disturbances depended significantly on both age and gender. For children aged 4 to 11 years, the prevalence rate was higher among boys (19.5%) than among girls (13.5%), whereas for adolescents aged 12 to 16 years, the picture was nearly the reverse (18.8% in boys, 21.8% in girls). Similar prevalence rates have been reported by Wittchen, Essau, von Zerssen, Krieg, and Zaudig (1992) and by Essau, Karpinski, Petermann, and Conradt (1998) on German children and adolescents. Epidemiological studies using a longitudinal design have further revealed that these are true age effects, not just cohort differences induced by the cross-sectional design. Esser et al. (1992) examined the longitudinal course of various psychological disorders in a representative sample from the city of Mannheim, Germany. The subjects were interviewed three times, at 5-year intervals. The prevalence rates for psychological disorders were 16.2% in the 8-year-olds (boys 22.2%, girls

10.2%), 17.8% in the 13-year-olds (boys 13.0%, girls 19.7%), and 16.0% in the 18-year-olds (boys 14.8%, girls 17.2%).

In most studies, symptomatology peaked in early adolescence. Like Esser et al. (1992) and Essau et al. (1998), Rozario, Kapur, and Kaliaperumal (1990) found the highest rates of psychological disturbances in younger adolescents around 13 years of age (11.7%). The percentage of adolescents with psychological disturbances declined by about 2 to 4% annually. Overall, the findings indicate that the gender ratio of psychopathology reverses in mid-adolescence. Whereas more boys than girls are diagnosed as having psychological disturbances in childhood, the situation is reversed in adolescence, when more females are diagnosed as suffering from psychopathology. In addition, early adolescence seems to be a particularly vulnerable time.

Like the general prevalence rates of psychopathology in adolescence, gender effects have been reported for particular symptoms and disorders. Male adolescents more frequently exhibit externalizing behavior syndromes (e.g., aggression, antisocial behavior, hyperactivity, or delinquency); female adolescents show higher prevalence rates for internalizing disorders (e.g., depression and anxiety) as well as eating disorders. Lewinson, Hops, Roberts, Seeley, and Andrews (1993) studied the distribution of psychological disorders in a sample of 1,508 high school students in the United States. Depression, anxiety, and eating disorders were more commonly diagnosed in girls, whereas adolescent boys had twice the girls' rate of externalizing behavior problems. Above all, these consisted of attention and hyperactivity disorders and aggressive, socially disruptive behaviors. The second most common diagnosis among male adolescents was substance abuse or dependence. These gender-specific rankings of psychological disorders were also found in a study by McGee et al. (1990) on a representative sample of 15-year-old adolescents. The prevalence rates for depression and anxiety disorders were twice as high in girls as in boys, whereas those for attention disorders were twice as high in boys. Aggressive behavioral problems occurred exclusively in male adolescents. Such gender differences have also been reported for clinically referred adolescents (Seiffge-Krenke, 1998a).

In summary, epidemiological studies reveal a relatively uniform picture. In general, adolescence is not a developmental phase of increased psychopathology. Rather, there are clear age and gender effects in the observed forms of disturbances. These patterns are also reflected in various clinically referred sample populations.

Psychopathology in Chronically Ill Adolescents

The question of whether chronically ill children and adolescents show increased psychopathology has been the focus of numerous research efforts for over 20 years (see summaries by Magan, 1990; Perrin & MacLean, 1988; Pless & Nolan, 1991). As early as the beginning of the seventies, Pless and Roughman (1971, p. 354) considered psychopathology in adolescents with chronic physical illness as a "secondary handicap caused by physical disorders." Although this suggestion was seldom explicitly stated, most of these studies were based on the assumption that such a strong nonnormative stressor during the transition to adulthood must have a negative impact on mental health.

The epidemiological study of Rutter and co-workers (Rutter, Tizard, & Whitmore, 1970b; Rutter, Graham, & Yule, 1970a) represents one of the earliest attempts to study the relationship between chronic disease and psychopathology. From 1964 to 1970, these investigators studied the entire population of 9- to 12-year-old children on the Isle of Wight ($N = 1,279$) and found a twofold increase in the prevalence rate of psychiatric disorders in chronically ill children ($N = 186$) in comparison with their physically healthy peers. Parents', teachers', and children's own responses in interviews and questionnaires showed that in chronically ill children, the rate of psychopathology was 17.2%, whereas it was only 6.6% in their healthy peers. Very similar findings were obtained in two other epidemiological studies corresponding to this time period, namely, the Rochester Child Health Survey (Pless & Roughman, 1971; Pless, Roughman, & Haggerty, 1972), conducted on representative samples of children and adolescents aged 6 to 16 years, and the National Survey (Douglas, 1964). The Rochester study reported behavioral disturbances in 23% of the chronically ill children compared with 16% of the physically healthy children. The ratio was 25% to 17% in the National Survey, which followed same-age cohorts longitudinally up to age 16 years.

These three epidemiological studies were the first to empirically document an increased risk of psychopathology in chronically ill children and adolescents, thereby laying the foundations for more research efforts in this area. Subsequent studies investigating considerably smaller samples confirmed these initial findings (e.g., Boyle, di Sant' Agnese, Sack, Millican, & Kulcyski, 1976; McCollum & Gibson, 1970; Tropauer, Franz, & Dilgard, 1970). However, the majority of these studies diagnosed psychopathology according to clinical impressions and did not include healthy control groups.

A study conducted by Tavormina, Kastner, Slater, and Watt (1976) represented a turning point in research on this topic. Using standardized measurements, they were unable to document an increased incidence of psychopathology in children and adolescents suffering from various chronic illnesses. In fact, they observed a "normalcy rather than a deviance of this sample" (p. 108). This finding was later confirmed in other studies on chronically ill children and adolescents using standardized methods of data collection. For example, Bedell, Giordani, Amour, Tavormina, and Boll (1977), who studied 6- to 16-year-old children and adolescents with asthma, diabetes, or cystic fibrosis, as well as Kellerman, Zeltzer, Ellenberg, Dash, and Rigler (1980), who studied adolescents with various chronic illnesses, were unable to observe any increase in psychopathology in these patient groups. Similarly, in a more recent study on a nationally representative sample of over 12,000 youths aged 12 to 21 years, Gortmaker, Perrin, Weitzman, Halmer, and Sobol (1993) found that although adolescents with chronic physical illness were at a slightly higher risk of developing psychological problems in early adult life, these effects were overshadowed by an "unexpected success story" (p. 317).

The Ontario Child Health Study (Cadman et al., 1987) is the most recent epidemiological study in the field. In contrast to the three studies mentioned so far, this study also differentiated between children and adolescents, so it warrants more detailed examination. The population included all children born between 1966 and 1976 living in Ontario; from these, a representative sample of 1,869 families was selected, which included a total of 3,294 children and adolescents aged 4 to 16. Cadman et al. (1987) used a modified form of the Child Behavior Checklist (CBCL) (Achenbach, 1991a), which assesses the psychological health of children and adolescents according to the diagnostic categories of the Diagnostic and Statistical Manual of Mental Disorders (DSM)-III-R. Three categories of psychological disturbances were distinguished: neurotic disorders (anxiety disorders, depression, and compulsive disorders), disturbances of social behavior, and attention and hyperactivity disorders. Two sources were used to evaluate each subject's psychological health. For children aged 4 to 11 years, the parents and a teacher were the informants; for 12- to 16-year-olds, the adolescents themselves provided reports, along with their parents. The participants were also classified into three groups according to their physical health: physically healthy (82% of the sample), chronically ill without disability (14%), and chronically ill with one or more disabilities (4%).

Each type of psychological disorder was close to twice as prevalent in the chronically ill sample as in the healthy control subjects and even more prevalent in the children and adolescents with disabilities in addition to chronic illnesses. Overall prevalence rates of psychological diagnoses were 14.1% in the healthy group, 23.4% in the chronically ill group, and 32.6% in the group of chronically ill with disabilities. The results of the Ontario Child Health Study thus indicate that the risk of psychopathology in chronically ill children and adolescents may be as high as twice that in their healthy peers. In contrast to the group with various disabilities, no age or gender differences could be identified in the group of chronically ill children and adolescents without disabilities.

In summary, although it has been suggested that physical illness in adolescence is associated with a significant risk of developing psychological disturbances, there is controversy about the existence and nature of such a relationship. This is probably related to weaknesses in the research methods employed but also to the theoretical foundations of these studies. Salient problems include (1) incomplete assessment of disease characteristics, such as type, severity, and duration of illness; (2) a lack of control for variables that might contribute to variance in chronic illness and psychopathology, such as age, gender, and SES; (3) limited sensitivity to the effects of sources of information on the outcome measure; (4) possible bias in interpreting data concerning physical symptoms; (5) problems in recruitment of samples; (6) a lack of longitudinal studies that connect phases of diseases with impact on psychopathology; and (7) a lack of theoretically based research. In the assessment of chronically ill adolescents' psychopathological symptoms, it is particularly important to clarify the overlap between psychosomatic symptoms and bodily complaints resulting from the chronic illness (Perrin, Stein, & Drotar, 1991).

Psychopathology in Diabetic Adolescents

A long-standing discussion has concerned the issue of whether diabetes places adolescents at greater risk for psychiatric disturbances. Controversial findings were already evident at the beginning of research in the 1960s and early 1970s. The findings obtained in an early study conducted by Swift, Seidman, and Stein (1967) are often presented as proof that psychopathology occurs disproportionately in diabetic adolescents. In this study, 7- to 17-year-old diabetic patients had a higher rate of psychiatric disorders (60%) than healthy control subjects (16%). This comparably high proportion was based on ratings by a psychologist and a psychiatrist in a semistructured interview carried out with the subjects' mothers. In contrast, Olatawura (1972) found no difference between a group of diabetic children and adolescents aged 5 to 13 years and an equally large group of healthy control subjects. In this study, psychopathology was assessed in various ways: through general information provided by the mother, by means of a behavioral inventory (also based on the mother's responses), and by various questionnaires for the teachers, which allowed neurotic and antisocial behavior to be distinguished. No significant differences between the groups' symptoms were revealed by any of these sources. According to Olatawura, these results contradict those of Swift et al. (1967) because the sample in the latter study was so heterogeneous. Similarly, Simonds (1977) criticized the study by Swift et al., pointing out that the diabetic participants varied greatly with respect to adjustment to the illness. Simonds also found age-typical levels of psychopathology among diabetic adolescents.

In their longitudinal study, Jacobson, Hauser and co-workers (Jacobson et al., 1986) came to similar conclusions. They analyzed compliance using the Diabetic Adjustment Scale (DAS) and assessed psychopathology based on responses of mothers in the Child Behavior Checklist (CBCL) and of adolescents in the Youth Self Report (YSR) (Achenbach, 1991b). Their subjects were 64 adolescents with recent onset of diabetes (mean age 12.7 years) and a same-age group of 68 acutely ill adolescents. The mean of the diabetic sample fell within the range of a nonpsychiatric sample. In addition, no significant group differences emerged on the measures of symptomatology, leading the authors to suggest that the majority of adolescents "were not consciously overwhelmed by the onset of the diabetes" (p. 326). However, the DAS total score was strongly correlated ($r = -.60$) with psychopathology, indicating that fewer symptoms were associated with better adjustment to the illness.

Even in the most recent research, contradictions surround the issue of whether diabetic adolescents have more psychopathology. Divergent results also exist with respect to specific forms of disturbances. For example, Thompson, Kronenberger, and Curry (1989) have reported that diabetic children and adolescents primarily develop internalizing symptoms. In their study, symptomatology belonging to this category was observed in 59% of the sample, with 22% showing purely internalizing and 31% showing a mixed pattern of internalizing and externalizing symptoms. None of the diabetic patients displayed exclusively externalizing symptoms, although 3% of the physically healthy control subjects did. Similarly, in a study by Kokkonen and Kokkonen (1993), diabetic subjects in late adolescence differed from healthy control subjects in their level of depressive symptoms, as measured by a standardized psychiatric interview. Seigel et al. (1990) found that 70% of 12- to 18-year-old diabetic adolescents exhibited symptoms of depression, compared with only 13% in the control group. These differences remained stable even when psychological and somatic items were evaluated separately. In contrast to these results, Engström (1992) was unable to reveal any differences in externalizing and internalizing symptoms between diabetic adolescents and their healthy peers, based on maternal assessments of symptomatology using the CBCL. Some studies found no increase in depression among diabetic adolescents. For example, Capelli et al. (1989) assessed diabetic adolescents' self-reports of depressive symptoms at a mean age of 14 years. Although the adolescents were concerned about their health and future and reported high levels of stress caused by fathers and siblings, they did not differ from their healthy peers in symptoms of depression.

With respect to the coexistence of diabetes and eating disorders, however, the findings are more equivocal. Several studies have confirmed an increase of anorexia nervosa and bulimia in diabetic females between the ages of 16 and 25 years (Spurdle & Giles, 1990; Streel, Young, Lloyd, & Macintyre, 1989). There is evidence that dietary restrictions, a major part of the treatment in diabetes, predisposes females to binge eating and other types of abnormal food consumption. Abnormal eating attitudes in diabetic females has been frequently associated with high HbA_1 levels, suggesting a relationship between poor metabolic control and the tendency to develop abnormal eating patterns.

Several studies in the past have revealed low cross-informant consistency in assessing adolescents' symptomatology (Achenbach et al., 1987; Seiffge-Krenke & Kollmar, 1998). In these studies, interparental agreement was substantial (mean $r = .60$), whereas agreement between parents' reports and adolescents' self-reports was much lower (mean $r = .28$). Consequently, in our longitudinal study, we explored adolescents' psychopathology from both the parents' and the adolescents' perspectives. Mothers and fathers filled out the Child Behavior Checklist (CBCL) (Achenbach, 1991a), which records the parents' views of their child's symptomatology. In addition, the adolescents' perspectives were explored by administering the Youth Self Report (YSR). Both questionnaires consist of 114 items, from which five narrow-band syndromes and two global broadband syndromes (internalizing and externalizing) can be derived.

In the first year of our study, when the adolescent mean age was 13.9 years, symptomatology in healthy and ill adolescents differed in an unexpected manner. The healthy girls reported that they had more somatic complaints and described themselves as being more depressive, less popular, more aggressive, more delinquent, and more confused in their thoughts than the diabetic girls did, resulting in significantly higher scores for internalizing and externalizing syndromes. Healthy adolescent boys' scores were significantly higher on two scales, resulting in a significantly higher score in externalizing syndromes. Healthy boys described themselves as being more aggressive and more delinquent than did diabetic boys.

The very positive evaluation made by diabetic adolescents, that is, a low level of symptoms, did not apply to one subgroup, namely, the diabetic adolescents with poor metabolic control ($HbA_1 > 9.5$). Female adolescents with poor metabolic control differed from the better adjusted females by showing higher values for depression, unpopularity, and somatic complaints, leading to increased scores for the broad-band internalizing and externalizing syndromes. In males with poor metabolic control, higher levels of psychopathology were also found, although the differences were not statistically significant. Rather unexpectedly, illness duration did not affect symptomatology. Thus, the majority of well or satisfactorily adjusted diabetic adolescents reported low levels of symptoms.

The adolescents' perspectives were not supported by the parents' reports. This finding was substantiated by the low cross-informant correlation between parents and adolescents. Fathers' and mothers' evaluations of their adolescents' symptoms in the CBCL correlated highly for daughters ($r = .67$) and sons ($r = .59$), whereas the agreement between parents and children was less (mean $r = .39$). Parents of girls in both groups described their daughters' symptomatology as highly similar. However, differences on some scales emerged in families with male diabetic adolescents. Mothers of diabetic adolescents described more somatic complaints in their sons, whereas fathers perceived their sons as being more hyperactive and having more thought disorders, as compared with parents of healthy male adolescents. In families with a diabetic adolescent, parental assessments did not differ according to illness duration and metabolic control. The sole difference was that fathers of adolescent boys with poor metabolic control described their sons as being more hyperactive and withdrawn.

Changes in Symptomatology over Time

The overall level of behavioral and emotional problems perceived by diabetic adolescents was low in our study. This was the case not only in comparison with the previously mentioned findings on symptomatology in chronically ill adolescents but also relative to our and other healthy comparison groups (Döpfner et al., 1998; Lösel, Bliesener, & Köferl, 1991;

Seiffge-Krenke & Kollmar, 1998). This raises the possibility of the existence of defense and denial processes, which have been observed several times in studies of diabetic adolescents (see chapter 6). We examined this possibility using the social desirability scale of Schmidt's (1981) Multidimensional Personality Test, which revealed that diabetic adolescents were significantly more likely to conform and to behave in a socially desirable manner than were the healthy control subjects. This tendency was noticeable in adolescents with poor metabolic control but was particularly strong in adolescents with good metabolic control. Perhaps the hidden, invisible nature of diabetes and the adolescent's simultaneous desire to belong to and share in the social activities of the peer group (e.g., eating junk food) encouraged the adolescents to trivialize or deny the illness. Indeed, adolescents strongly avoided admitting their own supposed deficiencies and weaknesses; under no circumstances did they want to stand out and be excluded by peers. This tendency was reflected in other findings, too, such as their answers on the DAS (detailed in chapter 4) as well as in their low reported levels of physical complaints (chapter 5) and everyday stressors (see chapter 6).

We initially expected that the normative façade observed at the beginning of our study might crack and that diabetic adolescents would describe behavioral or emotional problems more openly as they developed a more trusting relationship with the researchers. The longitudinal analysis, however, did not reveal a substantial decrease on the social desirability scale in diabetic adolescents.

The longitudinal analysis of the YSR further revealed that the basic discrepancies between healthy and diabetic adolescents hardly changed over time. This effect was significant with respect to externalizing and internalizing syndromes, despite a minor convergence in scores. The differences between healthy and ill female adolescents on almost all scales remained largely the same. As illustrated in Figure 9.3, the basic discrepancies remained stable until the fourth survey, when the female adolescents had a mean age of 16.9 years. Diabetic adolescent girls still thought they were much less burdened by symptoms than their healthy peers. Furthermore, the significant time effect found for all adolescent girls demonstrates that, as time went by, they reported fewer and fewer symptoms. This was true for somatic complaints, depression, unpopularity, and aggression, resulting in significant time effects for the broad-band internalizing syndromes and tendentially also for the broad-band externalizing syndromes.

A similar trend emerged in the male sample. As illustrated in Figure 9.4, which shows a comparison between diabetic and healthy male adolescents, the significant differences in the broad-band externalizing syndromes

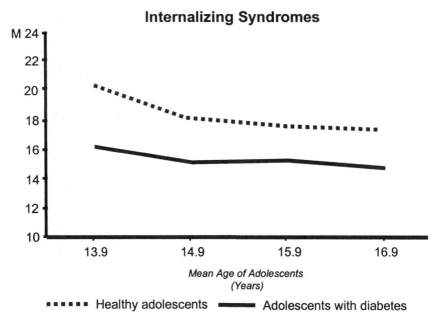

Figure 9.3. Changes over time in the levels of internalizing syndromes in female adolescents (diabetic: $N = 45$; healthy: $N = 62$).

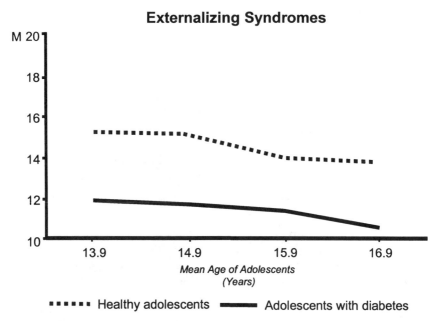

Figure 9.4. Changes over time in the levels of externalizing syndromes in male adolescents (diabetic: $N = 46$; healthy: $N = 45$).

largely remained constant from age 13.9 to 16.9 years. For all males, a main effect of time indicated a decrease in externalizing syndromes.

As already mentioned, social desirability was also examined across time. Diabetic adolescents continued to present themselves in a more socially desirable light than their healthy peers, despite slight increases in disclosure. Reports made by parents of healthy as well as ill adolescents depicted a somewhat different picture. Overall, no differences between healthy and diabetic female adolescent symptomatology were found in the parents' reports, but parents of diabetic adolescent boys rated their sons' symptomatology higher than did parents of healthy boys. With respect to time effects, however, parental assessments corresponded closely to their children's assessments. Mothers and fathers perceived a distinct decrease in their children's somatic complaints, depression, and hostility, thereby describing decreases in internalizing and externalizing behaviors over time. In the families with a diabetic adolescent, hardly any differences over time were found with respect to illness duration and metabolic control.

In summary, parents and adolescents in our study quite uniformly described a decrease in symptomatology over time, confirming the findings of Esser et al. (1992), Essau et al. (1998), and Rozario et al. (1990) of a peak in early adolescence, at about the ages of 13 or 14 years, and a decrease thereafter. This decrease emerged consistently across informants in all families, irrespective of health status. However, informants differed in the frequency of symptoms they reported.

The Problem of Denial in Chronically Ill Adolescents

Two points become clear on integrating the diverse findings from our study. In comparison with their healthy peers, diabetic adolescents reported much lower levels of psychopathology. These levels changed little over the course of the study and the different phases of the illness. Considering the diabetic adolescents' substantially higher scores on the social desirability scale, this may be interpreted as denial of symptoms. Other findings obtained in the diabetic sample uphold this view, in particular, the low perceived everyday stress, the low frequency of bodily complaints, and the strong wish expressed in the interviews to be as normal as possible. Second, the perceptions of diabetic adolescents' parents did not exactly parallel those of their children; for example, the parents described higher levels of symptoms in their sons. In addition, as is consistent with this divergence, parents described considerably more everyday burdens and stressors than did the diabetic adolescents over time.

Indications of denial tendencies have also been found in patients with other chronic illnesses. For instance, Haag, Graf, and Jost (1991) reported that adolescents with cancer presented themselves as being unusually free of psychological symptoms. This turned out to be independent of the specific type of cancer or therapy. The sample consisted of 6- to 17-year-old patients who were currently being treated for either leukemia or a malignant tumor. Comparison groups were drawn from children and adolescents who were receiving outpatient or short-term treatment for other illnesses at a pediatric clinic. Patients with malignant tumors indicated substantially less anxiety in various areas than the healthy or outpatient comparison groups. The most notable finding was that children and adolescents with cancer reported significantly less anxiety in precisely those areas that were most closely related to their illness (death and separation from the parents). Their reduced fears were interpreted by the authors to be a consequence of an "intrapsychic form of coping" in that "...the life-threatening nature of the situation is denied by the children and adolescents" (p. 82). A similar argument was put forward by Worchel et al. (1988), who investigated depression in oncological patients in the treatment phase. Once again, the ill children and adolescents reported far fewer depressive symptoms than their healthy peers. Another finding confirmed the supposition of denial processes: 96% of the participants said their condition had improved, although a much smaller proportion of their physicians (46%) were able to make this claim. Just like adolescents with cancer, patients with other illnesses, such as cystic fibrosis (Simmons et al., 1985; Cowen, et al., 1984; Boyle et al., 1976) or bronchial asthma (Kashani et al., 1988), have shown denial tendencies. Thus, forms of defense in chronically ill adolescents do not appear to be restricted to diabetic patients.

An interesting question here is whether the need for social desirability made our diabetic adolescents reluctant to express their symptoms in the research situation or whether a true defense mechanism was at work, preventing the adolescents from perceiving their own psychopathological symptoms. The clinical observations of Erlich (1987) argue in favor of the defense hypothesis. In describing the defense processes found in chronically ill adolescents, he mentioned a twofold suppression of aspects related to the body. When conflict is aroused around the time of physical maturity, bodily signals tend to be suppressed by some adolescents. The onset of a chronic illness in adolescence during a time of physical change may then lead to a double suppression of physical signals. Not only did our diabetic adolescents express a strong wish to be normal, but they were constantly aware of the fact that the family and their physicians expected them to cope effectively with the illness, thereby encouraging them to achieve good or normal health. Lazarus (1985, p. 41) has aptly described this situation as "trivialization of distress."

Furthermore, diabetic adolescents with good metabolic control in our study portrayed themselves as particularly nonstressed and almost asymptomatic, whereas those with poor metabolic control readily named their behavioral and emotional symptoms. Several studies have shown a higher rate of psychopathology in poorly adjusted diabetic patients (e.g., Gath, Smith, & Baum, 1980; Grey et al., 1980; Mayou et al., 1991; Simonds, 1976). Other authors have reported that diabetic adolescents with good metabolic control named fewer psychological symptoms than healthy adolescents (Gilbert, 1992; Simonds, 1977). In the light of these findings, it is questionable whether poor metabolic control is a general feature of those diabetic adolescents who show psychological disturbances (see, e.g., Johnson, 1980) or whether defense processes are more common among better adjusted diabetic patients. This may, as in our study, be a question of differences in how openly adolescents express their symptoms rather than evidence of actual denial in well adjusted diabetic adolescents. Despite the unusually carefree life described by our diabetic adolescents with good metabolic control, however, such defense processes cannot be ruled out.

10

Pathways for Resolving the Dilemma between Developmental Progression and Adaptation to the Illness

In chapter 9 we pointed out that coping with a chronic illness must be considered within the developmental context. Many developmental tasks must be solved within the relatively limited period of 5 to 10 years. In his research work on healthy adolescents, John Coleman was impressed by their enormous coping abilities and surprised that so few adolescents failed in coping with the abundance and diversity of developmental tasks with which they were confronted. In an attempt to explain these observations, he put forth his focal theory of development (Coleman, 1978), according to which successful development occurs through a process of continually focusing on and tackling relevant developmental tasks. Adolescents focus on the most urgent tasks and work sequentially through the tasks that appear most important at each developmental stage. The process of adaptation is extended over several years, so that different tasks come into focus and are dealt with at different times.

As has been detailed throughout this book, however, illness-related stressors and developmental tasks occur simultaneously, not sequentially. Chronically ill adolescents cannot wait until they have successfully dealt with the illness before tackling important developmental tasks: They must strive to maintain a delicate balance between following the course of normative developmental progression and maintaining good physical health (Seiffge-Krenke, 1998c). The previous chapter demonstrated that diabetic adolescents focus on achieving professional competence, in which they make enormous progress over the 4 years, compared with other developmental tasks. Their family context (typically marked by a very structured and achievement-oriented family climate) and their personality characteristics (low self-esteem, negative body concept, and deficiencies in beginning or maintaining close relationships) may help to explain why adolescents focus on this task so much and why they do so in this sequence. Family functioning, together with the ill adolescent's developmental history, clearly influence the delicate balance between attempting to follow and achieve developmental progression and coping with the illness.

As the following case studies demonstrate, the challenge of balancing the requirements involved in adhering to the diabetes regimen and of pursuing developmental tasks is approached in a variety of ways. We found essentially five different pathways according to which adolescents attempted to resolve this dilemma.

Adolescents Who Cope by Postponing Developmental Tasks

Most of the ill adolescents approached the dilemma between adhering to the therapeutic regimen and tackling developmental tasks by postponing development. Although these adolescents failed to achieve many important developmental tasks, they mostly adjusted well to the illness in a medical sense; that is, they maintained satisfactory to good metabolic control and showed good compliance. This solution was highly endorsed by the parents. However, as the case of Monika shows, it did affect adaptation to the illness in the long term.

Veronika

When the interviewer met Veronika for the first time in 1991, she was nearly 14 years old. She had long, straight hair tied back in a childlike ponytail and a pretty, elegantly proportioned face. Yet, she was extremely thin (1.58 m, 41 kg). Veronika was obviously very afraid and nervous; she sat stock-still for the entire interview. She reported that she had hardly any friends, and in the questionnaires, she skipped all questions about dating. She came across as helpless and overwhelmed. Questions on coping with illness were answered only sparingly. Veronika had little recollection of the time before, during, and after the diagnosis, although it had only been made in the previous year. Overall, the interview was very slow moving and difficult. When it was over, Veronika relaxed noticeably. Her parents seemed quite old and had very conservative attitudes. The mother was often close to tears in the interview; she found it difficult to accept their fate and directed many accusations toward herself. In contrast, the father was cheerful and optimistic; he took the illness lightly and tried to reassure his wife. Both were very talkative and eager to disclose their feelings. The parents repeatedly emphasized how good Veronika's metabolic adjustment had been in the hospital after diagnosis; they were pleased with the good treatment she was receiving at the clinic they had chosen.

By the time of the second interview in 1992, Veronika had gained some weight but was still quite thin. Her clothing was very old-fashioned. She appeared as frightened and anxious as before. Her mother "mothered" the interviewer in an unpleasant manner, encouraging her to drink coffee and eat cake while Veronika tensely sat opposite the interviewer. In this second interview it became clear that Veronika still had no friends. She reported that the other girls in her class wore makeup, dyed their hair, and had already started to have relationships with boys. Veronika dissociated herself completely from these girls and thought only of school and her future career. Her parents felt this was appropriate and praised her motivation. They reported an incident that Veronika would have preferred to conceal but that was quite typical for her. One day after school, Veronika experienced an episode of hypoglycemia. Although she had not sensed the warning signs, the rest of the family, even her brother, noticed them and pointed them out. Yet, Veronika did not react. She then lost consciousness, and her brother went for help. Veronika felt very uncomfortable discussing the incident; she was close to tears and protested that she truly had not noticed anything. In this regard, the information about her physical health was highly relevant: Despite her attempts to comply strictly with the therapeutic regimen, her blood glucose levels were constantly fluctuating. Veronika said that she was simply unable to "get them under control." She was so reserved yet obviously under so much psychological pressure that the interviewer was quite concerned. Unfortunately, Veronika indicated that she perceived the interviewer as an intruder and a threat and that she did not want to discuss her problems with her.

The interviewer had hoped that Veronika might have developed to a level typical for her age by the third interview in 1993, but this hope was not fulfilled. Although initially friendlier and wearing her hair more fashionably, her clothes were still very outdated (even her mother thought so). Veronika seemed even more anxious than in the previous interviews. In addition, she was quite unwilling to engage in conversation, and in the family interview she let her parents do all the talking. This year, too, tension was evident between Veronika and her parents. When they made jokes at her expense, Veronika could only defend herself by glaring at her parents and kicking them under the table. According to her parents, although their daughter was nearly 16 years old, she was practically friendless and still frowned on boys as a 10 year old would. Problems also seemed to have cropped up with regard to her physical development: When she had menstruated for the first time that year, she had lost a lot of blood and needed to take strong hormone medication. The large loss of blood had resulted in a temporary increase in her blood glucose levels.

In the fourth interview in 1994, Veronika still seemed stuck at the developmental level of a much younger girl. Her clothing was extremely childlike and she barely uttered a word of greeting. Her mother was lively yet cool, and she was very preoccupied with offering the interviewer coffee and cakes, among which was a variety that Veronika could also eat. The ensuing conversation was very labored. When the interviewer invited them to speak about the family's coping with the illness, the family members insisted that nothing had changed. Veronika sat silently throughout the entire interview with downcast eyes, saying little more than "yes" and "no." When her parents reported that they had found candy wrappers under her bed, Veronika cast angry looks at them and tried to silence them, but in vain. In the meantime, the interviewer felt that Veronika was about to break into tears from pure helplessness and rage but was able, with some effort, to control the impulse. When the time came for the parents to be interviewed in their daughter's absence, Veronika left the room with considerable relief. Whereas in the previous years the parents had been critical of their daughter's delayed development, they now beamed with pride over their intelligent, well-behaved daughter, who "didn't do anything stupid." They emphasized that Veronika did not hang around in bad company as other girls did and were proud that she was sensible enough not to join in with "all that nonsense" (discos, boys, etc.). Veronika was again very shy in her individual interview, responding almost entirely with "yes" or "no." She was very closed but still conveyed an impression of suffering, almost as if every question were too much for her. She often remained silent, evading the questions completely. The interviewer left the family feeling unhappy about Veronika's further development. Above all, the most troublesome issue was her parents' failure to develop any awareness of their child's problem. They were happy that Veronika seemed to be functioning perfectly well with regard to her achievements and managing the therapeutic regimen.

Moritz

In 1991, Moritz was 14 years old. He had suffered from diabetes for 8 years. His metabolic adjustment was good. His appearance in the first interview was not striking: He had short hair and wore jeans and a sweatshirt. He was generally quite open and sometimes a little precocious. Only his mother took part in the family discussion, explaining that the father's work and health were so strained that he could not take part in the study on this or future occasions. Moritz's mother was very nervous and frequently laughed with embarrassment. During the family discussion, Moritz's relationship with his mother came across as fraught with conflict, although the specific issues could not be named.

Moritz had barely changed by the second interview. He seemed a little inhibited about talking openly about many topics; for example, his answers to questions about girlfriends or girls in general were evasive and unclear. His mother confirmed that he had no contact with girls. Moritz had no problems with managing the illness. His sole concerns involved his career plans. Above all, he was afraid of unreasonable employers. The interviewer had the impression that Moritz was not a typical adolescent, especially since he described neither escapades nor daydreams. He had almost no friends, had no contact with peers, and was very withdrawn. In contrast, his parents seemed much more socially active; they especially liked to meet their friends at a camping ground on the weekend. In the interview, the mother and son agreed on almost every topic. The mother expressed many fears about her son's illness. Long periods of separation from Moritz caused her great concern, and she also worried about the little contact her son had with peers.

The third interview took place in 1993. Moritz was 16 years old and had grown up considerably. He had a slight mustache and appeared stronger than in the previous year. He behaved a little precociously in the interview. He was proud to be the first member of his family to have attended Gymnasium (the highest level of German high schools) and was already talking about obtaining a doctorate degree in some field of natural science. However, he also seemed lonely. He said that he dealt with his problems alone, since the only people he could talk to were much too busy. Moritz believed he managed his diabetes very well, and he claimed to know more than the physicians did. He confessed that he did not strictly follow his physician's advice. At the end of the interview, Moritz gave the interviewer a few suggestions on how he would run the kind of research study we were conducting.

Moritz's mother had grown more relaxed since the last meeting. She was generally eager and willing to talk. Although she told what she knew about Moritz, it was very little. As an explanation, she said that her son had become very closed.

As soon as the fourth interview began in 1994, Moritz exclaimed that everything was going wonderfully at school. Although he reported occasional conflicts with his father, he got along well with his mother. His career plans had changed; now he hoped to study another subject with more career opportunities. He admitted that he did not have a large circle of friends at the moment. It turned out that the boy he had called his best friend for the past 3 years was a neighbor whom he only saw at school. In contrast to the previous year, he openly acknowledged having no contact with girls, saying he had no time for them anyway. When asked about his current hobbies, he named weekend camping trips with his parents. He ("naturally") had no problems at all with the illness. Moritz's mother described him as being a completely easy and agreeable boy. She reported that he complied perfectly with his diabetes regimen and kept his distance from peers who smoked and drank. There were no problems with school. However, she did remark that Moritz liked to show off his academic superiority in the family, especially in front of his brother.

Monika

Monika was 15 years old at the time of the first interview in 1991. She had been diagnosed with diabetes 18 months earlier. Her one older sister no longer lived at home. Monika appeared to be typically developed for her age. She was somewhat chubby, had acne problems, wore her hair in a ponytail, and was dressed casually in jeans and a T-shirt. Although a little shy and inhibited in the interviewer's presence, she generally came across as a good-natured and friendly girl. She answered the questions readily, if not expansively. The biggest problem she named concerned her classmates at school, who teased and taunted her about having diabetes, often trying to tempt her into eating candy. These problems had twice encouraged her to change schools. In her current class she felt that she was treated normally and felt content. Monika's parents greeted the interviewer cordially. They were at first a little tense, as they were unsure what the interviewer had in store for them, but they were very willing to discuss their daughter's medical condition. The family seemed to be under a lot of stress. They reported that if any problems with diabetes cropped up, the entire family was involved in dealing with them.

At the second interview in 1992, Monika was a little chubbier than the year before. She chatted freely and with much more self-confidence. Her parents were again open and welcoming but seemed disinclined to discuss the conflicts that arose from their daughter's entrance into adolescence, especially with respect to her attempts to increase her autonomy. Their denial and trivialization of the problems in this area gave the interviewer the feeling that they were not being entirely honest. In contrast, they were much more open in discussing the difficulties of living with diabetes.

The father was not present for the beginning of the third interview, although he later returned home after a long trip. The first phase of the interview was characterized by a slight yet unmistakable atmosphere of aggression, which was initially hard to explain. Monika, now 17 years old, was as talkative, self-assured, and somewhat impudent as she had been the previous year. Since the middle of the year, she had been training to become a gymnastics instructor; this training was now her main occupation. Despite her athletic activities, she was remarkably unfit and overweight (she weighed 72 kg and was 160 cm tall). She reported that once she had accepted having diabetes, she coped with it well. Her blood glucose levels had always been kept in check and had never undergone major fluctuations. She maintained that she had no problems at all. As in the year before, Monika could not name a best friend or a group of friends. Since leaving school, she had rarely seen her former classmates and had no contact with boys. She seemed to be quite isolated. The only person she ever went out with was a 13-year-old girl she knew from her jazz dance class. In their interview, the parents also said they were convinced Monika had no problems with the diabetes.

By the time of the final interview in 1994, Monika had gained a considerable amount of weight. She looked so alarmingly round and childlike that the interviewer had to consciously remind herself that Monika was an 18-year-old adult and not a child. There had barely been any changes in Monika's pattern of friendships. What she glossed over was later made plain by her parents – she had no real friends. The only person she described as a friend was the same girl she had mentioned in the previous interview, who was 4 years younger. Monika spent almost all of her free time watching television or playing computer games. She rarely went out at all anymore, contrasting strongly with her sister, who at the same age had pursued many very different interests. Monika did not have a steady boyfriend nor did she go out with boys. The mother did not seem to be worried about her daughter's development, claiming that Monika had adjusted well to the diabetes overall. The interviewer disagreed, pointing out Monika's overtly childlike behavior, impudent manners, and physical appearance, which altogether gave the impression that her development had stagnated in the past year. In truth, some problems had arisen: The mother said that Monika could never be left alone anymore because unless she was supervised, she would purchase and eat huge quantities of candy and other forbidden foods. At first, Monika contested the claim but then confessed to often breaking the rules of her diet. In light of her poor compliance with the diabetes therapeutic regimen and her delayed psychosocial development, the interviewer's impression of Monika's situation had become quite negative. On conclusion of the interview with her mother, Monika was already sitting at the computer and could hardly draw herself away from the game she was playing to utter a sullen good bye.

These cases demonstrate quite vividly how an overly narrow focus on the illness can have negative consequences for overall development. Adaptation to the illness was essentially good in these adolescents; they exhibited good adherence to the therapeutic regimen, good compliance, and good to moderate levels of metabolic control. However, by pursuing one particular developmental task, for example, developing occupational competence, they narrowed their emotional and social lives. Their strong dependence on their parents was alarming, as was the fact that their parents encouraged achievement orientation and seemed to lack insight into the possible dangers of such an unbalanced development.

Denial and Trivialization of the Illness: A Way Out?

Our sample of diabetic adolescents also contained cases in which the clear presence of defense processes in relation to the illness raised doubts as to whether development was proceeding or would proceed successfully. Such adolescents stressed their normality excessively and denied or trivialized the illness. It is interesting to note that the defense response is almost always sustained by the entire family. These families deny their psychological suffering. For the adolescent, true developmental progression becomes impossible because the illness is not integrated into his or her everyday life.

Matthias

Twelve-year-old Matthias was an only child living with his parents. At the start of the first interview in 1991, the father was very cold to the interviewer and barely made eye contact. This changed over the course of the conversation as the father became more emotional. Both parents were very eloquent; they talked a lot, often at the same time. The main impression they made on the interviewer was that they were bitter and sad about their fate. Matthias suffered not only from diabetes but also from another chronic illness and had already undergone several operations since his birth. Matthias himself appeared very ill and pale, and the conversation seemed to physically exhaust him. His behavior was conforming; he denied any problems, saying he had accepted everything. He saw the diabetes as the lesser evil. He came across as a melancholy child, affected by his many stays in the hospital and by having to be alone in his experiences. He had neither friends nor hobbies. The family emanated a contagious despondency, and the interviewer began to feel especially sorry for Matthias. The parents themselves reported that Matthias comforted and strengthened them, not the other way around. As an example, they described how Matthias coped with his illnesses: He viewed everything in a positive way and had never once complained or cried about his difficult lot in life. The parents asserted how much they could still learn from him about accepting the illness without complaint. One of the illnesses had been inherited from the father, leading the father to feel deeply guilty and to look after Matthias a great deal, especially in illness-related matters.

During the second interview, the parents again talked about Matthias's operations, reporting that it had been a difficult year. The atmosphere was very uncomfortable and full of unspoken aggression. The interviewer felt uncomfortable with the mother's apparent envy of the interviewer, who in the mother's terms led an "easy life." Matthias's speech was slow and indifferent; he again denied that anything caused him difficulty, and he repeatedly stressed his happiness. He still had no friends or hobbies, and his life seemed dreary.

By the third interview in 1993, the aggressiveness and hostility within the family, especially between the parents, had escalated. The parents no longer talked to one another; rather, they seemed to use the interviewer as a medium for sending messages to each other. Both were full of reproach and hatred. Matthias' diabetes was moderately adjusted, and he had needed fewer operations in the past year. As in previous years, his mother reported a great deal about her own illnesses, often with a dramatic and almost unbelievable touch; the father noted this with satisfaction. The many soft toys in Matthias' room made it look more like a child's bedroom than one of a nearly 15-year-old boy. Again, his insistence that he was completely happy struck the interviewer as implausible, given the clear loss of physical strength and mobility due to his illnesses. Matthias had obviously taken on the difficult task of keeping his parents together. In doing so, he tried to act as if he were a completely untroubled child. This had became a grotesquely inappropriate responsibility, given the facts that he suffered from two serious illnesses and that the tension between his parents was inordinately extreme. There was no space in the family for Matthias's own problems, fears, and difficulties.

After observing the escalated aggression and hostility in the third interview, the interviewer was unsure how the family would receive her a year later. In 1994, the mother's appearance had completely changed: She had colored her hair, was smartly dressed in slacks and a fashionable T-shirt, and looked much younger. The atmosphere between the parents was unusually relaxed. This time, the mother did not talk endlessly about her own illnesses. Most importantly, the parents talked to one another and no longer used the interviewer as a go-between. The interviewer was puzzled at first, but over the course of the conversation she recognized what had reunited the two, namely, a devaluation of the outside world. This not only included all physicians and clinics but our research project as well. The parents made it quite clear how little they thought of medical professionals and scientific researchers. Aside from this, nothing new was discussed. The parents reported that the course of Matthias's diabetes had not changed; in fact, Matthias himself was barely mentioned. Their son seemed to be only a peripheral factor in their lives. In the interview with Matthias, he appeared even more delayed than in the previous year. His speech had grown less comprehensible. He was unable to identify any problems and called himself the happiest person on earth. Given his desolate family situation, as well as his own poor physical and psychological conditions, the interviewer found this to be a completely incongruous evaluation.

David

At the time of our first interview in 1991, David was 13 years old. He was powerfully built and appeared to be bright and a good student, which indeed was later revealed to be the case. To the interviewer, he portrayed his life as uncomplicated and entirely normal. There were, he said, no problems or arguments in the family. He got along well with both his parents, had no favorite, and felt equally well understood by both. He also got along well with his friend. David was one of the best students at school. His hobbies were tennis, music (he played the violin), skiing, and swimming. When the conversation turned to the topic of his illness, he immediately became taciturn and reluctant to speak. It was nearly impossible to encourage him to talk about any-thing associated with the illness, and his thoughts on coping and expe-riences with the illness remained vague and unclear. He continually responded to questions with fixed phrases, saying his life was com-pletely normal, nothing had changed, and no problems had resulted from his illness. He replied to almost every question by saying "I'm totally normal." He no longer recalled his reaction to the diagnosis, although it had been made only 10 months before the first interview. The discussion of coping with the illness was most unsatisfying for the interviewer, since David remained obscure not only in describing how he dealt with the illness but in discussing other matters pertaining to the rest of his life, that is, his friendships. His mother, a small, slightly chubby but pretty woman, was bubbly and very eloquent. She was a schoolteacher. She was divorced, and she complained that David's father barely looked after the children at all. She said that David was always pleased to hear from his father, noting that he particularly depended on him and needed him as a role model. David's mother became visibly depressed when asked to talk about her own life. She had resigned herself to having a terribly difficult and stressful life as a single parent. She reported that David coped very well with his illness, better than she did. She declared the greatest sympathy for him. If it were possible, she said, she would swap her health for his illness in an instant. Nevertheless she was proud to state that David managed the illness entirely by himself; she did not need to help him with anything. As such, the illness caused the family very little stress. However, she mentioned that he was reluctant to discuss his illness and did not want anybody else to know about it.

By the time of the second interview, David's outward appearance had barely changed. He had, however, become even less commu-

nicative. He responded to questions about coping with terse, often one-word answers, for example, "nothing," "no problems," "everything is normal," or "nothing has changed." He seemed to have no concerns whatsoever; he stated that there was nothing difficult about the illness, nor could he think of anything distinctly unusual about the rest of his life. Much was still unclear, for example, his relationships with his parents, whom he had idealized in the first interview. He continued to deny his parents' divorce. In speaking of his father, he only mentioned that visiting rights were every 2 weeks and that he enjoyed seeing him. Once again, the interviewer felt that she had not connected with David at all and that he himself was unclear about his own life and feelings and tended to ignore them. The mother's mood had changed considerably since the last interview; she felt much happier, almost euphoric. She had struck up new friendships and had emotionally profited from having a new circle of friends. She reported that David was now going through puberty, and, as such, had become much more difficult. He was very concerned about his physical development but avoided answering his mother's questions about girls. He had no true best friend. She repeated that she, but particularly David, coped very well with the illness; in fact, he did so all alone. She still felt the illness to be a significant burden on their lives, one which she could not handle so well. David concealed his illness from his friends and always administered injections in private.

David had grown up more and become more self-conscious by the time of the third interview in 1993. He was more articulate than before but still spoke very little about the illness. There had been some new developments in his life. He had started taking dancing lessons and occasionally went to parties. In addition, he had gone on vacation without his mother for the first time; instead he had gone with a friend and his family. Although he did not have a girlfriend, he was certainly interested in girls. His mother was very talkative in this interview, discussing her new friends and her attempts to develop a new partnership. As in previous years, she described David's younger brother as a problem child.

In the last interview, David was more relaxed. He still claimed that he had no problems. However, he repeatedly stressed that school and diabetes were the most important things in his life. This was considerable progress from the earlier years, when he had totally denied the importance of his illness. He also expressed the importance of complying more strictly with his therapeutic regimen if he was to avoid later damage. David was very cold and distant toward his mother in the discussion of coping with the illness. She complained that he did not report his true blood glucose levels to her and that she had to secretly look in his record book to find them out. Both of them seemed quite bitter toward one another. David seemed to have a strong need to become autonomous from his mother; yet, she could not understand or accept this.

Although denial and trivialization can be important ways of coping, Lazarus (1985) has already suggested that their efficacy is short-lived. Continuous denial and trivialization can become dangerous when applied over a long time, as was the case in the families presented above. The most problematical aspect is that because of these defense processes, the illness cannot be integrated into the life of the family and even more importantly, into the life of the adolescent. Clearly, the consequence of this failure will be the inhibition of the adolescent's development.

Overemphasizing Adolescent Development at the Expense of Metabolic Control

Finally, there were some among our ill adolescents who ruthlessly pressed on with important developmental tasks to the detriment of their metabolic control. The majority of these adolescents either were poorly adjusted or had initially had good or satisfactory metabolic control, which had considerably deteriorated. Notably, their development showed typical yet greatly subdued characteristics of adolescence. These adolescents caused concern to their physicians and parents, not only because of their poor or strongly fluctuating HbA_1 values but also because of their "acting out" and conspicuous social behavior. It was as if they were demanding to have access to adolescent development.

Milena

In the first interview in 1991, Milena came across as a very bright 12 year old who was developed in accordance with her age. She had had diabetes for only a few months and had successfully come to grips with the illness. She was a pretty girl with strong charisma and winning charm. It was noticeable that she had trouble keeping still: She stood up often during the conversation and would not tolerate being looked at steadily. Milena's mother had remarried after a divorce and had a younger son from this new marriage, so Milena was growing up in a family with a stepfather and half brother. Both parents made a very happy, harmonious impression. The conversation was lively, and the interviewer was impressed by how well the family had coped with all the many changes, for example, divorce, creating a new family, and the onset of diabetes. It appeared to be a perfect fairy-tale family that had taken all these changes in its stride, actively and without discord. The only striking negative features in this meeting were, as mentioned, Milena's restlessness and tendency to avoid direct gazes. Furthermore, she tended to give evasive responses to the interviewer's questions.

A year later, in 1992, the situation had changed completely. The parents began by informing the interviewer that Milena would only be living in the house for a few more days. She had expressed the wish to move to her biological father's house in northern Germany, and the move was due to take place shortly. Milena's school grades had deteriorated dramatically. Owing to her rebellious and aggressive nature, she quarreled a great deal with her friends and classmates. Hence, no one seemed to like her anymore. Since she believed that a "change of climate" would be the only way to improve the situation, she had decided to move in with her father, who lived alone. Her mother and stepfather had agreed to this decision because Milena had become such a burden to the family in the past few months: She was untidy, unreliable, insolent, and her diabetes was very hard to keep under control. Above all, her mother complained about Milena's lack of hygiene and neglect of her body. All in all, she conveyed the image of a daughter in puberty who cared about and for nothing and just used everyone around her.

This impression was confirmed in the interview with Milena herself. She began by plopping her feet onto the table, professing in an arrogant tone that she would immediately use the participant's compensation of 50 DM (German marks) to buy herself a new pair of boots. The interview, she said, bored her to tears, and she had absolutely no idea what we wanted from her. She portrayed the move to her father's home as an ideal solution but made little reference to the current problems and conflicts she had been having with her school friends and family. She blamed the others rather than herself and was glad that soon she would not have to see them anymore. Milena's rude, condescending tone of voice added to the impression she made of wanting to disgust people. The interviewer was sorry that this typical yet unbridled adolescent self-centeredness had precluded the possibility of achieving a closer relationship with Milena. In addition, the interviewer sensed that behind Milena's loud, demonstrative demeanor lay a very thinly disguised depressive basic mood.

It became clear in the third interview, in 1993, that Milena had in no way solved her problems by moving to her father's home. She was very lonely (her parents stressed this as well) because her father was at work all day, and she was looked after by a nanny. She had not managed to find a foothold in her new class, and her situation was desolate. The mother and stepfather reported this with a mixture of worry and an "I told you so" attitude. They seemed to be relieved not to have to bear the burden of this very difficult daughter alone. Milena declared that she had no close ties to her mother and stepfather, although she continued to visit them quite regularly. (The interview took place while she was "at home" for one of these visits.) She complained that her old friends from home never wrote. The adolescent pattern of using crude language and striving to make an appearance designed to shock others was again very conspicuous. Additionally, her diabetes control had become worse. Milena reported that her mother, her stepfather, and her father were often uncertain what her actual HbA_1-values were. Milena insisted they were a secret between her and her physician and none of anyone else's business. This, too, was an attempt by Milena to maintain her autonomy and manage everything alone, even at the expense of achieving good metabolic control. Her depressive mood was more clearly apparent than in the previous interview, especially in the accusing tone of voice with which she reported that her former friends never tried to stay in touch.

The situation in Milena's family had changed again by the time of the fourth interview in 1994. Whereas previously the happiness of the married couple and the balanced relationship to the younger brother had been noticeable, more tensions had developed, and the harmonious atmosphere had been disrupted. Milena, the "lost daughter," only showed up at home now and then. She displayed a certain self-satisfaction about the crumbling of the fairy-tale family. She remained silent about her social life at her father's, just as she continued to keep her level of metabolic control secret from her mother.

Milena, like other adolescents in this group, showed an imbalance between adjustment to the illness and developmental progression. In many cases, a feeling of neglect and being pushed out of the family formed the basis for overemphasizing adolescent development. Milena seemed to force the development of her autonomy, which could be considered as pseudo-progressive at best. The conflicts with her parents and with her peers were "solved" by a self-imposed displacement (i.e., by deciding to move to her biological father's home). However, because she had not devoted much effort to understanding or honestly appraising the reasons for her conflicts in close relationships, her attempts to build new ones failed. Thus, no true developmental progression was possible.

Families That Broke Down

In our sample, there were only a few cases in which the adolescents neither achieved typical developmental tasks nor adjusted to the illness. In each of these cases, it was not so much the individual adolescent as the entire family situation that had been responsible for this. Some cases involved unsolved neurotic problems within the family, that is, preexisting problems that were exacerbated by the onset and course of the illness. In other cases, many additional stressors accumulated after our study began, overtaxing the family's coping capacity. In the latter circumstance, there was often some interaction with preexisting problems in the family situation. The following case is one such example. The child's family had broken up, and the child's illness was only one of many problems the family was faced with. In other families, we discovered problems related to an intense dependency between the mother and the child, which have been described in detail elsewhere as indicating the phenomenon of one body for two (see chapter 7 and Seiffge-Krenke, 1997a).

Susanna

At the time of the first interview in 1991, Susanna had just turned 12. She had had diabetes for about 10 years. Her metabolic control was very poor, and her blood sugar levels varied hugely. Her mother seemed helpless in this respect but also appeared to be waiting to see if anything would change. Her view of Susanna's poor diabetes adjustment was that it could be worse. The mother seemed to be the family member with whom Susanna had the most contact and whom she most trusted. At the same time, Susanna's mother was the one most burdened by her daughter's illness. The father was not talked about in the interview discussion; in fact, he was not even there for the beginning of the interview. Susanna said that he was too strict, that he was "the dumbest father in the world," and that he often hit her.

Susanna was still open and frank in the second interview in 1992. She wore jeans and a sweater, did not appear very feminine, and was generally childlike and clumsy. Neither she nor her mother made a secret of Susanna's continued poor metabolic control and highly variable HbA₁ values. They seemed to have resigned themselves to her situation, falling back on the mantra, "Susanna's diabetes was always difficult to control." Susanna confessed in this interview that she did not have any good friends and that her closest confidants were her pets (she kept rabbits and birds). Toward the end of the conversation, the father came home. He looked prematurely aged. Although he seemed interested in the interview, he appeared too exhausted to make any real contribution.

In the third interview in 1993, it was clear that Susanna's mother was, once again, prepared for the meeting and very eager to talk openly with us. However, she seemed emotionally unstable and was at times very condescending toward the interviewer ("I don't think much of this whole thing any more but come in anyway"). She wore no makeup, and her very red cheeks created a slightly neglected appearance. Life with Susanna, she related, was becoming ever more difficult, as she was very aggressive and reproachful toward the family. The mother spoke very extravagantly and at great length, without interruption. She referred to Susanna's childhood in an effort to make clear that Susanna could not adjust to her diabetes on account of her bad temper and moodiness. She complained extensively about the physicians who refused to accept that Susanna's diabetes was uncontrollable. Thus, given the facts that Susanna's HbA₁ values had always been unsatisfactory and that the physicians seemed to be incapable of correcting them, Susanna's mother no longer considered it worthwhile to have her daughter seen by physicians. The mother appeared not only very sober and distant but also angry and aggressive. During the course of the interview she became more emotional, and her cheeks became more flushed. Finally, she explained that Susanna was always accusing her of drinking too much but that it was, of course, not true, and she would not let her daughter accuse her of being alcohol dependent just because she liked a glass of wine now and then. During the conversation, Susanna came into the living room and noticeably disturbed the interview several times. She became involved in aggressive arguments with her mother. It was evident how angry the mother really was with her daughter; she declared that she had let Susanna get away with too much and had not hit her enough.

Susanna again seemed fired up for the meeting. She had kept the afternoon free and immediately began by complaining: her mother was an alcoholic, her father was never home and went out all the time with different women, her sister was an "arrogant cow," nobody was interested in her, and there were always fights going on. Her only point of reference was the world she shared with her pets, to which she could talk about her troubles. The interviewer expressed her concern about Susanna's situation and suggested that Susanna consider the option of seeking external support. The interviewer recommended a counseling center, but Susanna was hesitant, saying she had little confidence in others. On the other hand, she acknowledged that she was worried about her poor metabolic control and was afraid of long-term consequences, such as blindness and amputation. During the individual interview, Susanna's father returned home. He disrupted the interview repeatedly by offering the interviewer something to eat or drink and trying by any possible means to distract the interviewer's attention away from the topic of discussion at hand. It turned out that both parents were unemployed. In addition, Susanna was thinking of taking up an apprenticeship after finishing high school. Following the conversation, Susanna showed her pets to the interviewer, who admired them greatly, much to Susanna's obvious pride. The interviewer gave Susanna the telephone number of a nearby counseling center, explaining how much effort it had taken to get an appointment. Susanna accepted this with the promise to go there within the next few days. The distance, 20 minutes by streetcar, presented no problem. A few weeks later, Susanna returned the questionnaires with a brief letter stating that she had not gone to the center, explaining that it was too far away. However, she had instead found refuge with an older man, a neighbor with whom she had also celebrated New Year's Eve. She also reported not having seen her father for some weeks. He was in another town, probably with a girlfriend. The interviewer reminded Susanna that she could always write or call if she had any problems.

The interviewer was greeted for the fourth interview in 1994 by a large dog, which would be 16-year-old Susanna's only "conversation partner." Since the previous interview, the mother had found a job. The interviewer hoped that some of the family's problems would now take a turn for the better. Susanna, however, dashed these hopes completely, relating pertly that her mother still drank just as much as before, her father came and went when he felt like it, and the marriage was in ruins. She herself just used her father whenever possible. She claimed she had nothing to say to her mother, who was drunk all the time anyhow. She still thought her sister was a "dumb bitch." Susanna evidently had contacts with younger or disabled children in the neighborhood. Her school performance had clearly worsened, and she was afraid that her final grades would not be good enough for her to find an apprenticeship and realize her dream of becoming an animal caretaker.

The mother arrived somewhat late for the interview. She was quite chipper and very friendly, almost effusive. During the conversation she became more and more talkative. In her individual interview she did not need to be prompted to mention her marital problems; she stated that she and her husband lived separately, and for all practical purposes the marriage was over. She then spoke at length about her new office job and confessed she was scared that she would not make it through the trial period because the nature of office work had changed so much since she was last employed. There was so much new technology that she did not completely understand, and she felt humiliated and degraded when younger colleagues grasped everything so quickly. In the course of the interview, the mother abandoned her cheerfulness and adopted a sour demeanor. She depicted everything from environmental pollution to food allergies very bleakly, as if she were intent on demonstrating that life in this world was not worth living.

In Susanna's family, several nonnormative stressors occurred simultaneously and overtaxed the family's adaptive resources. Susanna had had diabetes since she was a child, and her continually poor metabolic control finally led to apathy and neglect in the family and withdrawal from medical support. In addition, family communication was impaired; the family relationships were detached and aggressive. The mother's dysfunction as well as the overly distant and unreliable father further contributed to a dramatic culmination of negative situations. Both parents were absorbed by their own problems and failed to carry out their parental roles effectively. Susanna was disappointed with everyone in the family, including her sister. The overall picture was that of a disengaged family, and it seemed that the family as a whole or some family members in particular needed support. We addressed this concern with Susanna first because she seemed to be highly motivated and openly asked for help. However, she did not pursue a concrete offer of help, although the barriers (a confirmed appointment, a short distance to a counseling center, no costs) seemed to be few. Instead, she tried to evade and attempt to solve the problem by establishing a relationship with a man old enough to be her father. This case most vividly demonstrates the difficulty of encouraging problem families to seek counseling.

Families That Adapted Well Overall

A substantial proportion of the diabetic adolescents and their families that we studied demonstrated successful adaptation to the illness. They were able to cope with the illness without causing the adolescent to become developmentally delayed. When there was developmental delay in certain tasks at the beginning of our study, owing to the focus on illness management, the adolescents were still able to make considerable developmental gains over the course of the 4 years (see chapter 9). The cases we have selected offer a clear insight into the protective factors that promote adaptation.

Sophie

Sophie was 14 years old at the time of the first interview and had suffered from diabetes for 7 years. She had no siblings. Her father, a skilled tradesman, did not take part in the first interview, nor did he fill out the questionnaires. He also declined to participate in the following years on the ground of being unable to spare the time.

In the first interview in 1991, Sophie was a very open-minded, lively girl with long, straight blonde hair tied back in a ponytail. She wore jeans and a denim shirt and still appeared very childlike. Her mother was quiet and unobtrusive. Both seemed interested in the study (albeit not overly), were cooperative, and responded to the questions readily. Sophie reported that her favorite hobby was horseback riding and that she had had her own horse for 6 months. She spent most of her free time with her horse, and sometimes her father, a talented equestrian, accompanied her. While she had no close friendships, she did have some friends at school, but she did not spend much of her free time with them. Sophie also felt that she and her parents understood each other and got along well. Since her mother was more often at home, she was Sophie's main partner for discussing problems. However, she was perhaps fonder of her father, because she spent her leisure time with him and he shared her passion for riding. This hobby tended to lead to familial conflict because Sophie's mother was not fond of horses. She criticized the amount of time Sophie and her father spent riding or caring for the horses. The mother described how, after Sophie's diagnosis 7 years before, she gave up working immediately to devote herself to the family. Sophie was appropriately grateful, expressing several times how supportive her mother was, how many worries she relieved her of, commenting that "some diabetics don't have it this good." On the other hand, the mother stressed her daughter's increasing independence. Both mother and daughter agreed that the diabetes was no longer a problem or a burden on the family; on the contrary, it had brought them all closer together. The interviewer perceived the mother–daughter interaction to be very harmonious; the two seemed to work as a team, especially when it came to the diabetes therapy. The mother showed understanding for her daughter and stressed the importance of patience and a peaceful environment.

Both Sophie and her mother welcomed the interviewer warmly for the second survey, in 1992. Slim, and with long, fair hair, Sophie still looked quite childlike. She was very direct, yet not pushy. Her mother was a little more self-confident than she had been the previous year. Her life still appeared to revolve almost entirely around the family. Sophie had begun to show some tendency towards separating herself from the family; for example, she now enjoyed going out to parties. On the other hand, she still spent a great deal of time at home and with her horse. Friends continued to play only a minor role in her life. Not much had changed since the previous interview. The family was maintaining the diabetes well under control; the mother, especially, kept a watchful eye on its course and concerned herself with looking after her daughter's health. She touched on the topic of secondary effects of diabetes, for example, the shortened life expectancy. Sophie and her mother continued to get on well and harmonized with each other, often making eye contact and never interrupting one another. Toward the end of the session, the interviewer also met the father, who seemed quiet and kind.

Sophie's mother had bought cakes and set the coffee table for the third interview in 1993. She was very open and friendly. She frankly reported the developments of the past year. Sophie now went out often (e.g., to discos and parties) and was rarely at home in the evenings. This had been difficult for the parents to get used to. There were frequent arguments, especially because the irregularities in Sophie's new daily schedule had also affected her diabetes. Since then, however, they had come to an agreement, and the parents knew they could trust their daughter completely. During this conversation, Sophie arrived home.

She was very casual, yet cheerful and lively, and she now looked more like a teenager than a child. She and her mother were genuinely friendly with one another. They joked together about their earlier quarrels and problems, which now appeared to be solved. In the individual interview, Sophie was also open and cooperative. She took care of her diabetes responsibly, bore the possibility of later damage in mind, and made an effort to keep her metabolism stable. Contrary to previous years, she now had three best friends, whom her mother called the "clover leaf." She often went out with them, and they did many things together. In her open, high-spirited way, she told of a quarrel she had had with one of these friends, who had started flirting with a boy Sophie liked. She described quite aggressively how much she wanted to put a stop to this. Like her mother, Sophie reported that upsetting her daily rhythm and going out frequently had negatively affected her metabolic control. Sophie now used an insulin pump, which had allowed her more freedom. However, she admitted, it had encouraged her to become more careless. She was quite self-critical, saying she wanted to check her blood sugar levels more often and maintain good metabolic control despite the changes in her life-style. Nevertheless, her HbA$_1$ values were still quite good. In comparison with the previous 2 years, Sophie had become somewhat more independent. Although her mother probably still kept an eye on her daughter's treatment regimen, Sophie now had full responsibility for the procedures, that is, she handled the insulin pump and performed the blood and urine tests herself.

The interviewer was again received most cordially for the fourth interview in 1994. Sophie had retained her open, cheerful nature; she laughed often. She seemed to be typically developed for her 17 years. The interview with her ran smoothly, humorously, and frankly. In spite of all the work Sophie devoted to school, she managed to have plenty of free time for her three friends and her horseback riding. She also had had a boyfriend for the previous 4 months. She enjoyed his company and they got on well, but their interests diverged, especially because they had different hobbies. For that reason, when asked if she thought the relationship would last, she replied that it was questionable. With much giggling she related the progress in the story begun the year before: Her friend had succeeded in luring away the boy Sophie had liked, but it had not ended well for the two of them. In the meantime, the two friends had made up, because, according to Sophie, "you can't quarrel forever." In general, Sophie spent her time like any normal teenager, going to many parties and discos. Since she had managed to coordinate her social life with her illness, her parents had accepted these activities, and they had great faith in her. The mother stressed how well Sophie coped with her illness, how responsible she was, and how good her metabolic control was. Sophie's independence had relieved her mother of a huge burden. Sophie confirmed this, reporting that she tested herself more frequently and treated herself openly even outside her normal circle of acquaintances. She reported with amusement how she handled critical situations when her friends were around.

Conny

Conny, an only child, was 14 years old at the time of our first interview in 1991. She had been diagnosed with diabetes at the age of 10. The family was remarkably motivated to help with the study and remained a very reliable, motivated family over the course of the following years. In the first interview, Conny's mother felt heavily overburdened. She was barely able to enjoy herself or accept emotional support; she had become used to assuming and independently completing tasks and responsibilities, often to the point of exhaustion. The mother experienced the onset of Conny's illness as a flashback to the early childhood of her own sister, during which life had been marked by much care and regularity. During Conny's kindergarten years, she had had difficulty fulfilling her emotional mother role and found her duty of care an irksome responsibility. Her daughter's illness now forced her to assume this role again. Although she did her best to fulfill this role responsibly, she seemed dissatisfied with her life-style. In contrast, her husband appeared to be a quiet man of leisure. Both parents mentioned that their marriage had been through a difficult period, during which the two separated, but the family ties had remained strong despite the separation. Their physical separation had enabled the family to stay together.

By the time of the second meeting in 1992, Conny had taken on illness management much more independently. Her metabolic adjustment was satisfactory, she was well integrated into her class, and she had a large circle of friends. This allowed her mother to feel more relaxed.

By the time of the third interview, Conny managed her diabetes almost completely independently. She explained that her parents were poorly informed about her HbA_1 values. Even when Conny made a measurement during the interview, they did not ask about the results. Conny gave herself injections according to a strict schedule. She had *been encouraged to eat as she wished and calculate her insulin dose accordingly. Her metabolic control continued to be satisfactory. She now found herself in a demanding phase of school, 1 year before her final examinations, but was nevertheless performing well. She talked a lot about her best friend. The two were from completely different kinds of families, which constantly challenged yet enriched them both. The parents' relationship had improved since the previous year, as their nonverbal signals to each other clearly revealed. Conny had become more autonomous in her life-style as well as in her management of the illness, and the parents now undertook more activities together.*

Conny had grown even more independent by the fourth interview, with respect to both her psychosocial development and her diabetes management. Her parents allowed and supported her freedom. Nevertheless, Conny's mother missed her daughter very much. Conny's father was better able to tolerate his daughter's many activities outside the household. Conny was a lively adolescent who was able to build very rewarding social relationships and obtain recognition from her friends. Despite her dissatisfaction with her body (she believed she was overweight), Conny was satisfied by her many social contacts. In the meantime, her mother had successfully returned to work, something that she had strongly wished to do years ago. However, she reported frankly that work exhausted her. The relationship between the parents had grown more positive: they approached each other more and undertook more activities with their daughter or with one another.

At the time of this interview, Conny was 18 years old and had become a young adult who was almost completely and independently the master of her illness and her life. Her metabolic control was still satisfactory to good. The illness was no longer the central concern of the family as it had been in the first interview, and the parents were very much in the background when it came to Conny's treatment of the illness. Conny's life was going through the transition from school to career planning. She said she would like to first learn foreign languages and then work for a year or two as an au pair in an English-speaking country. However, she had no concrete career plans. One aspect of her future about which she expressed certainty was her desire to have two children. She conveyed this wish very strongly. She now dated a boy on a steady basis and had begun a satisfying sexual relationship.

Both cases, although quite different, share similar features, which contributed to the adolescent achieving a good overall adaptation. In Sophie's case, the interviewer left the family at the fourth interview feeling positive and optimistic about Sophie's future. Somehow Sophie had succeeded in coping with her illness and achieving an age-appropriate developmental progression that included all the usual features of development in her age group, in particular, the step-by-step separation from the family, which both parents were willing to accept and enjoy. The strength of the family lay in discussing their problems freely and, at times, in animated debate. Whenever a change occurred for all of them, they were able to discuss it together. This was demonstrated in the third interview, when Sophie and her mother were able to laugh in retrospect at all the tricks and maneuvers of the first, aggressive phase of Sophie's detachment from her parents. Of course, it is still uncertain why the father did not take part in any of the surveys at all. However, the father–daughter relationship was close and friendly, as was continually shown in Sophie's accounts. The mother had probably taken on the classical home-based supportive role, whereas the father acted in a distinctive way as leisure-time partner.

In the case of Conny, the situation was much more difficult at the beginning of our study because the mother was unsatisfied with her situation as housewife and caregiver and because the marital relationship was considerably strained. However, the family was able to cope with these additional burdens quite successfully. Despite their conflicts, the parents cooperated in helping Conny to manage her illness. Conny became increasingly able to do so on her own. This and the development of her autonomy overall made it possible for her mother to pursue employment outside of the home. Altogether, these changes promoted individuality without compromising the closeness among the family members; in fact, they helped foster a more positive marital relationship. This suggests that a positive overall development is dependent not only on the presence of a harmonious, conflict-free family climate but also on the mutual commitment and continuous efforts of all family members.

Different Pathways for Solving the Dilemma

In this chapter the dilemma between achieving adaptation to the illness and accomplishing developmental progression has been the focal point of our conceptual approach in the analysis of how families cope with the special circumstances of living with a diabetic adolescent. As we have seen, over the course of 4 years, the families' adaptation to the illness and the parallel progression of the adolescents' development was generally positive. However, there were several possible approaches to resolving the dilemma, as the case studies in this chapter vividly demonstrate.

The most common pathway, which emerged in about 45% of our families, was to assign the highest priority to illness adaptation, while postponing developmental tasks. This pathway was most effective for immediate management of the illness and its short-term consequences, that is, in the earlier phases of our research. At later stages, however, the slow developmental progression or in more severe cases, the developmental arrest negatively affected adaptation to the illness. Thus, although the adaptation-promoting qualities of this approach were evident at the onset of diabetes and for some time after, it became clear that in the long run, continuing to rigidly follow this pathway was maladaptive.

A small proportion of our diabetic adolescents, about 12% of our sample, chose the opposite pathway. These adolescents adamantly pressed on with important developmental tasks to the detriment of their adaptation to the illness. Metabolic control worsened dramatically and hospital stays due to hypoglycemia and hyperglycemia became more frequent. Communication problems commonly arose among the family members and between the adolescent and the physician. In extreme cases, the family seemed to have rejected the adolescent. Analyses of attainment of developmental tasks did not indicate mature development. The onset of heterosexual relationships was early and appeared to compensate for deficits in close relationships with parents and friends. Thus, pseudoautonomy was achieved, but at the expense of coping with the illness.

About 35% of families adapted well overall; that is, the adolescents and their families were able to cope with the illness while encouraging the adolescent to attain age-specific developmental tasks. In analyzing these cases, we highlighted the capacities that those families used to deal with the divergent challenges of raising a chronically ill adolescent as well as maintaining positive family communication and warmth. These families were able to adjust flexibly to the illness and deal effectively with the adolescents' emerging needs for more autonomy. The fact that only about one-third of the families with a diabetic adolescent were able to deal successfully with these divergent tasks simultaneously underlines the nature of this challenge. Even families with healthy adolescents had difficulty in balancing independence and connectedness, but the task was all the more difficult with chronically ill adolescents.

In our sample, there were only a few cases (8%) in which the adolescents neither achieved typical developmental tasks nor adjusted to the illness. In each of these cases, it was not the individual adolescent and his or her illness so much as the entire family situation that led to the negative outcome. Families that broke down altogether either had experienced an accumulation of an unusually large number of severe major stressors after the onset of the illness or had exhibited very high levels of psychopathology before the onset of diabetes.

Denial and trivialization of the illness were common responses in many families. They were, however, restricted to the time before or shortly after diagnosis. The life-threatening character of the illness and the fatal consequences of noncompliance prevented extensive use of this defense mechanism in later years. Families were forced to decide definitively on following one pathway or another. Although few families prolonged the use of such defense mechanisms, they corresponded in many ways to the families that broke down completely. These families were burdened by additional problems, such as parental illness or dysfunction, and lacked the capacity to deal with the challenges of raising a diabetic adolescent. Consequently, the adolescent was unable to progress developmentally.

In summary, although most families adapted positively overall, there were also families whose coping processes failed. In analyzing these cases, we have highlighted those processes and variables responsible for following one pathway or another. The cases led us to the conclusion that most families, for reasons of urgency and simplicity, chose to focus on coping with the illness, placing a lower priority on developmental progression. Only about one-third of the families were able to balance adaptation to the illness and following a normal developmental progression. A few families broke down altogether; these families exhibited severe forms of psychopathology or had experienced an unusually high number of severe stressors after the onset of diabetes.

11

Implications for Prevention and Intervention

This book is based on the results of a longitudinal study of diabetic adolescents, their families, and their physicians. Although the study focused on a single illness, the findings are applicable to a much greater range of issues, including those pertaining to other chronic illnesses involving similar characteristics and long-term stress. This was confirmed by comparisons of our findings with those obtained in other studies. In this chapter, the possibilities for prevention and intervention are considered. To this end, some of the more consistent findings obtained in our longitudinal study are discussed. In view of the fact that our sample of diabetic adolescents was highly representative, the suggestions offered here are certainly appropriate for other adolescents suffering from diabetes or even other chronic illnesses. As this book has shown, diabetes is a challenge not only for the affected adolescents, but also for their parents, siblings, and friends and the physicians who monitor their health status. The complex interactions between medical, psychological, social, and family factors must be included in any consideration of interventions. It must be asked *who* needs psychological help and support, *when* this should be given, and *how* it should be organized. The limits of psychological intervention should also be taken into account. As a first step, universal and illness-specific aspects of chronic illness as they relate to developmental progression are compared, after which the appropriateness of some theoretical models for planning interventions is evaluated. In each of the following sections, the question of whether the suggested prevention and intervention strategies are also appropriate for dealing with other chronic illnesses is addressed.

Do Chronic Illnesses Share Similar Characteristics?

The dilemma between adaptating to the illness and proceeding with developmental progression forms the conceptual approach for the longitudinal study on diabetic adolescents and their families presented in this volume. As detailed in chapter 1, most chronic illnesses share the following characteristics: the necessity for expensive treatment, the intermittent need for medical intervention, the experience of pain and physical complaints, and the possibility of slow physical degeneration and perhaps premature death. The degree to which a characteristic exists and the preponderance of one characteristic relative to the others makes each type of chronic illness unique. The visibility of the illness as well as individual variations in illness severity or course of illness represent additional characteristics, which preclude attempts to subsume different disorders under the global concept of chronic illness. In accordance with Pless and Perrin (1985) and Rolland (1984), our research has been characterized by a partial categorical approach, which allows illnesses with similar characteristics to be considered within one category (see chapter 1). For example, all illnesses characterized by a gradual beginning and progressive course, which, however, cause no severe impairment to the affected adolescents, form one group. Although diabetes belongs to this category, it must be remembered that it has some unique characteristics.

Compared with other chronic illnesses, such as arthritis and cancer, diabetes places relatively few restrictions on adolescents: They may participate in nearly all athletic and leisure-time activities and are mostly able to pursue the occupation of their choice. Although diabetic adolescents may not show overt signs of being afflicted with the illness, diabetes management requires that they constantly exercise extreme self-control. The nonobvious nature of this illness as well as the limitations and dangers associated with the afflicted adolescent's control of the illness are unique both in themselves and, of course, with respect to how the diabetic adolescent approaches the dilemma between adapting to the illness and proceeding with overall development. Given the validity of a partial categorical approach, it is reasonable to assume that adolescents suffering from illnesses with similar characteristics may follow comparable developmental pathways. In contrast, adolescents suffering from life-threatening illnesses associated with visible disabilities and severe restrictions on their life-styles will need to resolve the dilemma in different ways. Because of the restrictive and life-threatening nature of such illnesses, management of the illness must be given the utmost priority. Naturally, this applies to diabetic adolescents whose illness exhibits a more dramatic course, for example, in showing a condition of prolonged and highly unstable metabolic control.

The Need for a Developmentally Oriented Model

Some models have been developed to explain why some people fall ill whereas others remain healthy or why some people show compliance and others do not. The best known of these is the Health Belief Model (Becker, 1974). According to this model, health-related behaviors (preventive and curative) are dependent on both the subjectively perceived seriousness of an illness and the susceptibility to it. Other important factors are the perceived benefits of preventive or curative behavior as well as the perceived barriers to health-related behavior. Thus, the higher the perceived vulnerability associated with an illness, the more likely a person will be to take preventive measures. Another central assumption of this model is that the apparent threat posed by the illness will lead to preventive behavior and compliance with medical regimen.

This model appears to be more appropriate for more immediately threatening illnesses, perhaps owing to their higher mortality rates, or for illnesses with a more dramatic, life-threatening, and restrictive course. Although diabetes can result in severe short- and long-term damage, the behaviors of the diabetic adolescents in our study cannot be adequately described by the model. This may be because most of the more severe consequences were not visible until after a certain time has elapsed. In analyzing data obtained from diabetic adolescents, we found that the risk connected with the illness was realistically perceived, whereas the use of preventive and curative measures was rather restricted during the labile developmental phase of puberty. It should be recalled that at the height of puberty, blood glucose values are difficult to control. The adolescents in our study, who consistently desired to develop in a normal, expected manner, perceived the barriers to complying with the medical regimen to be quite formidable. We also learned that the adolescents approached the accomplishment of tasks in the sequential manner that best allowed them to cope with the illness as well as to continue developing. Some typical adolescent activities, such as eating fast food, drinking alcohol, and smoking, are generally health-damaging behaviors, but for the diabetic adolescent, they also represent a constant challenge to compliance. The temptation to join in with the others can be hard to resist, because these activities reinforce autonomy and are seen as demonstrating adult status. Some adolescents in our study showed evidence of defense mechanisms, indicating possible limitations and distortions in their perceptions. These mechanisms arose from the adolescents' strong (and understandable) wish to be normal. However, according to the Health Belief Model, these could also decrease the perceived seriousness and personal risks associated with the illness. Thus, it has become clear that models of health and illness must acknowledge and accommodate for the influence that developmentally related variables may exert on the health and health-related behaviors of chronically ill adolescents.

Although the Health Belief Model is concerned with identifying and describing individual factors that determine preventive and curative behaviors, it does not adequately explain how individuals cope with illness or how certain coping behaviors can lead to adaptation. The process model of stress and coping designed by Coyne and Smith (1991) is currently the most comprehensive model of stress, coping, and adaptation and seems to be suitable for explaining coping with chronic illness in adolescence. This model adopts a realistic view of stress. First of all, it does not assume that every problem is mastered. Second, the model acknowledges that a situation is only stressful if it is appraised as such. The appraisal process is also influenced by internal resources. Finally, coping is simply defined as the mobilization of efforts, irrespective of the outcome. This model is more appropriate for explaining our findings in diabetic adolescents, namely, their emotional, cognitive, or behavioral efforts to manage illness-related stressors even if these did not always lead to adjustment to the illness in terms of stable metabolic control.

As demonstrated throughout this book, the coping efforts of chronically ill adolescents are embedded in the family context. Family system models (Olson et al., 1983b) and models of family stress and adaptation (McCubbin & Patterson, 1982) also have to be considered. Although these models have offered important insight into the dynamics of family life and the ways families react in times of stress, they are limited in a number of ways. For one, coping is incorporated only in terms of strategies that seek to maintain family stability. Thus, the outcome of coping is defined in terms of family, as opposed to individual well-being. However, our findings indicate that diabetic adolescents are able to accomplish developmental progression despite a comparably rigid and developmentally inhibiting family climate. Focusing on the family thus would tell us only half of the story.

In summary, each of these models loses its explanatory power by overemphasizing one particular aspect of adaptation to the illness. These aspects must be integrated if one is to arrive at a truly comprehensive conceptualization of how adolescents and their families cope with chronic illness. For our study of diabetic adolescents, we created a developmental model of coping with diabetes (see Figure 3.2). Considerable evidence has been furnished in this book to uphold the claims that knowledge of the illness and compliance are necessary but not sufficient conditions for achieving successful medical adaptation and that developmental factors play an enormous role in successful coping with diabetes. The model is, of course, based on diabetes-specific factors and outcomes, such as metabolic control. However, the general framework of this model may apply equally well to other chronic illnesses sharing similar characteristics. As mentioned in the previous section, the partial categorical approach would place diabetes together with other illnesses characterized by a gradual beginning and showing, after a labile pubertal phase, a more stable course that poses no severe risk of impairment for the affected adolescent. Thus, although the illness is progressive in that long-term damage may occur, the affected adolescent may experience a certain stability. Our model also acknowledges that the impact of stress and coping and the buffering effect of internal and social resources, as well as the interaction among medical, social, and psychological factors are universal for several illnesses sharing these same characteristics. The relationships among these factors will naturally vary according to illness-specific characteristics. Unique characteristics of diabetes include the emphasis on the adolescent's control and the invisibility of the illness, which despite its developmental advantages may contribute to the burden on the adolescent. Our diabetic adolescents' overwhelming need to appear more normal than normal may originate from these features.

Deficits in Internal Resources but Also Improvements with Time

As our study demonstrated, diabetic adolescents were very active in coming to terms with their chronic illness. They almost independently managed a complex therapeutic regimen and tried to comply with the physician's instructions about blood and urine testing, insulin injections, diet, and physical exercise. Their coping competence was outstanding, which usually resulted in the achievement of good to satisfactory metabolic control (as seen in two-thirds of the diabetic adolescents in our study). Health professionals, such as physicians, nurses, and counselors, need to acknowledge efforts such as these. At the same time, they should be aware that diabetic adolescents can be considered as a risk group because of their negative body image and their more negative attitude toward physical maturity.

Overall, the importance of the body image has been sorely neglected in research on chronically ill adolescents. A further important finding of our study was that diabetic adolescents tended to be very cautious in coping with everyday stressors, as compared with their healthy peers. In addition, diabetic adolescents often relied too heavily on their own resources; they had difficulty seeking and accepting support.

Noticeable improvements occurred over time in several developmental fields. The negative body image became more positive and adult; that is, it lost its childlike connotations. Furthermore, the adolescents increased their active coping and reflection about possible solutions, showing that these deficits do eventually disappear. This increase in competence over time should be emphasized. Too much research on chronically ill adolescents has focused on negative outcomes, thereby ignoring the positive changes over time. Health care professionals should acknowledge the possibility that despite the illness, changes in other domains may take place over time, which in the long run can be considered as resources for dealing with the disease. This viewpoint, so evident in our sample, also applies to adolescents with many other chronic illnesses. Adaptation to the illness is all too often the focus of attention, and the ill adolescent's considerable developmental achievements are overlooked or inadequately respected.

Focusing on the Illness and Sequencing of Developmental Tasks

Clearly, the low degree of freedom that chronically ill adolescents have in their life-styles can negatively influence their coping efforts. How then, do chronically ill adolescents respond to this limitation? For the chronically ill adolescent, the most important issue is dealing with the requirements of the illness. This is particularly true in cases of adolescents with illnesses of a life-threatening nature or with a severe, dramatic progression. The chronically ill adolescents in our study suffered from an illness of moderate severity, which, given good compliance, has a relatively stable course. We found that although the majority of diabetic adolescents assigned the utmost priority to illness management, they adopted the strategy of approaching developmental tasks sequentially. Developmental tasks related to school, friends, leisure, and their future careers were addressed according to their subjectively perceived levels of priority. The cautious style in approaching certain aspects of developmental progression displayed by many adolescents was understandable, considering that in exerting so much effort to succeed in illness management, they might have exhausted their resources used to cope with these developmental tasks. Although the strategy of approaching developmental tasks in sequence was initially considered to be a developmental delay, it became clear that it should be considered as representing functionally adaptive behavior, not as failure. In this regard, it is worth stressing that diabetic adolescents subsequently made enormous efforts to catch up to the development norms. Their success varied depending on the individual adolescent-typical task. The majority of diabetic adolescents in our study preferred to focus their efforts on achievement-oriented areas (e.g., school and career) first, followed by social interactions (friends and romantic relationships). A strong focus on achievement and career applied to the entire group of diabetic adolescents but was even more pronounced among those with good metabolic control. This sequence was related to the overall developmental context and family variables in our study, but it is nevertheless an "unexpected success story," as Gortmaker et al. (1993, p. 317) put it.

The capacity to balance achieving and maintaining physiological adaptation with following the course of developmental progression is perhaps more obvious in adolescents suffering from diabetes or other chronic illnesses sharing similar features. Nevertheless, the following basic questions underlying our approach are appropriate ones to ask in studying adolescents afflicted with various chronic conditions: Do chronically ill adolescents share the same developmental goals as their healthy peers? Do chronically ill adolescents, even those with severe handicaps and life-threatening conditions, strive to achieve these developmental goals? Are chronically ill adolescents able to progress developmentally, and, if so, what particular sequence is chosen? Is this sequence dependent on illness-specific characteristics? Is there any indication of a developmental delay in their achievement of age-typical developmental tasks? And how does the developmental context contribute to success or failure in achieving developmental tasks? These questions are important ones for most chronically ill adolescents, and they need to be addressed openly and carefully.

Understanding the Parents' Perspectives

The parents must also recognize the enormous coping competence that their ill child may possess. They should, in addition, try to understand their child's dilemma of being confronted with the challenge of meeting illness-related demands and pursuing developmental progression. Unfortunately, not all families are able to be flexible or to make adjustments in their interactions with their adolescent children who are seeking autonomy. As demonstrated in this book, increasing adolescent autonomy may put an additional strain on the parents, especially if their child suffers from severe health impairments. Many diabetic adolescents' parents also find it difficult to make the distinction between illness-specific and development-related problems. This may explain the rather unexpected finding in our study that despite good reasons for consulting psychological services, actual rates for utilizing such services were quite low.

The protective function of supportive and cohesive family relations and the development-inhibiting influence of high parental control and low warmth have been frequently demonstrated in the literature and were also important issues in this book. Health care professionals must recognize the challenges involved for both parties and take the parents' worries and concerns seriously. Indeed, the parents themselves may also need counseling during specific phases of the illness, for example, around the time immediately following diagnosis, the phase during which the adolescent's condition deteriorates, or during the terminal phase. The diabetic adolescents' parents in our sample needed more support particularly in the initial phase of the illness or at later stages when compliance worsened or when the adolescent's developmentally normal separation process made management of the illness increasingly difficult. Moreover, chronically ill adolescents' parents may need the support of counselors if the marital relationship is strained or when family duties need to be shared and/or parental roles clarified. This was also an issue in our families caring for a diabetic adolescent.

Parents as Coping Models

Other issues that might call for implementing strategies of prevention and intervention involve the discrepancies between maternal and paternal coping behaviors, both in illness-related and in more general family matters. Noteworthy here are the different efforts parents make, depending on the child's gender. In our study, parents assumed a more active approach in dealing with ill sons than with ill daughters. These interesting results may also emerge in families caring for adolescents suffering from other illness. If so, it may be of interest to determine whether such a discrepancy may result in more conflicts between the parents. In addition, it is unclear to what extent adolescents will later incorporate this discrepancy in modeling their parents' coping behaviors. Should this be the case, then preventive and intervention strategies may be developed to counteract these developments.

In some respects, the role of the health expert in supporting chronically ill adolescents is similar to that of the parents. Adolescents frequently struggle with feelings of being rejected by their families, which may create diffi-culties in their relationships with counselors, physicians, and nurses (Weissman & Appleton, 1995). Consequently, many difficulties in the treat-ment of adolescents emerge as a result of the health care provider's insecu-rity about his or her roles and functions. While it is important for care providers, for example, to understand and acknowledge the parents' per-spectives about their child's illness, they cannot always act in the interests of two parties. In this case, it is advisable to encourage separate meetings with the parents. Such an approach allows the provider to obtain informa-tion to supplement that offered by the adolescent.

Strengthening the Resources of Adolescents and Their Families

Approaches to strengthening the resources of individual adolescents and their families assume an adequate "self-helping capacity" (Baranowski, Nada, Dunn, & Vanderpool, 1982). Adolescents from risk groups and mul-tiproblem families require stronger initiatives because these adolescents often have a cumulative deficit of internal as well as social resources. However, this approach would also be appropriate for most of the diabetic adolescents in our study even though they did not, as a rule, report elevated levels of everyday stress in addition to the illness and did not exhibit extreme deficits in internal resources as compared with healthy adolescents.

It is important to bear in mind that the majority of diabetic adolescents and their families in our study interacted under special conditions. Their social isolation was noticeable; in many cases, it might have been self-imposed. Yet, the parents might have been unable to maintain friendships owing to the physical and mental exhaustion that results from caring for a chronically ill child and being overwhelmed by chronic sorrows, as was found, for example, by Gough, Li, and Wroblewska (1993). The type of social support most frequently used in our families caring for diabetic ado-lescents was support derived from family members. However, the family often undergoes a "shrinking process," so that the bulk of family interaction is limited to the adolescent–mother dyad. Siblings do have a role in the cop-ing process and are addressed by chronically ill adolescents more fre-quently than by healthy adolescents. Relative to other forms of social support, support for the parent from the spouse is perhaps the most impor-tant (Beresford, 1994). However, in our study, fathers of diabetic adoles-cents provided almost no emotional or instrumental support to their spouses. Over the years, only between 3 and 9% of mothers reported receiv-ing spousal support in illness-related or other family-related matters. In addition, the overall level of activity by fathers of diabetic adolescents' in coping with family problems was clearly less than in families with healthy adolescents. Fathers of healthy adolescents were much more involved in family activities.

This particular aspect of family dynamics may similarly arise in families with adolescents afflicted with other chronic illnesses. For prevention and intervention purposes, it is important to break the close alliance between mother and ill adolescent and promote the father's importance and function in helping the adolescent to deal with the illness, as well as in assisting the adolescent in making the transition to adulthood (Shulman & Seiffge-Krenke, 1997). This would help to relieve the mother's burden, thereby indirectly strengthening the entire family's resources. In a similar vein, increased paternal involvement may also relieve the adolescent of his or her support-giving responsibilities. Indeed, often the adolescent, not the husband, supports the mother. Finally, the adolescents' siblings might profit from the increased availability and attention of another parent. Intervention strategies should thus attempt to reverse a "parentification" of the adolescent's support, thereby reinstating or augmenting the father's role as support provider in the family. Moreover, his role in increasing the ill adolescent's independence must be emphasized. In addition, both parents should be encouraged to invest more time and energy in their marital relationship and to extend their support networks. As was evident in the later years of our study, diabetic adolescents became increasingly responsible and autonomous, leaving their parents more room to fulfill their own needs. This could also apply to adolescents suffering from other chronic illnesses.

The Coping Potential Offered by the Broader Social Network

Research has frequently demonstrated that orientation toward the peer group is a developmental marker for adolescence. In their coping behavior, adolescents do not just orient themselves to the family; in early and mid-adolescence, same-sex friendships are seen as increasingly supportive and become models for coping (Cotterell, 1992; Seiffge-Krenke, 1995), whereas in late adolescence, romantic relationships became increasingly important (Furman & Buhrmester, 1992). Generally, it would be desirable for chronically ill adolescents to utilize this social network more than they currently appear to do. However, various obstacles stand in the way. First, as was found in our study, diabetic adolescents' friendships are characterized by less companionship, less affection, and less intimacy, qualities that are generally found to be central in adolescents' friendships. Consequently, they do not entirely fulfill the requirements for appearing attractive to their peers. Additionally, the diabetic adolescents in our study tended to strongly "functionalize" their relationships, as was particularly obvious in their romantic relationships. This restricts the romantic partner's and the diabetic adolescent's possibilities for growth in the relationship. Furthermore, owing to the diabetic adolescent's strong need for harmony, they may have avoided experiencing conflict in their relationships with friends and romantic partners. Thus, they may have had little chance of learning how to deal with discord, which would be important for the development of these and other relationships over time.

Consequently, prevention and intervention should encourage chronically ill adolescents to use social support from friends and romantic partners and focus on helping the adolescent to improve the quality of these close relationships. In designing strategies for prevention and intervention, it is very important to explore the reasons for these developments and to integrate the perspectives of healthy peers. It should be emphasized, for example, that it is a general social rule that individuals in threatening situations avoid social comparison with those in better circumstances (Harlow & Cantor, 1995). In addition, because of the diabetic adolescents' stronger bonds to their families, particularly to their mothers and siblings, as well as the support they provide to their mothers, a situation may ensue that limits extrafamilial social contact and interaction. In addition, healthy adolescents may have trouble identifying with chronically ill adolescents and can therefore feel inadequate at empathizing with their problems. In a similar vein, healthy people may stigmatize and exclude ill adolescents. In our study, we learned that some teachers overtly expressed their irritation at having a diabetic pupil in their class, which sometimes reached the level of a shocking exclusion of diabetic adolescents, both in the classroom and in school-organized leisure activities. Since this behavior may be caused by a lack of understanding of the illness, there is clearly a need to provide better information to those directly involved with the chronically ill child or adolescent. We observed that over 30% of the diabetic adolescents in our study felt rejected by healthy peers, and about 20% thought they were less attractive in the eyes of healthy romantic partners. Consequently, experiences of exclusion and stigmatization probably contribute to ill adolescents' hesitance in separating themselves from family bonds and leading more independent lives. This complex interplay of motives, expectations, and experiences, from the perspectives both of the ill adolescents and of their friends and romantic partners, must be integrated into approaches for prevention and intervention.

Phases of the Illness and the Desire to Receive Professional Help

Chronic illness is rarely experienced as a static state. Most chronically ill individuals, including the diabetic adolescents in our study, perceived the illness in terms of phases marked by the highs and lows of their illness progression or their adjustment to it. For understandable reasons, more attention has been devoted to describing the phases of more life-threatening illnesses, such as cancer (Cole & Reiss, 1993). In such cases, the onset of the illness casts the family into an initial state of crisis, which is followed by a phase of assisting the patient as he or she undergoes intensive therapies or learns to meet demands related to illness management. Furthermore, the terminal period of illness is associated with a period of severe stress and loss. Most chronic illnesses, however, have a stable and nonprogressive course, and most of the time the family learns to accept and live with the chronic aspects of the condition. Nevertheless, the feature of chronicity is particularly important because it may take years for the ill adolescent and the family to accept and understand the implications of being chronically ill.

The demands that chronic illness places on families change over time. As was seen in our diabetic sample, the diagnosis was typically a major shock for patients and their parents. This frequently ignited the desire to obtain further information and psychological support. This observation certainly holds true for patients with other illnesses. As such, it would certainly be helpful to these families if they were provided with as much information about the illness as possible, not only with the intent of preparing them for what may come but to thwart any possibility that the parents begin to blame themselves or their partners for their child's illness. Even in the treatment phase, ill adolescents have different feelings about how much of the illness's course they will be able to influence or control. Some have more difficulty than others in solving practical problems and integrating the treatment into everyday life. It is often important to motivate adolescents and their parents to work together actively and to help them to mobilize emotional and social resources. In phases in which the illness deteriorates, various strategies can be pursued. These include establishing potential emotional reserves for treatment, reviving and strengthening a sense of responsibility, recalling and attempting to mirror the ways in which previous critical periods were mastered, anticipating future problems, and demonstrating possible solutions.

According to our experience with the diabetic adolescents in our study, the best time to offer intervention is during the phase after diagnosis. The case studies presented in chapter 6 demonstrated that even a large amount of stress does not necessarily imply a willingness to accept help. Intervention and support were most desired immediately after the onset of the illness; some time later, this wish for assistance was much less fervent, and help was not readily accepted. This may have been partly a result of emerging or existing defense processes or may have been due to an enormous mobilization of family resources, whereby the family tried to cope with the illness together. For families such as these, accepting help would have meant appearing weak, dependent, and needy, which they might have considered to be unacceptable qualities.

Rather unexpectedly, we did not find a direct effect of illness duration on coping behavior, family climate, or the adolescent's symptomatology. At best, the effect of illness duration was confounded by physical maturation. That is, even when the diabetic adolescents had been ill for a longer time, the changes associated with the beginning of puberty and its consequences for metabolic control encouraged the development of a more rigidly organized family climate such as that commonly exhibited in families of newly diagnosed adolescents. Nevertheless, it cannot be assumed that even if an adolescent has had diabetes for years, the illness will be more easily managed in puberty. Rather, the illness may make the adolescent's development a more difficult process. The links invoked here between phases of the illness and acceptance of help are of a very general nature and may be observed in many different chronic illnesses.

Improving the Relationship between Adolescent Patients and Their Physicians

The results obtained in our study highlight the importance of the relationship between the chronically ill adolescent and the physician responsible for monitoring the adolescent's health status. Important findings were related to the changes in this relationship over the course of adolescence. Most of the diabetic adolescents reported very good relationships with their physicians at the beginning of the study. The physicians initially enjoyed a great deal of trust and were credited with much competence. However, patient–physician relationships clearly worsened over time, and a change of physicians was frequently reported. Research has suggested that confidentiality is crucial to the patient–physician relationship. The quality of this relationship and perceptions of a physician's competence also play a role (Ginsburg et al., 1995). Some investigators have found that adolescents who are satisfied with their health care providers keep appointments more consistently; furthermore, providers who are skilled in adolescent care are more likely to experience better patient compliance.

In our study, diabetic adolescents' compliance decreased over time for a variety of reasons. First, the adolescents may have felt more independent and become less careful about adhering to their therapeutic regimen. Second, the initially high expectations of patient–physician relationships may not have corresponded to reality. Third, because half of the diabetic adolescents in our study changed physicians at some point, this may have reduced their commitment. Fourth, there were indications that communication problems between adolescent patients and their physicians led to decreased compliance and hence unfavorable metabolic control. In the later stages of our longitudinal study, the contact between the adolescents and their physicians seemed to be less regular and less close. One explanation for this finding might be that many pediatricians continued to interact with their adolescent patients in the same manner used for younger children. If the physicians are committed to continuing a good relationship with their adolescent patients, it is necessary for them to understand the effects that the developmental transitions in adolescence may have on patient compliance. This may entail attempting to demonstrate to the adolescents that they are recognized as adults or encouraging them in their efforts to gain autonomy, especially with respect to managing their illness. This may take more time and effort than busy physicians are otherwise able to offer their patients, but the benefits are no doubt worth the cost. In any case, if an adolescent is certain that he or she will benefit from seeking health care elsewhere, the physician must respect the adolescent's wish.

Understanding Noncompliance and the Function of Cheating

Much research has focused on investigating the noncompliant behavior of adolescent patients. In a review of studies on patient compliance, Cromer and Tarnowksi (1989) found that 30 to 50% of adolescents with various types of chronic illness showed poor compliance. The problem of noncompliance cannot be separated from the central issue of the adolescent's struggle to achieve independence. In this book, it has been demonstrated that there are considerable developmental barriers that hinder diabetic adolescents' compliance. The invisibility of the illness functions here as a disadvantage. In other words, others may not know that the adolescent is ill and may interpret the adolescent's efforts to exert self-control as a reluctance to "follow the crowd." Unfortunately, almost all peer-group activities either implicitly or explicitly result in noncompliance. Prevention and intervention programs designed to enhance compliance would profit greatly from taking such developmental factors into account. It is quite likely, for example, that the developmentally related changes in parent–adolescent relationships bear on physician–adolescent relationships. Furthermore, one must not overlook the dangers associated with "hypercompliance," for example, the risk of learned dependency.

Being well informed about one's illness does not always mean good compliance, as several studies, including our own, have shown. Chronically ill adolescents typically know quite a lot about their disease, but this knowledge implies being aware of having to depend on others. This dependence is all the more intolerable because it is unavoidable. According to Marcelli and Alvin (1994), adolescents frequently solve this conflict by cheating, for example, they report false results of self-performed blood tests. By cheating they may be attempting to preserve some measure of autonomy, or they may be trying to forget or make others forget that they are sick. Health experts have to understand that cheating is a functional compromise between having knowledge and avoiding unbearable dependence.

Physicians often maintain that poor compliance is the adolescent's fault. This negative judgment can only reinforce the patient's already heightened guilt. Guilt may increase anxiety and thus increase defense mechanisms. Therefore, health care providers should try to understand the chronically ill adolescent's dilemma. In this regard, it is important to be aware of the aggressive nature inherent in many noncompliant behaviors. Noncompliance may thus also represent the expression of aggressive or self-destructive tendencies.

Education about Unstable Blood Glucose Levels in Puberty

The medical aspects of any illness are of great significance. They determine its further course and interact with social and psychological variables. Therefore, the medical parameters of the illness received much attention in our study on diabetic adolescents. We found that they vary strongly with the course of puberty. Despite their good compliance, diabetics in early and mid-adolescence found it difficult to achieve stable blood glucose levels. This fact, combined with the adolescents' increasing tendency to spend much of their time away from home, caused even more concern for their parents. Unable to continually supervise the adolescents, they anticipated further deterioration in their adolescent's metabolic control. A longitudinal analysis of metabolic control revealed, however, that the HbA$_1$ and HbA$_1$c values stabilized again in mid- to late adolescence, leading to a more stable course of the illness. Information of this type would be of great value to the adolescents and their parents. It might relieve the adolescents of unnecessary worry about the fluctuations in their blood sugar levels and help rid their parents of the corresponding guilt and worry about being unable to monitor their children because of their stronger extrafamilial orientation.

Are Adolescents Unmotivated Patients?

When discussing psychological interventions for chronically ill adolescents, it is important to consider their motivation for seeking counseling. In research on psychotherapy, adolescents have often been stigmatized as "unmotivated patients" (Rogers, 1970). However, a distinction between conscious and unconscious motivation must be made. Adolescents who appear indifferent might well have a high latent motivation. A lack of understanding about what advantages counseling may offer the adolescent is not sufficient to explain adolescents' aversion to counseling. Furthermore, a lack of pressure cannot explain this behavior, because a worsening of the illness does not correspond to an increased tendency to seek advice. Rather, a whole series of factors are related to fostering this aversion. These include often ambivalent attitudes about being ill, interacting with the physician or therapist, and approaching the institutions associated with providing counseling. An analysis of aversion to counseling in adolescents with high or low stress (Seiffge-Krenke, 1998a) revealed that adolescents with high stress tended to be more willing to accept psychotherapy and counseling, but this was overshadowed by their need to protect their privacy. In particular, adolescents were afraid that a therapist might have too much insight into their lives, that they could not defend themselves well enough, or that they might not be taken seriously. They also had had experiences that they did not want to discuss with anyone.

These results clearly indicate the adolescents' ambivalence about accepting professional assistance: They want help but simultaneously feel distrustful, vulnerable, and in need of protection. Their desire to express themselves is balanced by inhibition about disclosing personal information to others. Similar observations were made in our group of diabetic adolescents. They made a tremendous effort to build a façade of supernormality, expressed far fewer problems and concerns than their healthy peers, and consistently affirmed that they managed well and needed no help. In view of the adolescents' insistence on having no problems, we must ask ourselves: Do they really need our help? (Nadler, 1978). Based on our findings, it became clear that the need for help was not always easy to identify, nor was it a simple matter to decide what kind of problem had generated this need. For example, the negative, childlike body image observed in many diabetic adolescents reflected deficits in self-awareness, such that the body was perceived as damaged and underdeveloped. Furthermore, having diabetes was perceived by diabetic adolescents as a barrier in their interactions with close friends and romantic partners. Generally, the diabetic adolescents were not openly motivated to accept offers of psychological counseling. Nevertheless, they talked about many everyday problems with their physicians, which indicated, albeit indirectly, their need for discussion, explanation, and support. However, the adolescent–physician relationship typically deteriorated over time. We attributed this to the physician being unable to meet the high demands for emotional assistance imposed by the adolescent. Although the adolescents were understandably disappointed, they seemed unwilling to turn to other health professionals for fulfillment of these needs. In considering this and the comments about the developmental function of noncompliance and cheating, not asking for psychological help can have the function of preserving some measure of autonomy. Consequently, caution must be exercised in attempting to determine if an adolescent needs psychological counseling. In other words, it is important that the adolescent not perceive being offered, seeking, or receiving counseling as a sign of personal weakness.

What Sorts of Intervention are Available to Diabetic Adolescents and Their Families?

Although research on psychosocial intervention for diabetic adolescents has increased over the past decade, a broad base of research data is not yet available. In a review of the pediatric intervention literature, Hauser et al. (1997) pointed out that the majority of studies have focused on group interventions with adolescents and their families. This does not imply that families necessarily cause problems related to illness management or that diabetes inevitably disrupts individual or family adjustment. Often what is most critical is a redistribution of responsibilities for illness management within the family, particularly when the course of illness is deteriorating. Many adolescents and their parents have difficulty in coping both with the lability of metabolic control characteristic of this age group and with the constant need to renegotiate responsibilities for treatment. In particular, when the course of illness is unstable, these families are virtually tyrannized by repeated hospitalizations, debilitating symptoms of chronic poor metabolic control, concomitant school problems, and family conflicts over treatment responsibilities. Yet, services for promoting self-care and effective family problem solving after initial diagnosis are lacking.

Some intervention efforts have focused on fostering coping skills in training group programs with afflicted adolescents. In a series of well controlled group interventions, Marrero et al. (1982) focused specifically on adolescents with chronic poor metabolic control. The efficacy of their group model, emphasizing the development of coping skills, was demonstrated for a wide range of psychosocial variables. Several counseling programs feature the combination of offering adolescent clients knowledge, helping them to change attitudes, and training them to improve their social skills (Barglow et al., 1983). Some intervention programs for diabetic adolescents offer group sessions (such as a 2-hour theater or music group), which appear highly suitable for this group since the atmosphere is less structured and creative. In the group counseling program designed by Blum and Galatzer (1982), small groups initially discuss illness-related themes, then personal topics are integrated into the discourse. Some counselors deal with newly diagnosed diabetic patients in their group and try to cushion the particularly strong stress of the initial phase. Other concepts of intervention start by focusing on shaping illness-related attitudes and encouraging compliance. Hamburg and Inoff (1982) proposed a broad-ranging model of therapeutic intervention designed to help the patient cope with the illness by introducing problem-specific psychological counseling over the entire course of the illness. Aside from acknowledging the developmental perspective, this model considers the course of diabetes and its critical phases, from before diagnosis to the period of insulin adjustment and right through to the period when apprehensions about permanent physical damage begin to emerge.

The realm of therapeutic interventions includes individual, group, and family therapy. Most approaches focus on identifying concrete compliance problems in the diabetic patient and helping the patient to learn new behaviors to correct these problems. Because the patients often stay only for a short time, behavior therapy has been applied most frequently. However, this may encourage the patient to fixate on achievement and structure. Moreover, the psychological background related to noncompliance is rarely incorporated. Whereas behavior therapy and family dynamic approaches dominate interventions with diabetic adolescents, very little is known about how psychoanalytic treatment works. Psychoanalytic therapy may be demanding in terms of time and expense; nevertheless, it is definitely indicated for the adolescent patient whose motivation is high. In an interesting study, Moran and Fonagy (1987) compared the weekly course of metabolic control in adolescent patients with the course of psychoanalytic therapy. One of the impressive results was that the medical values improved rapidly over the course of the individual therapy, although the processes of emotional maturation and problem resolution took much longer.

Intervention for Few – Prevention for All?

While a disrupted course of illness is not seen in all diabetic adolescents, many experience a cycle of dysfunction, with medical and interpersonal crises closely intertwined. Only a small group of diabetic adolescents in our study required and accepted psychological help. These were largely the poorly adjusted diabetic adolescents, who named more everyday problems and illness-related stressors and had more difficulty in simultaneously dealing with these stressors. They also experienced more deficits in internal and social resources. It is remarkable how openly adolescents with poor metabolic control named their problems and expressed their desire for help. Without sufficient motivation for treatment, psychological intervention would not have been possible. It was also clear that the diabetic adolescents' parents, particularly the mothers, required special help and support. They were overwhelmed by chronic worries and felt extraordinarily stressed. Our 4-year longitudinal study revealed that the stressors in various areas did not decrease over time; only their relative significance varied. Whereas concrete illness management became less difficult, there was an increase in stress related to the child's future in private and professional domains. Considering how little support most diabetic adolescents' mothers receive from their husbands, it would be advisable to offer counseling or supportive psychotherapy to the family, particularly to those families of adolescents with chronic poor metabolic control. This could occur in the form of a mothers' or a family discussion circle as well as in individual, partner, or family therapy.

Diabetic adolescents' emotional problems are not necessarily manifested in overt psychological symptoms as much as in subclinical disturbances, such as an impaired self-concept and body image. Preventive measures are highly recommended in these cases. Indeed, various approaches in pediatric developmental psychology call for intervention not only after the first symptoms have emerged, but preemptively, for all children at risk and at a relatively early stage. Compas et al. (1993) have even recommended compulsory participation in fundamental preventive courses for early adolescents. According to their proposals, selected participants in these courses should attend follow-up courses for specific risk groups, based on the outcome of the earlier courses. The advantage of this general prevention program is that it helps adolescents not only to anticipate and correctly identify stressors but also to learn what methods of coping they may apply to deal with these stressors most appropriately. All chronically ill adolescents, especially diabetic adolescents, must learn how to increase and apply their social competence, delegate tasks, and accept help. They should also learn that anticipating stressors may help them to cope with them later. In addition, specific preventive measures for highly stressed chronically ill adolescents or those with consistently maladaptive functioning (such as poor metabolic control) over a longer time span could, for example, rectify deficits in perceiving problems and coping with stress and also promote suitable skills in using social and institutional resources. It is also important to ensure that creative, relaxing, and physical activities are encouraged.

Taken together, all of these prevention and intervention efforts indicate that by buffering some of the adverse effects of strict illness management and by building on emerging coping abilities, adolescents can be encouraged to participate more actively and effectively in their own health care. It is also obvious that more intensive intervention is needed for families with adolescents who are experiencing more serious metabolic and psychosocial dysfunction.

Revising the Treatments Offered

Most current intervention programs for the chronically ill, especially for diabetic adolescents, are oriented to illness management. Based on our findings, it is clear that some revision of the therapies commonly offered to adolescents is warranted. For example, given the developmental barriers responsible for the adolescents' aversion to seeking professional help, especially as it is offered in traditionally institutionalized counseling centers, more unconventional forms of providing assistance, such as at-home counseling for school and family problems or drop-in counseling centers, may be more attractive to the adolescent (Seiffge-Krenke, 1998a). Counseling in these environments is more private and easier for the adolescent to approach. Furthermore, the emphasis is more treatment-related and less verbal, which may encourage adolescents in certain problem groups to make use of counseling services. Physical proximity, reduced obligations, easy accessibility, and a more symmetrical pattern of relationships between counselor and client certainly reduce the "costs" of using the service, not only for adolescents but also for their parents. An evaluation of the clients who frequented a drop-in counseling center revealed that spontaneity and constancy in attendance do not exclude one another (Seiffge-Krenke, 1998a). The majority of clients used the services offered by the drop-in counseling center on a regular basis, although they were under no obligation to do so. Clearly, this kind of psychosocial care is only suitable for a limited population. It is not appropriate if the illness or disturbance is so severe that regular care or inpatient treatment is needed because of life-threatening circumstances, danger to the patient or others, or urgent health problems.

The questions of when, who, and how introduced at the beginning of this chapter may now be answered as follows:

> *When:* An intervention should be implemented as soon as possible after the onset of illness and its diagnosis, that is, ideally in the initial phase of the illness, or at least whenever adolescents or their parents display motivation to seek treatment. It is important to remember that this motivation may not be overtly expressed. Thus, one should be careful not to overlook or disregard superficial signs of motivation inherent in behavior that might initially be considered as reflecting a lack of motivation. Often such adolescents and their families showing signs that apparently indicate borderline motivation are indeed highly motivated to begin treatment and work through their problems with the help of a therapist or counselor.
>
> *Who:* Parents seem to need treatment even more than the ill adolescents do. Particularly mothers seemed to be highly stressed by caring for a chronically ill adolescent. Still, it must be recalled that adolescents, because of their developmental level, maintain a façade of normalcy and thus try to appear unmotivated. One exception is seen in the diabetic adolescent with poor metabolic control, who typically expresses problems and a desire for help and support openly.
>
> *How:* It appears sensible to integrate as many different interaction partners as possible into the intervention program. Apart from conveying knowledge and changing attitudes, the program should address a series of pressing, important psychological problems relevant to the ill adolescents and their parents, siblings, close friends, and romantic partners. These include the adolescent's dilemma

between adhering to the strict diabetes regimen and attempting to accomplish developmental tasks. The parents' chronic worries must be relieved, and the father needs to be better integrated into family life. Furthermore, the ill adolescent's siblings must be assisted in learning to accept their changed roles. For the physician, the adolescent's developmental dynamics along with the family dynamics may represent problems that profit from open discussion.

Of course, the individual form of intervention will depend on various criteria. The overall goal should be to achieve satisfactory compliance and physiological adaptation, while still allowing adolescents to develop appropriately in all important areas. In this regard, even classical psychoanalysis may help in achieving this goal. These principles, although formulated with diabetic adolescents in mind, could certainly be applied to many other chronic illnesses in adolescence that exhibit similar characteristics and long-term stress.

References

Abramovitch, R., Pepler, D., & Corter, C. (1982). Patterns of sibling interaction among preschool age children. In M. E. Lamb & B. Sutton-Smith (Eds.), *Sibling relationships: Their nature and significance across the lifespan* (pp. 61–86). Hillsdale, NJ: Lawrence Erlbaum Associates.

Achenbach, T. M. (1991a). *Manual for the Child Behavior Checklist and 1991 Child Behavior Profile.* Burlington, VT: University of Vermont, Department of Psychiatry.

Achenbach, T. M. (1991b). *Manual for the Youth Self-Report and 1991 YSR Profile.* Burlington, VT: University of Vermont, Department of Psychiatry.

Achenbach, T. M., McConaughy, S. H., & Howell, C. T. (1987). Child and adolescent behavioral and emotional problems: Implications of cross-informant correlations for situational specificity. *Psychological Bulletin, 101,* 213–232.

Adams, B. N. (1972). Birth order: A critical review. *Sociometry, 34,* 411–439.

Adler, A. (1926). Menschenkenntnis Kap. 8: Geschwister [Knowledge of People. Chap. 8: Siblings] (pp. 117–124). Leipzig: Hirzel.

Ahmed, P. I., & Ahmed, N. (Eds.) (1985). *Coping with juvenile diabetes.* Springfield, IL: Charles C Thomas.

Aimez, P., Tutin, M., Guy-Grand, B., Desme, F., & Bour, H. (1971). Étude psychosociologique des contraintes thérapeutiques du diabète sucré [Psychosociological study of the limitations of diabetes therapy]. *La Presse Médicale, 79,* 1149–1152.

Alvin, P., Rey, C., & Frappier, J. Y. (1995). Therapeutic compliance in adolescents with chronic disease. *Archives of Pediatry, 2,* 874–882.

Amon, T. (1989). Psychosomatik und Diabetes mellitus? Überlegungen zu einem Thema, das noch wenig Gegenliebe findet. [Psychosomatics and diabetes mellitus? Thoughts on a topic that still finds little acceptance] In

G. Bergmann (Ed.), *Psychosomatische Grundversorgung* [Basic care of the psychosomatic patient] (pp. 61–69). Berlin: Springer.

Anderson, B. J., Auslander, W., Jung, K. C., Miller, J. P., & Santiago, J. V. (1990). Assessing family sharing of diabetes responsibilities. *Journal of Pediatric Psychology, 15,* 477–492.

Anderson, B. J., Darling, C., Davidson, J. K., & Passarello, L. C. (1992). The mystique of first intercourse among college youth: The role of partners, contraceptions, and psychological reactions. *Journal of Youth and Adolescence, 21,* 97–117.

Anderson, B. J., Miller, J. P., Auslander, W., & Santiago, J. V. (1981). Family characteristics of diabetic adolescents: Relationship to metabolic control. *Diabetes Care, 4,* 586–594.

Anthony, J. E. (1970). The impact of mental and physical illness on family life. *American Journal of Orthopsychiatry, 127,* 138–146.

Antonovsky, A. (1981). *Health, stress, and coping.* San Francisco, CA: Jossey-Bass.

Argyle, M. (1986). Social behavior problems in adolescence. In R. K. Silbereisen, G. Rudinger, & K. Eyferth (Eds.), *Development as action in context* (pp. 55–86). Berlin: Springer.

Auslander, W., Anderson, B. J., Bubb, J., Jung, K. C., & Santiago, J. V. (1990). Risk factors to health in diabetic children: A prospective study from diagnosis. *Health and Social Work, 15,* 133–142.

Badura, B. (Ed.) (1971). *Soziale Unterstützung und chronische Krankheit. Zum Stand sozialepidemiologischer Forschung* [Social support and chronic illness. State of socio-epidemiological research]. Frankfurt a.M.: Suhrkamp.

Band, E. E., & Weisz, J. R. (1990). Developmental differences in primary and secondary control coping and adjustment to juvenile diabetes. *Journal of Clinical Child Psychology, 19,* 150–158.

Baranowksi, T., Nader, P. R., Dunn, K., & Vanderpool, N. A. (1982). Family self-help: Promoting changes in health behavior. *Journal of Communication, 32,* 161–172.

Barglow, P., Edidin, E. V., Budlong-Springer, A. S., Berndt, D., Phillips. D., & Dubrow, E. (1983). Diabetic control in children and adolescents: Psychosocial factors and therapeutic efficacy. *Journal of Youth and Adolescence, 10,* 77–94.

Baumrind, D. (1991). Effective parenting during the early adolescent transition. In P. A. Cowan & M. Hetherington (Eds.), *Family transitions* (pp. 111–163). Hillsdale, NJ: Lawrence Erlbaum Associates.

Becker, H. M. (1974). *The health belief model and personal health behavior.* Thorofare, NJ: Slack.

Becker, R. D. (1979). Adolescents in the hospital. *Israel Annals of Psychiatry and Related Disciplines, 17,* 328–352.

Bedell, J. R., Giordani, B., Amour, J. L., Tavormina, J., & Boll, T. (1977). Life stress and the psychological and medical adjustment of chronically ill children. *Journal of Psychosomatic Research, 21,* 237–242.

Ben-Sira, Z. (1984). Chronic illness, stress and coping. *Social Science and Medicine, 18,* 725–736.

Beresford, B. (1994). Resources and strategies: How parents cope with the care of a disabled child. *Journal of Child Psychology and Child Psychiatry, 35,* 171–209.

Berman, J. S. (1983). *The effects of perceived control on adolescent coping with hospitalization and major illness.* Ann Arbor, MI: Temple University.

Berndt, T. J. (1982). The features and effects of friendship in early adolescence. *Child Development, 53,* 1447–1460.

Berndt, T. J., Hawkins, J. A., & Hoyle, S. G. (1986). Changes in friendship during a school year: Effects on children's and adolescents' impressions of friendship and sharing. *Child Development, 57,* 1284–1297.

Billings, A. G., & Moos, R. H. (1982). Family environments and adaptation: A clinically applicable typology. *American Journal of Family Therapy, 10,* 26–38.

Billings, A. G., Moos, R. H., Miller, J. J., & Gottlieb, J. E. (1987). Psychosocial adaptation to juvenile rheumatic disease: A controlled evaluation. *Health Psychology, 6,* 343–359.

Binger, C. M., Ablin, A. R., Feuerstein, R. C., Kushner, J. H., Zoger, S., & Mikkelson, C. (1969). Childhood leukemia: Emotional impact on patient and family. *New England Journal of Medicine, 280,* 414–418.

Bird, H. R., Canino, G., Rubio-Stipec, M., Gould, M. S., Ribera, J., Sesman, M., Woodbury, M., Huertas-Goldman, S., Paga, A., Sanchez-Lancay, A., & Moscoso, M. (1988). Estimates of the prevalence of childhood maladjustment in a community survey in Puerto Rico. *Archives of General Psychiatry, 45,* 1120–1126.

Blanz, B., Rensch-Riemann, B., Fritz-Sigmund, D., & Schmidt, M. H. (1993). Zur Rolle erkrankungsbezogener kognitiv-emotionaler Faktoren als Determinanten der Compliance bei Jugendlichen mit Diabetes mellitus [The role of illness-specific cognitive and emotional factors in determining compliance in adolescents with diabetes mellitus]. *Zeitschrift für Klinische Psychologie, 22,* 264–275.

Blos, P. (1973). *Adoleszenz. Eine psychoanalytische Interpretation* [Adolescence. A psychoanalytic interpretation]. Stuttgart: Klett-Cotta.

Blum, A., & Galatzer, A. (1982). Group counseling for diabetic patients. In Z. Laron & A. Galatzer (Eds.), *Psychological aspects of diabetes in childhood and adolescence* (pp. 230–234). Basel: Karger.

Blum, R. W. (1992). Chronic illness and disability in adolescence. *Journal of Adolescent Health, 13,* 364–368.

Blyth, D. A., Simmons, R. G., & Zakin, D. F. (1985). Satisfaction with body image for early adolescent females: The impact of pubertal timing within different school environments. *Journal of Youth and Adolescence, 14,* 207–225.

Bobrow A., & Avkuskin, B. C. (1985). Communication and interaction in families with chronically ill adolescents. *Family Process, 23,* 127–149.

Bowman, M. (1985). Doctor-patient relationship. In P. J. Ahmed & N. Ahmed (Eds.), *Coping with juvenile diabetes* (pp. 295–305). Springfield, IL: Charles C Thomas.

Boyce, M. M. (1998). Chronic illness in adolescence. *Adolescence, 33*, 927–939.

Boyle, I. R., di Sant' Agnese, P. A., Sack, S., Millican, F., & Kulcyski, L. L. (1976). Emotional adjustment of adolescents and young adults with cystic fibrosis. *The Journal of Pediatrics, 88*, 318–326.

Boyle, M. H., Offord, D. R., Racine, Y. A., Szatmari, P., Fleming, J. E., & Links, P. S. (1992). Predicting substance use in late adolescence: Results from the Ontario Child Health Study follow-up. *American Journal of Psychiatry, 149*, 761–767.

Brähler, E. (Ed.). (1988). *Body experience.* Berlin: Springer.

Brand, A. H., Johnson, J. H., & Johnson, S. B. (1986). Life stress and diabetic control in children and adolescents with insulin-dependent diabetes. *Journal of Pediatric Psychology, 11*, 481–496.

Bremer, H. J. (1990). Stoffwechsel [Metabolism]. In D. Palitzsch (Ed.), *Pädiatrie* (3. neu bearb. Aufl.) [Pediatrics, 3rd ed., rev.] (pp. 97–137). Stuttgart: Enke.

Breslau, N. (1982). Siblings of disabled children: Birth order and age-spacing effects. *Journal of Abnormal Child Psychology, 10*, 85–96.

Brody, G. H., Stoneman, Z., & Burke, M. (1987). Child temperaments, maternal differential behavior, and sibling relationships. *Developmental Psychology, 23*, 354–362.

Brook, J. S., Whiteman, M., Gordon, A. S., & Brook, D. W. (1990). The role of older brothers in younger brothers' drug use viewed in the context of parent and peer influences. *Journal of Genetic Psychology, 151*, 59–75.

Brooks-Gunn, J., & Petersen, A. C. (1991). Studying the emergence of depression and depressive symptoms during adolescence. *Journal of Youth and Adolescence, 20*, 115–119.

Brooks-Gunn, J., & Reiter, E. O. (1990). The role of pubertal processes in the early adolescent transition. In S. Feldman & G. Elliott (Eds.), *At the threshold. The developing adolescent* (pp. 16–53). Cambridge, MA: Harvard University Press.

Brown, R. T., Doepke, K. J., & Kaslow, N. J. (1993a). Risk-resistance-adaptation model for pediatric chronic illness: Sickle cell syndrome as an example. *Clinical Psychology Review, 13*, 119–132.

Brown, R. T., Kaslow, N. J., Doepke, K., Buchanan, I., Eckman, J., Baldwin, K., & Goonan, B. (1993b). Psychosocial and family functioning in children with sickle cell syndrome and their mothers. *Journal of the American Academy of Child and Adolescent Psychiatry, 32*, 545–553.

Brown, R. T., Kaslow, N. J., Hazzard, A. P., Madan-Swain, A., Sexson, S. B., Lambert, R., & Baldwin, K. (1992). Psychiatric and family functioning in children with leukemia and their parents. *Journal of the American Academy of Child and Adolescent Psychiatry, 31,* 495–502.

Buhrmester, D., & Furman, W. (1987). The development of companionship and intimacy. *Child Development, 58,* 1101–1113.

Buhrmester, D., & Furman, W. (1990). Age differences in perceptions of siblings relationships in childhood and adolescence. *Child Development, 61,* 1387–1398.

Bukowski, W. M., Hoza, B., & Boivin, M. (1993). Popularity, friendship, and emotional adjustment during early adolescence. In B. Laursen (Ed.), *Close friendships in adolescence* (pp. 23–38). San Francisco: Jossey Bass.

Bulcroft, R. A. (1991). The value of physical change in adolescence: Consequences for the parent-adolescent exchange relationship. *Journal of Youth and Adolescence, 20,* 89–105.

Bundesminister für Familie und Senioren (Ed.) (1994). *Datensammlung zu Formen und Strukturen des familiären Zusammenlebens und zur Geburtenentwicklung* [Data on forms and structures of family life and population rates]. Bonn: Bouvier.

Bundesminister für Gesundheit (Ed.) (1991). *Daten des Gesundheitswesens. Ausgabe 1991* [Data on health services. 1991]. Baden-Baden: Nomos.

Bundeszentrale für gesundheitliche Aufklärung (BZgA) (Ed.) (1992). *Aktionsgrundlagen 1990 der Bundeszentrale für gesundheitliche Aufklärung* [Foundations of the Federal Agency for Health Awareness, 1990]. Cologne: BZgA.

Burbach, D. J., & Peterson, L. (1986). Children's concepts of physical illness: A review and critique of cognitive-developmental literature. *Health Psychology, 5,* 307–325.

Burns, K. L., Green, P., & Chase, H. P. (1986). Psychosocial correlates of glycemic control as a function of age in youth with insulin-dependent diabetes. *Journal of Adolescent Health Care, 7,* 311–319.

Cadman, D., Boyle, M. H., Szatmari, P., & Offord, D. R. (1987). Chronic illness, disability, and mental and social well-being: Findings of the Ontario Child Health Study. *Pediatrics, 79,* 805–813.

Cadman, D., Rosenbaum, P., Boyle, M., & Offord, D. R. (1991). Children with chronic illness: Family and parent demographic characteristics and psychosocial adjustment. *Pediatrics, 87,* 884–889.

Cain, A. C., Fast, I., & Erickson, M. E. (1964). Children's disturbed reactions to the death of a sibling. *American Journal of Orthopsychiatry, 34,* 741–752.

Campbell, T. L. (1986). Family's impact on health: A critical review. *Family Systems Medicine, 4,* 135–200.

Canning, E. H., Hanser, S. B., Shade, K. A., & Boyce, W. T. (1993). Maternal distress and discrepancy in reports of psychopathology in chronically ill children. *Psychosomatics, 34,* 506–511.

Cantor, N., Acker, M., & Cook-Flanagan, C. (1992). Conflicts and preoccupation in the intimacy life task. *Journal of Personality and Social Psychology, 63,* 644–655.

Cappelli, M., McGrath, P. J., Heick, C. E., MacDonald, N. E., Feldman, W., & Rowe, P. (1989). Chronic disease and its impact – the adolescents' perspective. *Journal of Adolescent Health Care, 10,* 283–288.

Carlson, K. P., Gesten, E. L., McIver, L. S, DeClue, T., & Malone, J. (1994). Problem solving and adjustment in families of children with diabetes. *Children's Health Care, 23,* 193–210.

Centers for Disease Control and Prevention (1996). Asthma mortality and hospitalization among children and young adults – United States, 1980–1993. *Morbidity and Mortality Weekly Report, 45,* 350–353.

Chaney, J. M., Mullins, L. L., Frank, R. G., & Peterson, L. (1997). Transactional patterns of child, mother, and father adjustment in insulin-dependent diabetes mellitus: A prospective study. *Journal of Pediatric Psychology, 22,* 229–244.

Chase, H. P., & Jackson, G. G. (1981). Stress and sugar control in children with insulin dependent diabetes mellitus. *The Journal of Pediatrics, 98,* 1011–1013.

Cicirelli, V. G. (1973). Effects of sibling structure and interaction on children's categorization style. *Developmental Psychology, 9,* 132–139.

Cicirelli, V. G. (1975). Effects of mother and older sibling on the problem-solving behavior of the younger child. *Developmental Psychology, 11,* 749–756.

Cicirelli, V. G. (1976). Mother-child and sibling-sibling interactions on a problem-solving task. *Child Development, 47,* 588–596.

Cicirelli, V. G. (1982). Sibling influence throughout the life span. In M. E. Sutton-Smith (Ed.), *Sibling relationships: Their nature and significance across the life-span.* Hillsdale, NJ: Lawrence Erlbaum Associates.

Claes, M. (1994). Friendship characteristics of adolescents referred for psychiatric treatment. *Journal of Adolescent Research, 9,* 180–192.

Clark-Lempers, D. S., Lempers, J. D., & Ho, C. (1991). Early, middle, and late adolescents' perceptions of their relationships with significant others. *Journal of Adolescent Research, 6,* 296–315.

Clement, U., Schmidt, G., & Kruse, M. (1984). Changes in sex-differences in sexual behavior: A replication of a study on West German students (1933–1981). *Archives of Sexual Behavior, 13,* 99–120.

Cohen, S., & Wills, T. A. (1985). Stress, social support and the buffering hypothesis. *Psychological Bulletin, 98,* 310–357.

Cole, R. E., & Reiss, D. (1993). *How do families cope with chronic illness.* Hillsdale, NJ: Lawrence Erlbaum Associates.

Coleman, J. C. (1978). Current contradictions in adolescent theory. *Journal of Youth and Adolescence, 7,* 1–11.

Coleman, J. C. (Ed.) (1980). *The nature of adolescence.* London: Methuen.

Coleman, J. C. (1984). Eine neue Theorie der Adoleszenz [A new theory of adolescence]. In E. Olbrich & E. Todt (Eds.), *Probleme des Jugendalters. Neuere Sichtweisen* [Problems in adolescence. Recent perspectives] (pp. 49–67). Berlin: Springer.

Collins, W. A., & Russel, G. (1991). Mother-child and father-child relationships in middle childhood and adolescence: A developmental analysis. *Developmental Review, 11,* 99–136.

Compas, B. E., Davis, G. E., Forsythe, C. J., & Wagner, B. M. (1987). Assessment of major and daily stressful events during adolescence: The Adolescent Perceived Events Scale. *Journal of Consulting and Clinical Psychology, 55,* 534–541.

Compas, B. E., Orosan, P. G., & Grant, K. E. (1993). Adolescent stress and coping: Implications for psychopathology during adolescence. *Journal of Adolescence, 16,* 331–349.

Condon, S. L., Cooper, C. R., & Grotevant, H. D. (1984). Manual for the analysis of family discourse. *Psychological Documents,* No. 2616.

Cook, J. A. (1984). Influence of gender on the problems of parents of fatally ill children. *Journal of Psychosocial Oncology, 2,* 71–91.

Cooper, C. R., Grotevant, H. D., & Condon, S. M. (1982). Methodological challenges of selectivity in family interaction: Assessing temporal patterns of individuation. *Journal of Marriage and the Family, 44,* 749–754.

Cooper, C. R., Grotevant, H. D., & Condon, S. M. (1983). Individuality and connectedness in the family as a context for adolescent identity formation and role-taking skills. In H. D. Grotevant & C. R. Cooper (Eds.), *Adolescent development in the family: New directions for child development* (pp. 43–59). San Francisco: Jossey Bass.

Cotterell, J. L. (1992). School size as a factor in adolescent's adjustment to the transition to secondary school. *Journal of Early Adolescence, 12,* 28–45.

Cowen, L., Corey, M., Simmons, R., Keenan, N., Robertson, J., & Levison, H. (1984). Growing older with cystic fibrosis: Psychologic adjustment of patients more than 16 years old. *Psychosomatic Medicine, 46,* 363–376.

Coyne, J. C., & Anderson, B. J. (1988). The psychosomatic family reconsidered: Diabetes in context. *Journal of Marriage and Family Therapy, 14,* 113–124.

Coyne, J. C., & Smith, D. A. (1991). Couples coping with a myocardial infarction: A contextual perspectives on wives' distress. *Journal of Personality and Social Psychology, 61,* 404–412.

Cozby, P. C. (1973). Self-disclosure: A literature review. *Psychological Bulletin, 2,* 73–91.

Crain, A. J., Susman, M. B., & Weil, W. B. (1986). Effects of a diabetic child on marital integration and related measurements of family functioning. *Journal of Health Behavior, 7,* 122–127.

Cromer, B. A., & Tarnowski, K. J. (1989). Noncompliance in adolescents: A review. *Developmental Behavioral Pediatrics, 10,* 207–215.

Csikszentmihalyi, M., & Larson, L. (1984). *Being adolescent: Conflict and growth in the teenage years.* New York: Basic Books.

Dacey, J. (1979). *Adolescents today.* Glennville, IL: Scott, Foresman & Co.

Daniels, D., Moos, R. H., Billings, A. G., & Miller, J. J. (1987). Psychosocial risk and resistance factors among children with chronic illness, healthy siblings and healthy controls. *Journal of Abnormal Child Psychology, 15,* 295–308.

Davies, E., & Furnham, A. (1986a). The dieting and body shape concerns of adolescent females. *Journal of Child Psychology and Psychiatry, 27,* 417–428.

Davies, E., & Furnham, A. (1986b). Body satisfaction in adolescent girls. *British Journal of Medical Psychology, 59,* 279–287.

Delamater, A. M., Kurtz, S. M., Bubb, J., White, N. H., & Santiago, J. V. (1987). Stress and coping in relation to metabolic control of adolescents with type I diabetes. *Journal of Developmental Behavior Pediatrics, 8,* 136–140.

Delbridge, L. (1975). Educational and psychological factors in the management of diabetes in childhood. *Medical Journal of Australia, 2,* 737–739.

Deschamps, J. P. (1983). Zur Gesundheit der Jugendlichen [Adolescent health], *Kinderarzt, 14,* 473–476.

Deusinger, J. (1992). *Die Frankfurter Körperkonzeptskalen* [The Frankfurt body image scales]. Unpublished manuscript. Frankfurt a. M.

DiGirolamo, A. M., Quittner, A. L., Ackerman, V., & Stevens, J. (1997). Identification and assessment of ongoing stressors in adolescents with a chronic illness: An application of the behavior-analytic model. *Journal of Clinical Child Psychology, 26,* 53–66.

Döpfner, M., Plück, J., Berner, W., Englert, E., Fegert, J. M., Huss, M., Lenz, K., Schmeck, K., Lehmkuhl, G., Lehmkuhl, U., & Poustka, F. (1998). Psychische Auffälligkeiten und psychosoziale Kompetenzen in den neuen und alten Bundesländern [Psychological disturbances and psychosocial competence in the new and old German federal states]. *Zeitschrift für Klinische Psychologie, 27,* 9–19.

Douglas, J. W. B. (1964). *The home and the school.* London: Macgibon and Kee.

Dreher, E., & Dreher, M. (1985). Entwicklungsaufgaben im Jugendalter: Bedeutsamkeit und Bewältigungskonzepte [Developmental tasks in adolescence: Significance and coping concepts]. In D. Liepmann & A. Stiksrud (Eds.), *Entwicklungsaufgaben und Bewältigungsprobleme in der Adoleszenz* [Developmental tasks and problems of coping in adolescence] (pp. 56–70). Göttingen: Hogrefe.

Drotar, D. (Ed.) (1998). *Measuring health-related quality of life in children and adolescents: Implications for research and practice* (pp. 3–24). Mahwah, NJ: Lawrence Erlbaum Associates.

Drotar, D., & Crawford, P. (1985). Psychological adaptation of siblings of chronically ill children: Research and practice implications. *Developmental and Behavioral Pediatrics, 6,* 355–361.

Drotar, D., Owens, R., & Gotthold, J. (1981). Personality adjustment of children and adolescents with hypopituitarism. *Annual Progress in Child Psychiatry and Child Development, 14,* 304–306.

Dubow, E. F., Lovko, K. R., & Kausch, D. F. (1990). Demographic differences in adolescents' health concerns and perceptions of helping agents. *Journal of Clinical Child Psychology, 19,* 44–54.

Dunn, J., & Kendrick, C. (1981). Social behavior of young siblings in the family context: Differences between same-sex and different-sex dyads. *Child Development, 52,* 1265–1273.

Dunn, S. M., & Turtle, J. R. (1981). The myth of diabetic personality. *Diabetes Care, 4,* 640–645.

Dusek, J. B., & Flaherty, J. F. (1981). The development of the self-concept during the adolescent years. *Monographs of the Society for Research in Child Development, 4.*

Eiser, C. (1985). *The psychology of childhood illness.* New York: Springer.

Eiser, C. (1990a). *Chronic childhood disease.* Cambridge, U.K.: Cambridge University Press.

Eiser, C. (1990b). Psychological effects of chronic disease. *Journal of Child Psychology and Psychiatry, 31,* 85–98.

Eiser, C. (1992). Psychological consequences of chronic disease in children. In S. Maes, H. Leventhal, & M. Johnston (Eds.), *International Review of Health Psychology* (Vol. 1, pp. 145–165). New York: Wiley.

Eiser, C., & Berrenberg, J. L. (1995). Assessing the impact of chronic disease on the relationship between parents and their adolescents. *Journal of Psychosomatic Research, 39,* 109–114.

Eiser, C., Havermans, T., Kirby, R. Eiser, J. R., & Pancer, M. (1993). Coping and confidence among parents of children with diabetes. *Disability and Rehabilitation, 15,* 10–18.

Engel, U., & Hurrelmann, K. (1989). *Psychosoziale Belastung im Jugendalter. Empirische Befunde zum Einfluß von Familie, Schule und Gleichaltrigengruppe* [Psychosocial stress in adolescence. Empirical findings on the influence of family, school, and peers]. Berlin: Walter de Gruyter.

Engström, I. (1992). Mental health and psychological functioning in children and adolescents with inflammatory bowel disease: A comparison with children having other chronic illnesses and with healthy children. *Journal of Child Psychology and Psychiatry and Allied Disciplines, 33,* 563–582.

Erikson, E. H. (1968). *Jugend und Krise: Die Psychodynamik im sozialen Wandel* [Adolescence and crisis. The psychodynamics in social change]. Stuttgart: Klett.

Erlich, H. S. (1987). Denial in adolescence. *Psychoanalytic Study of the Child, 42,* 315–336.

Essau, C. A., Karpinski, N. A., Petermann, F., & Conradt, J. (1998). Häufigkeit, Komorbidität und psychosoziale Beeinträchtigung von depressiven Störungen bei Jugendlichen: Ergebnisse der Bremer Jugendstudie [Frequency, comorbidity, and psychosocial impairment of depressive disorders in adolescents: Results from the Bremen Adolescent Study]. *Zeitschrift für Klinische Psychologie, Psychiatrie und Psychotherapie, 46,* 316–329.

Esser, G., Schmidt, M. H., Fätkenheuer, B., Fritz, A., Koppe, T., Laucht, M., Rensch, B., & Rothenberger, W. (1992). Prävalenz und Verlauf psychischer Störungen im Kindes- und Jugendalter [Prevalence and course of psychological disturbances in childhood and adolescence]. *Zeitschrift für Kinder- und Jugendpsychiatrie, 20,* 232–242.

Evans, C. A., Stevens, M., Cushway, D., & Houghton, J. (1992). Sibling response to childhood cancer: A new approach. *Child: Health, Care and Behavior, 18,* 229–244.

Fällström, K. (1974). On the personality structure in diabetic school children, aged 7–15 years. *Acta Paediatrica Scandinavica, 251,* 8–9.

Faust, J., Baum, C. G., & Forehand, R. (1985). An examination of the association between social relationships and depression in early adolescence. *Journal of Applied Developmental Psychology, 6,* 291–297.

Fentner, S., & Seiffge-Krenke, I. (1997). Die Rolle des Vaters in der familiären Kommunikation: Befunde einer Längsschnittstudie an gesunden und chronisch kranken Jugendlichen [The role of the father in family communication. Results of a longitudinal study of healthy and chronically ill adolescents]. *Praxis für Kinderpsychologie und Kinderpsychiatrie, 46,* 36–52.

Ferrari, M. (1984). Chronic illness: Psychosocial effects on siblings – I. Chronically ill boys. *Journal of Child Psychology and Psychiatry, 25,* 459–476.

Fielding, D., Moore, B., Dewey, M., Ashley, P., McKendrick, T., & Pinkerton, P. (1985). Children with end-stage renal failure: Psychological effects on patients, siblings, and parents. *Journal of Psychosomatic Research, 29,* 457–465.

Fife, B., Norton, J., & Groom, G. (1987). The family adaptation to childhood leukemia. *Social Science and Medicine, 24,* 159–168.

Finck, H. (1994). Soziale und berufliche Diskriminierung des Typ-I-Diabetikers [Social and vocational-occupational discrimination of type-I diabetics]. In F. Petermann (Ed.), *Diabetes mellitus* (pp. 31–48). Göttingen: Hogrefe.

Fishbein, H. A., La Porte, R. E., Orchard, T. J., Drash, A. L., Kuller, L. H., & Wagener, D. K. (1982). The Pittsburgh insulin-dependent diabetes mellitus registry: Seasonal incidence. *Diabetologica, 23,* 83–85.

Frankel, K. A. (1990). Girls' perceptions of peer relationship, support, and stress. *Journal of Early Adolescence, 10,* 69–88.

Franz, J. M., & Crystal, R. M. (1985). A career developmental model for the juvenile diabetic: Implications for rehabilitation practice. *Journal of Applied Rehabilitation Counseling, 17,* 24–27.

Freedman, R. (1989). *Die Opfer der Venus* [The victims of Venus]. Zürich: Kreuz.

Freeman, G. K., & Richards, S. C. (1994). Personal continuity and the care of patients with epilepsy in general practice. *British Journal of General Practice, 44,* 395–399.

French, A. (1977). *Disturbed children and their families: Innovations in evaluation and treatment.* New York: Human Sciences Press.

Freud, S. (1905). Drei Abhandlungen zur Sexualtheorie [Three essays on sexual theory]. In A. Mitscherlich, A. Richards, & J. Strachey (Eds.) (1972), *Sigmund Freud. Studienausgabe* [Sigmund Freud. Studies] (Vol. 5, pp. 37–145). Frankfurt a.M.: Fischer.

Freund, E. E. S., & McGuire, M. B. (1991). *Health, illness and the social body.* Englewood Cliffs, NJ: Prentice-Hall.

Fröhlich, F. (1986). *Die seelische Verarbeitung lebensbedrohlicher Krankheit im Jugendalter* [Psychological coping with life-threatening illness in adolescence]. Basel: Schwabe.

Frydenberg, E., & Lewis, R. (1993). Boys play sport and girls turn to others: Age, gender and ethnicity as determinants of coping. *Journal of Adolescence, 16,* 253–266.

Furman, W., Brown, B. B., & Feiring, C. (Eds). (1999). *The development of romantic relationships in adolescence.* New York: Cambridge University Press.

Furman, W., & Buhrmester, D. (1985). Children's perceptions of the personal relationships in their social networks. *Developmental Psychology, 21,* 1016–1024.

Furman, W., & Buhrmester, D. (1992). Age and sex differences in perceptions of networks of personal relationships. *Child Development, 63,* 103–105.

Furman, W., & Wehner, E. A. (1994). Romantic views: Toward a theory of adolescent romantic relationships. In R. Montemayor, G. R. Adams, & T. P. Gullotta (Eds.), *Personal relationships during adolescence.* Thousand Oaks, CA: Sage.

Gagnon, J., Lindenbaum, S., Martin, J. L., May, R. M., Menken, J., Turner, C. F., & Zabin, L. S. (1989). Sexual behavior and AIDS. In C. F. Turner, H. G. Miller, & J. E. Moses (Eds.), *AIDS, sexual behavior and intravenous drug use.* Washington, DC: National Academy Press.

Galambos, N. L., & Almeida, D. M. (1992). Does parent-adolescent conflict increase during early adolescence? *Journal of Marriage and the Family, 54,* 737–747.

Galambos, N. L., & Tilton-Weaver, L. (1996). *The adultoid adolescent: Too much, too soon.* Paper presented at the biennial meeting of the Society for Research on Adolescence, Boston, MA.

Gallo, A. M., Breitmeyer, B. J., Knafl, K. A., & Zoeller, L. H. (1992). Well siblings of children with chronic illness: Parents' report of their psychological adjustment. *Pediatric Nursing, 18,* 23–27.

Gamble, D. R. (1980). The epidemiology of insulin dependent diabetes with particular reference to the relationship of virus infection to its etiology. *Epidemiological Review, 2,* 49–70.

Garrison, W. T., Biggs, D., & Williams, K. (1990). Temperament characteristics and clinical outcomes in young children with diabetes mellitus. *Journal of Child Psychology and Psychiatry, 31,* 1079–1088.

Gath, A., Smith, M. A., & Baum, J. D. (1980). Emotional, behavioral, and educational disorders in diabetic children. *Archives of Disease in Childhood, 55,* 371–375.

Geleerd, E. R. (1972). *Kinderanalytiker bei der Arbeit* [Child analysts at work]. Stuttgart: Klett.

Giambra, L. (1974). Daydreaming across the life-span. Late adolescence to senior citizen. *International Journal of Aging and Human Development, 5,* 115–140.

Gibbs, J. T., & Moskowitz Sweet, G. (1991). Clinical and cultural issues in the treatment of bisocial and bicultural adolescents. *Families in Society, 72,* 579–592.

Gilbert, B. O. (1992). Insulin-dependent diabetes control, personality and life stress in adolescents. *Personality and Individual Differences, 13,* 269–273.

Ginsburg, K. R., Slap, G. B., Cnaan, A., Forke, C. M., Balsley, C.-M., & Ronselle, D. M. (1995). Adolescents' perceptions of factors affecting their decisions to seek health care. *Journal of the American Medical Association, 273,* 1913–1918.

Givin, C. W., Given, B. A., Gallin, R. S., & Condon, J. W. (1983). Development of scales to measure beliefs of diabetic patients. *Research of Nursing and Health, 6,* 127–141.

Goertzel, L., & Goertzel, T. (1991). Health locus of control, self-concept, and anxiety in pediatric cancer patients. *Psychological Reports, 68,* 531–540.

Goldberg, S., Marcovitch, S., McGregor, D., & Lojkasek, M. (1986). Family responses to developmentally delayed preschoolers: Etiology and the father's role. *American Journal of Mental Deficiency, 90,* 610–617.

Gortmaker, S. L. (1985). Demography of chronic childhood diseases. In N. Hobbs & J. M. Perrin (Eds.), *Issues in the care of children with chronic illness* (pp. 135–154). San Francisco: Jossey-Bass.

Gortmaker, S. L., Perrin, J. M., Weitzman, M., Halmer, C. J., & Sobol, A. M. (1993). An unexpected success story: Transition to adulthood in youth with chronic physical health conditions. *Journal of Research on Adolescence, 3,* 317–336.

Gortmaker, S. L., Walker, D. B., Weitzman, M., & Sobol, A. M. (1990). Chronic conditions, socio-economic risks, and behavioral problems in children and adolescents. *Pediatrics, 85,* 267–276.

Gough, D., Li, L., & Wroblewska, A. (1993). *Services for children with a motor impairment and their families in Scotland.* Glasgow: University of Glasgow, Public Health Research Unit.

Greenberg, H. S., Kazak, A. E., & Meadows, A. T. (1989). Psychologic functioning in 8- to 16-year-old cancer survivors and their parents. *The Journal of Pediatrics, 114,* 488–493.

Grey, M. J., Boland, E. A., Yu, C., Sullivan-Bolyai, S., & Tamborlane, W. V. (1998). Personal and family factors associated with quality of life in adolescents with diabetes. *Diabetes Care, 21,* 909–914.

Grey, M. J., Cameron, M. E., & Thurber, F. W. (1991). Coping and adaptation in children with diabetes. *Nursing Research, 40,* 144–149.

Grey, M. J., Genel, M., & Tamborlane, W. V. (1980). Psychological adjustment of latency-aged diabetics. Determinants and relationship to control. *Pediatrics, 65,* 69–73.

Grotevant, H. D., & Cooper, C. R. (1985). Patterns of interaction in family relationships and the development of identity exploration in adolescence. *Child Development, 56,* 415–428.

Grotevant, H. D., & Cooper, C. R. (1986). Individuation in family relationships. A perspective on individual differences in the development of identity and role-taking skill in adolescence. *Human Development, 29,* 82–100.

Gutezeit, G. (1984). Erhebungen zur beruflichen Integration diabetischer Jugendlicher [Findings on the occupational-vocational integration of diabetic adolescents]. *Sozialpädiatrie, 6,* 71–78.

Gutezeit, G. (1987). Bemerkungen zur Eingliederung diabetischer Jugendlicher in das Berufsleben [Comments on the integration of diabetic adolescents in the work force]. *Zeitschrift für Personenzentrierte Psychologie, 6,* 239–249.

Gyolay, J. E. (1978). *The dying child.* New York: McGraw-Hill.

Haag, R., Graf, N., & Jost, W. (1991). Subjektiv erlebte Ängstlichkeit als Aspekt der Krankheitsverarbeitung bei Kindern mit bösartigen Erkrankungen [Subjectively perceived anxiety as an aspect of coping with illness in children with fatal illnesses]. *Praxis der Kinderpsychologie und Kinderpsychiatrie, 40,* 78–84.

Hall, G. S. (1904). *Adolescence.* New York: Appleton.

Hamburg, B. A., & Inoff, G. E. (1982). Relationships between behavioral factors and diabetic control in children and adolescents. *Psychosomatic Medicine, 44,* 321–339.

Hamburg, B. A., & Inoff, G. E. (1985). Coping behaviors in diabetes: Relationships between knowledge of diabetes, locus of control and metabolic control. In P. I. Ahmed & N. Ahmed (Eds.), *Coping with juvenile diabetes* (pp. 61–84). Springfield, IL: Charles C Thomas.

Hamlett, K. W., Pellegrini, D. S., & Katz, K. S. (1992). Childhood chronic illness as a family stressor. *Journal of Pediatric Psychology, 17,* 33–47.

Hammarström, A. (1990). Youth unemployment and health. Results from a five-year follow-up study. In K. Hurrelmann & F. Lösel (Eds.), *Health hazards in adolescence* (pp. 131–148). Berlin: de Gruyter.

Hanl, J. (1995). *Bewältigung chronischer Krankheiten im Jugendalter* [Coping with chronic illnesses in adolescence]. Diploma Thesis. Department of Psychology, University of Bonn, Germany.

Hanson, C. L., De Guire, M. J., Schinkel, A. M., Henggeler, S. W., & Burghen, G. A. (1992a). Comparing social learning and family systems correlates of adaptation in youths with IDDM. *Journal of Pediatric Psychology, 17,* 33–47.

Hanson, C. L., De Guire, M. J., Schinkel, A. M., & Kolterman, O. G. (1995). Empirical validation for a family-centered model of care. *Diabetes Care, 10,* 1347–1356.

Hanson, C., Harris, M., Relyea, G., Cigrang, J., Carle, D., & Burghen, G. (1989). Coping styles in youths with insulin-dependent diabetes mellitus. *Journal of Consulting and Clinical Psychology, 57,* 644–651.

Hanson, C. L., Henggeler, S. W., & Burghen, G. A. (1987). Social competence and parental support as mediators of the link between stress and metabolic control in adolescents with insulin-dependent diabetes mellitus. *Journal of Consulting and Clinical Psychology, 55,* 529–533.

Hanson, C. L., Henggeler, S. W., Harris, M. A., Burghen, G. A., & Moore, M. (1989). Family systems variables and the health status of adolescents with insulin-dependent diabetes mellitus. *Health Psychology, 8,* 239–253.

Hanson, C. L., Henggeler, S. W., Harris, M. A., Cigrang, J. A., Schinkel, A. M., Rodrigue, J. R., & Klesges, R. C. (1992b). Contributions of sibling relations to the adaptation to chronic disability and chronic illness. *Journal of Consulting and Clinical Psychology, 60,* 104–112.

Harlow, R. E., & Cantor, N. (1995). To whom do people turn when things go poorly? Task orientation and functional social contacts. *Journal of Personality and Social Psychology, 69,* 329–340.

Hartup, W. W. (1993). Adolescents and their friends. In B. Laursen (Ed.), *Close friendships in adolescence* (pp. 3–22). San Francisco: Jossey Bass.

Hasche, H. (1994). Die Leistungsfähigkeit des Diabetikers im Berufsleben [The performance of diabetics in the work force]. In F. Petermann (Ed.), *Diabetes mellitus* (pp. 49–66). Göttingen: Hogrefe.

Hauser, S. T. (1991). *Adolescents and their families.* New York: The Free Press.

Hauser, S. T., & Bowlds, M. K. (1990). Stress, coping and adaptation within adolescence: Diversity and resilience. In S. Feldman & G. Elliot (Eds.), *At the threshold: The developing adolescent* (pp. 388–413). Cambridge, MA: Harvard University Press.

Hauser, S. T., Di Placido, J., Benes, K., Jenkins, J., & Kim, K. (1993a). *Family Coping Processes Manual – Revision IV, 7/22/93.* Cambridge, MA: Harvard University Medical School, Massachussetts Mental Health Center, and Joslin Diabetes Center, Laboratory for Social Psychiatry.

Hauser, S. T., Di Placido, J., Jacobson, A. M., Willett, J., & Cole, C. (1993b). Family coping with an adolescent's chronic illness: An approach and three studies. *Journal of Adolescence, 16,* 305–329.

Hauser, S. T., Jacobson, A. M., Benes, K. A., & Anderson, B. J. (1997) Psychological aspects of diabetes mellitus in children and adolescents: Implications and interventions. In N. E. Alessi (Ed.), *Handbook of child and adolescent psychiatry* (Vol. 4, pp. 340–354). New York: Wiley.

Hauser, S. T., Jacobson, A. M., Lavori, P., Wolfsdorf, J. I., Herskowitz, R. D., Milley, J., Bliss, R., Gelfand, E., Wertlieb, D., & Stein, J. (1990). Adherence among children and adolescents with insulin-dependent diabetes mellitus over a 4-year longitudinal follow-up: Immediate and long-term linkages with the family milieu. *Journal of Pediatric Psychology, 15,* 527–542.

Hauser, S. T., Jacobson, A. M., Weiss-Perry, B., Vieyra, M. A., Rufo, P., Spetter, L., Wertlieb, D., Wolfsdorf, J., & Herskowitz, R. D. (1988a). *Family coping strategies: A new approach to assessment.* Cambridge, MA: Harvard University Medical School, Massachusetts Mental Health Center, and Joslin Diabetes Center.

Hauser, S. T., Jacobson, A., Wertlieb, D., Weiss-Perry, B., Follansbee, D., Wolfsdorf, J. I., Herskowitz, R. D., Houlihan, J., & Rajapark, D. C. (1986). Children with recently diagnosed diabetes: Interactions within their families. *Health Psychology, 5,* 273–296.

Hauser, S. T., Paul, E. L., Jacobson, A. M., Weiss-Perry, B., Vieyra, M. A., Rufo, P., Spetter, L. D., DiPlacido, J., Wertlieb, D., Wolfdorf, J. Y., Herskowitz, R. D. (1988b). How families cope with diabetes in adolescence. *Pediatrician, 15,* 80–94.

Hauser, S. T., & Pollets, D. (1979). Psychological aspects of diabetes mellitus: A critical review. *Diabetes Care, 2,* 227–232.

Hauser, S. T., & Solomon, M. L. (1985). Coping with diabetes: Views from the family. In P. I. Ahmed & N. Ahmed (Eds.), *Coping with juvenile diabetes* (pp. 234–266). Springfield, IL: Charles C Thomas.

Havighurst, R. J. (1953). *Human development and education.* New York: Longmans, Green & Co.

Havighurst, R. J. (1972). *Developmental tasks and education.* New York: McKay.

Hawton, K. (1986). *Suicide and attempted suicide among children and adolescents.* Beverly Hills, CA: Sage.

Hendry, L. B., Raymond, M., & Stewart, C. (1984). Unemployment, school and leisure: An adolescent study. *Leisure Studies, 3,* 175–187.

Hendry, L. B., Shucksmith, J., Love, J. G., & Glendinning, A. (1993). *Young people's leisure and lifestyles.* London: Routledge.

Herman-Stahl, M., Stemmler, M., & Petersen, A. C. (1995). Approach and avoidant coping: Implications for adolescent health. *Journal of Youth and Adolescence, 24,* 649–665.

Hetherington, E. M., Reiss, D., & Plomin, R. (1994). *Separate social worlds of siblings: The impact of nonshared environment on development.* Hillsdale, NJ: Lawrence Erlbaum Associates.

Hill, J. P. (1987). Research on adolescents and their families: Past and prospect. In C. E. Irwin (Ed.), *Adolescent social behavior and health* (pp. 13–31). San Francisco: Jossey-Bass.

Hill, J. P., & Holmbeck, G. N. (1986). Attachment and autonomy. *Annals of Child Development, 3,* 145–189.

Hinkle, L., & Wolf, S. (1952). Importance of life stress in the course and management of diabetes mellitus. *Journal of the American Medical Society, 148,* 513–520.

Hofmann, A. D., & Becker, R. D. (1973). Psychotherapeutic approaches to the physically ill adolescent. *International Journal of Child Psychotherapy, 2,* 492–511.

Howe, G. W., Feinstein, C., Reiss, D., Molock, S., & Berger, K. (1993). Adolescent adjustment to chronic physical disorders. I. Comparing neurological and nonneurological conditions. *Journal of Child Psychology and Psychiatry and Allied Disciplines, 34,* 1153–1171.

Hunter, F. T., & Youniss, J. (1982). Changes in functions of three relations during adolescence. *Developmental Psychology, 18,* 806–811.

Hurrelmann, K. (1987). The importance of school in the life course: Results from the Bielefeld study on school-related problems in adolescence. *Journal of Adolescent Research, 2,* 111–126.

Hurrelmann, K. (1990). Basic issues and problems of health in adolescence. In K. Hurrelmann & F. Lösel (Eds.), *Health hazards in adolescence. Prevention and intervention in childhood and adolescence* (pp. 1–24). Berlin: de Gruyter.

Hurrelmann, K. (1991). *Sozialisation und Gesundheit: somatische, psychische und soziale Risikofaktoren im Lebenslauf,* 2. Aufl. [Socialization and health: Somatic, psychological and social risk factors in the life span, 2nd ed.]. Munich: Juventa.

Hurrelmann, K. (1992). *Jugendgesundheitssurvey* [Survey on adolescent health]. Unpublished manuscript. University of Bielefeld, Bielefeld, Germany.

Hurrelmann, K., & Lösel, F. (1990). Basic issues and problems of health in adolescence. In K. Hurrelmann & F. Lösel (Eds.), *Health hazards in adolescence. Prevention and intervention in childhood and adolescence, 8,* 1–24. Berlin: de Gruyter.

Hurtig, A. L., Koepke, D., & Park, K. B. (1989). Relation between severity of chronic illness and adjustment in children and adolescents with sickle cell disease. *Journal of Pediatric Psychology, 14,* 117–132.

Jacobson, A. M., Hauser, S. T., Lavori, P., Wolfsdorf, J. I., Herskowitz, R. D., Milley, J. E., Bliss, R., Gelfand, E., Wertlieb, D., & Stein, J. (1990). Adherence among children and adolescents with insulin-dependent diabetes mellitus over a four-year longitudinal follow-up: I. The influence of patient coping and adjustment. *Journal of Pediatric Psychology, 15,* 511–526.

Jacobson, A. M., Hauser, S. T., Wertlieb, D., Wolfsdorf, J. I., Orleans, J., & Vieyra, M. (1986). Psychological adjustment of children with recently diagnosed diabetes mellitus. *Diabetes Care, 9,* 323–329.

Jamison, R. N., Lewis, S., & Burish, T. G. (1986). Psychological impact of cancer on adolescents: Self-image, locus of control, perception of illness and knowledge of cancer. *Journal of Chronic Disease, 39,* 609–617.

Jenny, J. (1983). A compliance model for diabetic instruction. *Rehabilitation Literature, 44,* 258–263.

Jessop, D. J., & Stein, R. E. K. (1985). Uncertainty and its relation to the psychological and social correlates of chronic illness in children. *Social Science and Medicine, 20,* 993–999.

Jessor, R., & Jessor, S. L. (1975). Transition from virginity to nonvirginity among youth: A social-psychological study over time. *Developmental Psychology, 11,* 473–484.

Johnson, S. B. (1980). Psychosocial factors in juvenile diabetes: A review. *Journal of Behavioral Medicine, 3,* 95–116.

Johnson, S. B. (1984). Knowledge, attitudes and behaviors: Correlates of health in childhood diabetes. *Clinical Psychology Review, 4,* 503–524.

Johnson, S. B., & Rosenbloom, A. L. (1982). Behavioral aspects of diabetes mellitus in childhood and adolescence. *Pediatric Clinics of North America, 5,* 357–369.

Joner, G., & Sovik, O. (1989). Increasing incidence of diabetes mellitus in Norwegian children 0–14 years of age, 1973–1982. *Diabetologica, 32,* 79–83.

Joy, A. E. (1987). Developmental aspects of children's strategies for coping with painful medical procedures. *Dissertation Abstracts International, 41* (1-B), 284.

Kager, V. A., & Holden, E. W. (1992). Preliminary investigation of the direct and moderating effects of family and individual variables on the adjustment of children and adolescents with diabetes. *Journal of Pediatric Psychology, 17,* 491–502.

Kammeyer, U. (1967). Birth order as a research variable. *Social Forces, 46,* 71–80.

Kaplan, R. M., & Chadwick, M. W. (1987). Training sozialer Kompetenz bei Typ-I-Diabetes [Training social competence in type-I diabetics]. In F. Strian, R. Hölzl, & M. Haslbeck (Eds.), *Verhaltensmedizin und Diabetes mellitus* [Behavioral medicine and diabetes mellitus] (pp. 309–325). Berlin: Springer.

Kashani, J., Carlson, G., & Beck, N. (1987). Depression, depressive symptoms and depressed mood among a community sample of adolescents. *American Journal of Psychiatry, 144,* 931–934.

Kashani, J. H., König, P., Sheppered, J. A., Wilfley, D., & Morris, D. A. (1988). Psychopathology and self-concept in asthmatic children. *Journal of Pediatric Psychology, 13,* 509–520.

Katz, S. J., Hofer, T. P., & Manning, W. G. (1996). Physician use in Ontario and the United States: The impact of socioeconomic status and health status. *American Journal of Public Health, 86,* 520–524.

Kaufman, R. V., & Hersher, B. (1971). Body image changes in teenage diabetics. *Pediatrics, 48,* 123–148.

Kavsek, M., & Seiffge-Krenke, I. (1996). The differentiation of coping traits in adolescence. *International Journal of Behavioral Development, 19,* 651–668.

Kellerman, J., Zeltzer, L., Ellenberg, L., Dash, J., & Rigler, D. (1980). Psychological effects in illness in adolescence. I. Anxiety, self-esteem, and perception of control. *Journal of Pediatrics, 97,* 126–131.

Kerek-Bodden, H. E. (1989). Ausgewählte Aspekte der Inanspruchnahme und der Versorgung [Selected aspects of use and availability]. In Zentralinstitut für die kassenärztliche Versorgung in der Bundesrepublik Deutschland (Eds.), *Die EVAS-Studie. Eine Erhebung über die ambulante medizinische Versorgung in der Bundesrepublik Deutschland* [The EVAS study. An assessment of ambulant medical care in the Federal Republic of Germany] (pp. 94–110). Cologne: Zentralinstitut für die kassenärztliche Versorgung in der Bundesrepublik Deutschland.

Kiecolt-Glaser, J. K., Fisher, L. D., Ogrocki, P., Stout, J. C., Speicher, C. E., & Glaser, R. (1987). Marital quality, marital disruption and immune function. *Psychosomatic Medicine, 49,* 13–34.

Kieselbach, T., & Svensson, P. G. (1988). Health and social policy response to unemployment in Europe. *Journal of Social Issues, 44,* 173–191.

Kirchler, E., Palmonari, A., & Pombeni, M. (1992). Auf der Suche nach einem Weg ins Erwachsenenalter. Jugendliche im Dickicht ihrer Probleme und Unterstützung seitens Gleichaltriger und der Familienangehörigen [Looking for a way to adulthood. Adolescents in the labyrinth of their problems and support from peers and family]. *Psychologie in Erziehung und Unterricht, 39,* 277–295.

Kirchler, E., Palmonari, A., & Pombeni, M. L. (1993). Developmental tasks and adolescents' relationships with their peers and their family. In S. Jackson & H. Rodriguez-Tomé (Eds.), *Adolescence and its social world* (pp. 145–168). Hillsdale, NJ: Lawrence Erlbaum Associates.

Klink, F., & Kieselbach, T. (1990). *Jugendarbeitslosigkeit als gesundheitlicher Risikofaktor.* Bremer Beiträge zur Psychologie. Reihe C: Forschungsberichte der wissenschaftlichen Einheit "Arbeit, Arbeitslosigkeit und Persönlichkeitsentwicklung," Bd. 91 [Adolescent unemployment as a risk factor to health. Bremen contributions to psychology. Series C: Research reports on "Work, unemployment, and personality development", Vol. 91]. Bremen: University of Bremen, Department of Psychology.

Kokkonen, J., & Kokkonen, E. R. (1993). Prevalence of mental disorder in young adults with chronic physical disease since childhood as identified by the Present State Examination and the CATEGO program. *Acta Psychiatrica Scandinavica, 87,* 239–243.

Koocher, G. P., & O'Malley, J. E. (Eds.). (1981). *The Damocles syndrome. Psychosocial consequences of surviving childhood cancer.* New York: McGraw-Hill.

Koski, M. (1969). The coping processes in childhood diabetes. *Acta Pediatrica Scandinavica Supplement, 189,* 1–82.

Koski, M. (1982). Formation of positive diabetes identity. In Z. Laron & A. Galatzer (Eds.), *Psychological aspects of diabetes in children and adolescents* (pp. 9–11). Basel: Karger.

Koski, M., & Kumento, A. (1975). Adolescent development and behavior: A psychosomatic follow-up study of childhood diabetes. In Z. Laron (Ed.), *Diabetes in juveniles.* Basel: Karger.

Kovacs, M., & Feinberg, T. (1982). Coping with juvenile onset of diabetes. In A. Baum & J. Singer (Eds.), *Handbook of psychology and health* (Vol. 2, pp. 165–212). Hillsdale, NJ: Lawrence Erlbaum Associates.

Kovacs, M., Feinberg, T. L., Paulaskas, S., Finkelstein, R., Pollock, M., & Crouse-Novak, M. (1985). Initial coping responses and psychosocial characteristics of children with insulin-dependent diabetes mellitus. *Journal of Pediatrics, 106,* 827–834.

Kovacs, M., Iyengar, S., Goldston, D., Obrosky, D. S., Stewart, J., Marsh, J. (1990). Psychological functioning among mothers of children with insulin-dependent diabetes mellitus: A longitudinal study. *Journal of Consulting and Clinical Psychology, 58,* 189–195.

Kulzer, B. (1992). Psychologische Interventionskonzepte bei Diabetes mellitus [Concepts of psychological intervention in diabetes mellitus]. In H. Weber-Falkensammer (Ed.), *Psychologische Therapieansätze in der Rehabilitation* [Psychological therapy in rehabilitation] (pp. 104–162). Stuttgart: Fischer.

La Greca, A. M. (1988). Children with diabetes and their families: Coping and disease management. In T. Field, P. M. McCabe, & N. Schneiderman (Eds.), *Stress and coping across development* (pp. 139–159). Hillsdale, NJ: Lawrence Erlbaum Associates.

La Greca, A. M. (1992). Peer influences in pediatric chronic illness: An update. *Journal of Pediatric Psychology, 17,* 775–784.

La Greca, A. M., Follansbee, D. M., & Skyler, J. S. (1990). Developmental and behavioral aspects of diabetes management in youngsters. *Children's Health Care, 19,* 132–139.

La Greca, A. M., Siegel, L. J., Wallander, J. L., & Walker, C. E. (Eds.) (1992). *Stress and coping in child health.* New York: Guilford Press.

Larson, R., & Richards, M. H. (1991). Daily companionship in late childhood and early adolescence: Changing developmental contexts. *Child Development, 62,* 284–300.

Laufer, M., & Laufer, M. E. (1984). *Adolescence and developmental breakdown.* New Haven: Yale University Press.

Laursen, B. (1993). Conflict management among close peers. In B. Laursen (Ed.), *Close friendships in adolescence* (pp. 39–54). San Francisco: Jossey Bass.

La Vecchia, C., Decarli, A., Negri, E., Ferraroni, M., & Pagano, R. (1992). Height and prevalence of chronic disease. *Revue d'épidémiologie et de santé publique, 40,* 6–14.

Lavigne, J. V., & Ryan, M. (1979). Psychologic adjustment of siblings of children with chronic illness. *Pediatrics, 63,* 616–627.

Lavigne, J. V., Traisman, H. S., Marr, T. J., & Chasnoff, I. J. (1982). Parental perceptions of the psychological adjustment of children with diabetes and their siblings. *Diabetes Care, 5,* 420–426.

Lazarus, R. S. (1985). The trivialization of distress. In P. Ahmed & N. Ahmed (Eds.), *Coping with juvenile diabetes* (pp. 33–60). Springfield, IL: Charles C Thomas.

Lazarus, R. S., Averill, J. R., & Opton, E. M. (1974). The psychology of coping: Issues of research and assessment. In G. V. Coelho, D. A. Hamburg, & J. E. Adams (Eds.), *Coping and adaptation* (pp. 249–316). New York: Basic Books.

Lazarus, R. S., & Folkman, S. (1984). *Stress, appraisal and coping.* New York: Springer.

Lee, H., Chan, D. W., & Yik, S. M. (1992). Coping style and psychological distress among Chinese adolescents in Hong Kong. *Journal of Adolescent Research, 7,* 494–506.

LePontois, J. (1975). Adolescents with sickle-cell anemia deal with life and death. *Social Work in Health Care, 1,* 71–80.

Lerner, R. M. (1987). A life-span perspective for early adolescence. In R. M. Lerner & T. T. Foch (Eds.), *Biological-psychosocial interactions in early adolescence: A life-span perspective* (pp. 9–34). Hillsdale, NJ: Lawrence Erlbaum Associates.

Lerner, R. M., & Foch, T. T. (Eds.) (1987). *Biological-psychosocial interactions in early adolescence: A life-span perspective.* Hillsdale, NJ: Lawrence Erlbaum Associates.

Lewinsohn, P. M., Hops, H., Roberts, R. E., Seeley, J. R., & Andrews, J. A. (1993). Adolescent psychopathology: I. Prevalence and incidence of depression and other DSM-III-R disorders in high school students. *Journal of Abnormal Psychology, 102,* 133–144.

Lewinsohn, P. M., Klein, D. N., & Seeley, J. R. (1995). Bipolar disorders in a community sample of older adolescents: Prevalence, phenomenology, comorbidity, and course. *Journal of the American Academy of Child and Adolescent Psychiatry, 34,* 454–463.

Lewis, J. M. (1986). Family structure and stress. *Family Process, 25,* 235–247.

Lewis, K. G. (1987). Bulimia as a communication to siblings. Special issue: Psychotherapy with families. *Psychotherapy, 24,* 640–645.

Litt, I. F., Cuskey, W. R., & Rosenberg, A. (1982). Role of self-esteem and autonomy in determining medication compliance among adolescents with juvenile rheumatoid arthritis. *Pediatrics, 69,* 15–17.

Lobato, D., Barbour, L., Hall, L. J., & Miller, C. T. (1987). Psychosocial characteristics of preschool siblings of handicapped and non-handicapped children. *Journal of Abnormal Child Psychology, 15,* 329–338.

Lobato, D., Faust, D., & Spirito, A. (1988). Examining the effects of chronic disease and disability on children's sibling relationships. *Journal of Pediatric Psychology, 13,* 389–407.

Lösel, F., Bliesener, T., & Köferl, P. (1991). Erlebens- und Verhaltensprobleme bei Jugendlichen: Deutsche Adaptation und kulturvergleichende Überprüfung der Youth Self Report Form der Child Behavior Checklist [Emotional and behavioral problems in adolescents: Comparison and Revision of the Youth Self Report Form in the Child Behavior Checklist for German populations]. *Zeitschrift für Klinische Psychologie, 20,* 22–51.

MacLean, W. E., Perrin, J. M., Gortmaker, S., & Pierr, C. B. (1992). Psychological adjustment of children with asthma: Effects of illness severity and recent stressful life events. *Journal of Pediatric Psychology, 17,* 159–171.

Magan, J. (1990). Psychiatric aspects of chronic disease in adolescence. *Journal of the American Osteopathic Association, 90,* 521–525.

Malhotra, S., & Malhotra, A. (1990). Psychological adjustment of physically sick children: Relationship with temperament. *Indian Pediatrics, 27,* 577–584.

Mansel, J., & Hurrelmann, K. (1989). Emotionale Anspannung als Reaktion auf Leistungsschwierigkeiten. Stabilität und Veränderung von psychosozialer Belastung während der schulischen Ausbildung [Emotional tension as reaction to performance deficits. Stability and change of psychosocial stress during the school years]. *Zeitschrift für Sozialisationsforschung und Erziehungssoziologie, 4,* 285–304.

Mansel, J., & Hurrelmann, K. (1991). *Alltagsstreß bei Jugendlichen* [Everyday stress of adolescents]. Weinheim: Juventa.

Marcelli, D., & Alvin, P. (1994). Submission or cheating in chronic illness in adolescence. The therapist's stand. *International Journal of Adolescent Medicine and Health, 7,* 65–71.

Marrero, D. G., Myers, G. L., Golden, M. P., West, D., Kershnar, A., & Lau, N. (1982). Adjustment to misfortune in the use of a social support group for adolescent diabetics. In Z. Laron & A. Galatzer (Eds.), *Psychological aspects of diabetes in children and adolescents* (pp. 141–146). Basel: Karger.

Marteau, T. M., Bloch, S., & Baum, J. D. (1987). Family life and diabetic control. *Journal of Child Psychology and Psychiatry, 28,* 823–833.

Mayou, R., Peveler, R., Davis, B., Mann, J., & Fairburn, C. (1991). Psychiatric morbidity in young adults with insulin-dependent diabetes mellitus. *Psychological Medicine, 21,* 639–645.

McCollum, A. T., & Gibson, L. E. (1970). Family adaptation to the child with cystic fibrosis. *Journal of Pediatrics, 77,* 571–578.

McCubbin, H. I., McCubbin, M. A., Patterson, J. M., Cauble, A. E., Wilson, L. R., & Warwick, W. (1983). CHIP – Coping Health Inventory for Parents: An assessment of parental coping patterns in the care of the chronically ill child. *Journal of Marriage and the Family, 45,* 359–370.

McCubbin, H. I., Olson, D. H., & Larsen, A. S. (1991). F-Copes. In I. Hamilton, H. I. McCubbin, & A. I. Thompson (Eds.), *Family assessment inventories for research and practice* (pp. 203–211). Madison, WI: The University of Wisconsin, Madison.

McCubbin, H. I., & Patterson, J. M. (1982). Family adaptation to crisis. In H. I. McCubbin, A. E. Cauble, & J. M. Patterson (Eds.), *Family stress, coping and social support* (pp. 26–48). Springfield, IL: Charles C Thomas.

McDougall, J. (1987). Ein Körper für zwei [One body for two]. *Forum Psychoanalyse, 3,* 265–287.

McGee, R., Feehan, M., Williams, S., Partridge, F., Silva, P. A., & Kelly, J. (1990). DSM-III disorders in a large sample of adolescents. *Journal of the American Academy of Child and Adolescent Psychiatry, 29,* 611–619.

McKay, M. M. (1977). Adolescent problems: An examination of the rank comparison of the latent categories of problems as defined and ordered by high school students. *Dissertation Abstracts International, 38,* 3193.

Miller, K. E. (1990). Adolescents' same-sex and opposite-sex peer relations: Sex differences in popularity, perceived social competence, and social cognitive skills. *Journal of Adolescent Research, 5,* 222–241.

Millstein, S. G., & Litt, J. J. (1990). Adolescent health. In S. S. Feldman & G. R. Elliott (Eds.), *At the threshold. The developing adolescent* (pp. 431–456). Cambridge, MA: Harvard University Press.

Minde, K. K. (1978). Coping styles of 34 adolescents with cerebral palsy. *American Journal of Psychiatry, 135,* 1344–1349.

Minuchin, P. (1985). Family and individual development: Provocatives from the field. *Child Development, 56,* 289–302.

Minuchin, S., Baker, L., & Rosman, B. (1975). A conceptual model of psychosomatic illness: Family organization and family therapy. *Archives of General Psychiatry, 32,* 1031–1038.

Minuchin, S., Rosman, B., & Baker, L. (1978). *Psychosomatic families: Anorexia nervosa in context.* Cambridge, MA: Harvard University Press.

Minuchin, S., Rosman, B. L., & Baker, L. (1989). *Psychosomatische Krankheiten in der Familie* [Psychosomatic illnesses in the family]. Stuttgart: Klett-Cotta.

Mönks, F. J. (1968). Future time perspective in adolescence. *Human Development, 11,* 107–123.

Montemayor, R. (1983). Parents and adolescents in conflict: All families some of the time and some families most of the time. *Journal of Early Adolescence, 3,* 83–103.

Moore, S., & Rosenthal, D. (1993). *Sexuality in adolescents.* London: Routledge.

Moos, R. H., & Moos, B. S. (1981). *Family Environment Scale. Manual.* Palo Alto, CA: Consulting Psychologists Press.

Moran, P. B., & Eckenrode, J. (1991). Gender differences in the costs and benefits of peer relationships during adolescence. *Journal of Adolescent Research, 6,* 396–409.

Moran, G. S., & Fonagy, P. (1987). Psychoanalysis and diabetic control: A single-case study. *British Journal of Medical Psychology, 60,* 357–372.

Mrazek, J. (1987). Das Gesundheitskonzept von Jugendlichen [The health concepts of adolescents]. *Brennpunkte der Sportwissenschaften, 1,* 83–103.

Murch, R. L., & Cohen, L. H. (1989). Relationships among life stress, perceived family environment, and the psychological distress of spina bifida adolescents. *Journal of Pediatric Psychology, 14*(2), 193–214.

Musa, K., & Roach, M. (1973). Adolescent appearance and self-concept. *Adolescence, 8,* 385–394.

Nadler, R. (1978). Are we helping? *Adolescence, 13,* 453–459.

Nathan, S. W., & Goetz, P. (1984). Psychosocial aspects of chronic illness: Group interactions in diabetic girls. *Children's Health Care, 13,* 24–30.

National Center for Health Statistics. (1993). Advance report of final mortality statistics, 1991. *Monthly Vitality Statistics Reports, 42* (2).

National Safety Council. (1993). *Accidents facts*. Itasca, IL: National Safety Council.

Needle, R., McCubbin, H., Wilson, M., & Reineck, R. (1986). Interpersonal influences in adolescent drug use: The role of older siblings, parents, and peers. *International Journal of the Addictions, 21*, 739–766.

Nelms, B. C. (1989). Emotional behaviors in chronically ill children. *Journal of Abnormal Child Psychology, 6*, 657–668.

Nelson, J., & Aboud, F. E. (1985). The resolution of social conflict between friends. *Child Development, 56*, 1009–1017.

Neubauer, G. (1990). *Jugend und Sexualität* [Adolescence and Sexuality]. Stuttgart: Enke.

Neugarten, B. L. (1979). Time, age, and the life cycle. *American Journal of Psychiatry, 136*, 887–894.

Neumark-Sztainer, D., Story, M., Resnick, M. D., Garwick, A., & Blum, R. W. (1995). Body dissatisfaction and unhealthy weight-control practices among adolescents with and without chronic illness: A population-based study. *Archives of Pediatry and Adolescent Medicine, 149*, 1330–1335.

Neumark-Sztainer, D., Story, M., Toporoff, E., Cassuto, N., Resnick, M. D., & Blum, R. W. (1996). Psychosocial predictors of binge eating and purging behaviors among adolescents with and without diabetes mellitus. *Journal of Adolescent Health, 19*, 289–296.

Newacheck, P. W., Budetti, P. P., & McManus, P. (1984). Trends in childhood disability. *American Journal of Public Health, 74*, 232–236.

Newacheck, P. W., Stoddard, J. J., & McManus, M. (1993). Ethnocultural variations in the prevalence and impact of childhood chronic conditions. *Pediatrics, 91*, 1031–1039.

Newacheck, P. W., & Taylor, W. R. (1992). Childhood chronic illness: Prevalence, severity, and impact. *American Journal of Public Health, 82*, 364–371.

Niemcryk, S. J., Speers, M. A., Travis, L. B., & Gray, H. E. (1990). Psychosocial correlates of hemoglobin Alc in young adults with type-I-diabetes. *Journal of Psychosomatic Research, 34*, 617–627.

Niethammer, D. (1993). Klinische Onkologie des Kindes- und Jugendlichenalters [Clinical oncology in childhood and adolescence]. In F. J. Schulte & J. Spranger (Eds.), *Lehrbuch der Kinderheilkunde, 27 Aufl.* [Textbook of Pediatric Medicine, 27th ed., rev.] (pp. 423–430). Stuttgart: Gustav Fischer.

Nordlohne, E., & Hurrelmann, K. (1990). Health impairment, failure in school and the use and abuse of drugs. In K. Hurrelmann & F. Lösel (Eds.), *Health hazards in adolescence* (pp. 149–166). Berlin: de Gruyter.

Norell, J. E. (1984). Self-disclosure: Implications for the study of parent-adolescent interaction. *Journal of Youth and Adolescence, 13*, 163–177.

Nurmi, J. E., Poole, M. E., & Kalakowksi, V. (1994). Age differences in adolescent future-oriented goals, concerns, and related temporal extension in different sociocultural contexts. *Journal of Youth and Adolescence, 23,* 471–487.

Nurmi, J. E., Poole, M. E., & Seginer, R. (1995). Tracks and transition: A comparison of adolescent future-oriented goals, explorations, and commitment in Australia, Israel, and Finland. *International Journal of Psychology, 30,* 355–375.

Offer, D., Ostrov, E., & Howard, K. J. (1981). *Adolescence: A psychological self portrait.* New York: Basic Books.

Offord, D. R., Boyle, M. H., & Racine, Y. (1989). Ontario Child Health Study: Correlates of disorder. *Journal of the American Academy of Child and Adolescent Psychiatry, 28,* 856–860.

Offord, D. R., Boyle, M. H., Szatmari, P., Rae-Grant, N. I., Links, P. S., Cadman, D. T., Byles, J. A., Crawford, J. W., Munroe Blum, H., Byrne, C., Thomas, H., & Woodward, C. A. (1987). Ontario Child Health Study. II. Six-month prevalence of disorder and rates of service utilization. *Archives of General Psychiatry, 44,* 832–836.

Ogura, Y. (1987). Examination hell: Japanese education's most serious problem. *The College Board Review, 144,* 8–11.

Olatawura, M. O. (1972). The psychiatric complications of diabetes mellitus in children. *African Journal of Medical Science, 3,* 231–240.

Olson, D. H., McCubbin, H. I., Barnes, H. L., Larsen, A. S., Muxen, M. J., & Wilson, M. A. (1983a). *Families. What makes them work.* Beverly Hills, CA: Sage.

Olson, D. H., Russell, C. S., & Sprenkle, D. H. (1983b). Circumplex model of marital and family systems: Theoretical update. *Family Process, 22,* 69–83.

O'Malley, J. E., Koocher, D., Foster, L., & Slavin, L. (1979). Psychiatric sequelae of surviving childhood cancer. *American Journal of Orthopsychiatry, 49,* 608–616.

Orr, D. P., Weller, S. C., Satterwhite, B., & Pless, I. B. (1984). Psychosocial implications of chronic illness in adolescence. *Journal of Pediatrics, 104,* 152–157.

Overstreet, S., Goins, J., Chen, S. R., Holmes, C. S., Greer, T., Dunlap, W. P., & Frentz, J. (1995). Family environment and the interrelation of family structure, child behavior, and metabolic control for children with diabetes. *Journal of Pediatric Psychology, 20,* 435–447.

Palentien, C., Settertobulte, W., & Hurrelmann, K. (1994). Jugendliche meiden Arztbesuch [Adolescents avoid consulting physicians]. *Psychomed, 6,* 52–55.

Palmonari, A., Pombeni, M., & Kirchler, E. (1990). Adolescents and their peer groups: A study on the significance of peers, social categorization processes and coping with developmental tasks. *Social Behavior, 5,* 33–48.

Parens, H. (1988). Siblings in early childhood: Some direct observational findings. *Psychoanalytic Inquiry, 8,* 31–50.

Parker, J. G., & Asher, S. R. (1987). Peer relations and later personal adjustment: Are low-accepted children at risk? *Psychological Bulletin, 102,* 357–389.

Parker, J. G., & Asher, S. R. (1993). Friendship and friendship quality in middle childhood: Links with peer group acceptance and feelings of loneliness and social dissatisfaction. *Developmental Psychology, 29,* 611–621.

Partridge, J. W., Garner, A. M., Thompson, C. W., Pullman, W., & Cherry, T. (1972). Attitudes of adolescents toward their diabetes. *American Journal of the Disabled Child, 124,* 226–229.

Patterson, J. M., Budd, J., Goetz, D., & Warwick, W. J. (1993). Family correlates of a ten-year pulmonary health trend in cystic fibrosis. *Pediatrics, 91,* 383–389.

Patterson, J. M., McCubbin, H. J., & Warwick, W. J. (1990). The impact of family functioning on health changes in children with cystic fibrosis. *Social Science and Medicine, 2,* 159–164.

Patton, W., & Noller, P. (1984). Unemployment and youth: A longitudinal study. *Australian Journal of Psychology, 36,* 399–413.

Pearlin, C. J., & Schooler, C. (1978). The structure of coping. *Journal of Health and Social Behavior, 19,* 2–21.

Perrin, E. C., Ayoub, C. C., & Willett, J. B. (1993). In the eyes of the beholder: Family and maternal influences on perceptions of adjustment of children with chronic illness. *Journal of Developmental and Behavioral Pediatrics, 14,* 94–105.

Perrin, E. C., Stein, R. E. K., & Drotar, D. (1991). Cautions in using the Child Behavior Checklist: Observations based on research about children with a chronic illness. *Journal of Pediatric Psychology, 16,* 411–421.

Perrin, J. M. (1985). Introduction. In H. Hobbs & J. M. Perrin (Eds.), *Issues in the care of children with chronic illness* (pp. 1–10). San Francisco: Jossey-Bass.

Perrin, J. M., & McLean, W. E. (1988). Children with chronic illness: The prevention of dysfunction. *Pediatric Clinics of North America, 35,* 1325–1337.

Petermann, F. (1991). Psychosoziale Faktoren des Diabetes im Kindes- und Jugendalter – eine Übersicht [Psychosocial factors of diabetes in childhood and adolescence: An overview]. In R. Roth & M. Borkenstein (Eds.), *Psychosoziale Aspekte in der Betreuung von Kindern und Jugendlichen mit Diabetes* [Psychosocial aspects in the care of children and adolescents with diabetes] (pp. 116–122). Basel: Karger.

Petermann, F. (Ed.) (1994). *Diabetes mellitus. Sozial- und verhaltensmedizinische Ansätze* [Diabetes mellitus. Social, behavioral, and medical aspects]. Göttingen: Hogrefe.

Petermann, F., Appunn, R., & Noeker, M. (1987a). Berufsfindungsprobleme bei jugendlichen Diabetikern [Difficulties in choosing a profession in diabetic adolescents]. *Sozialpädiatrie, 9,* 188–194.

Petermann, F., Bode, U., & Schlacker, H. G. (1990). *Chronische Krankheiten bei Kindern und Jugendlichen* [Chronic illnesses in children and adolescents]. Cologne: Deutscher Ärzte Verlag.

Petermann, F., Noeker, M., & Bode, U. (1987b). *Psychologie chronischer Krankheiten im Kindes- und Jugendalter* [Psychology of chronic illnesses in childhood and adolescence]. Weinheim: Psychologie Verlags Union.

Petermann, F., Pliske, A., & Seefried, B. (1993). Erlebte berufliche Benachteiligungen von Typ-I-Diabetikern [Perceived discrimination of type-I diabetics in the work force]. *Prävention und Rehabilitation, 5,* 139–145.

Petersen, A. C., & Crockett, L. (1985). Pubertal development and its relation to cognitive and psychosocial development in adolescent girls: Implications for parenting. In J. B. Lancaster & B. A. Hamburg (Eds.), *School-age pregnancy and parenthood. Biosocial dimensions* (pp. 147–175). New York: de Gruyter.

Petersen, A. C., & Ebata, A. T. (1987). Developmental transitions and adolescent problem behavior: Implications for prevention and intervention. In K. Hurrelmann, F. Kaufmann, & F. Lösel (Eds.), *Social intervention: Potential and constraints* (pp. 167–184). Berlin: de Gruyter.

Phinney, G. V., Jensen, L. C., Olsen, J. A., & Cundick, B. (1990). The relationship between early development and psychosexual behaviors in adolescent females. *Adolescence, 25,* 321–332.

Piaget, J. (1970). Piaget's theory. In P. H. Mussen (Ed.), *Handbook of Child Psychology* (pp. 103–128). New York: Wiley.

Plancherel, B., Bolognini, M., & Halfon, O. (1998). Coping strategies in early and mid-adolescence: Differences according to age and gender in a community sample. *European Psychologist 3,* 192–201.

Pless, I. B., Cripps, H. A., Davies, J. M. C., & Wadsworth, M. E. J. (1989). Chronic physical illness in childhood: Psychological and social effects in adolescents and adult life. *Developmental Medicine and Child Neurology, 31,* 746–755.

Pless, I. B., & Nolan, T. (1991). Revision, replication and neglect – Research on maladjustment in chronic illness. *Journal of Child Psychology and Psychiatry, 32,* 347–365.

Pless, I. B., & Perrin, J. M. (1985). Issues common to a variety of illnesses. In N. Hobbs & J. M. Perrin (Eds.), *Issues in the care of children with chronic illness* (pp. 41–60). San Francisco, Jossey-Bass.

Pless, I. B., & Pinkerton, P. (1975). *Chronic childhood disorder: Promoting patterns of adjustment.* London: Henry Kimptom Publishers.

Pless, I. B., & Roughman, K. J. (1971). Chronic illness and its consequences: Observation based on three epidemiologic surveys. *Journal of Pediatrics, 79,* 351–359.

Pless, I. B., Roughman, K. J., & Haggerty, R. J. (1972). Chronic illness, family functioning, and psychological adjustment: A model for the allocation of preventive mental health services. *International Journal of Epidemiology, 1,* 271–277.

Pulakos, J. (1989). Young adult relationships: Siblings and friends. *Journal of Psychology, 123,* 237–244.

Pumariega, A. J., Pearson, D. A., & Seilheimer, D. K. (1993). Family and childhood adjustment in cystic fibrosis. *Journal of Child and Family Studies, 2,* 109–118.

Raffaelli, M., & Duckett, E. (1989). "We were just talking…". Conversations in early adolescence. *Journal of Youth and Adolescence, 18,* 567–582.

Rakonen, O., & Lahelma, E. (1992). Gender, social class and illness among young people. *Social Science and Medicine, 34,* 649–656.

Rapoff, M. A. (1998). Adherence issues among adolescents with chronic disease. In S. A. Shumaker & E. B. Schron (Eds.), *The handbook of health behavior change* (pp. 377–408). New York: Springer.

Rauste-von-Wright, M. (1988). Body image satisfaction in adolescent girls and boys: A longitudinal study. *Journal of Youth and Adolescence, 18,* 71–83.

Reinhardt, D. (1993). Asthma bronchiale [Bronchial asthma]. In F. J. Schulte & J. Spranger (Eds.), *Lehrbuch der Kinderheilkunde,* 27. neu bearb. Aufl. [Textbook of Pediatrics, 27th ed., rev.] (pp. 642–647). Stuttgart: Gustav Fischer.

Reiser, L. W. (1987). Denial of physical illness in adolescence. *Psychoanalytic Study of the Child, 42,* 385–402.

Reiss, D., & Klein, R. (1987). Paradigm and pathogenesis. In T. Jacobs (Ed.), *Family interaction and psychopathology: Theories, methods and findings.* New York: Plenum.

Reiss, D., & Oliveri, M. E. (1980). Family paradigm and family coping: A proposal for linking the family's intrinsic adaptive capacities to its responses to stress. *Family Relations, 29,* 431–444.

Rice, K. G., Herman, M. A., & Petersen, A. C. (1993). Coping with challenge in adolescence: A conceptual model and psycho-educational intervention. *Journal of Adolescence, 16,* 235–252.

Riegel, K. F. (1976). The dialectics of human development. *American Psychologist, 31,* 689–700.

Rierdan, J., & Koff, E. (1980). Representation of the female body by early and late adolescent girls. *Journal of Youth and Adolescence, 9,* 339–346.

Rierdan, J., Koff, E., & Stubbs, M. L. (1987). Depressive symptomatology and body image in adolescent girls. *Journal of Early Adolescence, 7,* 205–216.

Ritchie, K. (1981). Research note: Interaction in the families of epileptic children. *Journal of Child Psychology and Psychiatry, 22*, 65–71.

Robinson, N., Busch, L., Protapapa, L. E., & Yateman, N. A. (1989). Employers' attitudes to diabetes. *Diabetic Medicine, 6*, 692–697.

Robinson, N., & Fuller, J. H. (1985). Role of life events and difficulties in the onset of diabetes mellitus. *Journal of Psychosomatic Research, 29*, 583–591.

Rodin, G. M., Daneman, D., Johnson, L. E., Kenshole, A., & Garfinkel, P. (1985). Anorexia nervosa and bulimia in female adolescents with insulin-dependent diabetes mellitus. A systematic study. *Journal of Psychosomatic Research, 19*, 381–384.

Rogers, R. (1970). The "unmotivated" adolescent patient who wants psychotherapy. *American Journal of Psychotherapy, 24*, 411–418.

Rolland, J. S. (1984). Towards a psychosocial typology of chronic and life-threatening illness. *Family Systems Medicine, 2*, 245–262.

Rolland, J. S. (1987). Chronic illness and the life cycle: A conceptual framework. *Family Process, 26*, 203–221.

Roth, R. (1986). Verhaltensmedizinische Aspekte des juvenilen Diabetes [Behavioral medical aspects of juvenile diabetes]. *Wiener Medizinische Wochenschrift, 136*, 522–524.

Roth, R., Borkenstein, M., & Otto, S. (1987a). Eine teststatistische Evaluation eines Wissens- und Einstellungsfragebogens für juvenile Diabetiker [A statistical test evaluation of a knowledge and attitudes questionnaire for patients with juvenile diabetes]. *Zeitschrift für Klinische Psychologie, 16*, 124–134.

Roth, R., Franthal, I., & Borkenstein, M. (1987b). Juveniler Diabetes mellitus. Krankheitserleben und Verhalten [Juvenile diabetes mellitus. Patient's perceptions of illness and behavior]. *Zeitschrift für personenzentrierte Psychologie und Psychotherapie, 6*, 225–237.

Roth, R., Neuper, C., & Borkenstein, M. (1988). Erprobung eines neu entwickelten Wissens- und Einstellungsfragebogens zum juvenilen Diabetes mellitus auf einem Diabetes-Sommercamp [Test of a new knowledge and attitudes questionnaire for patients with juvenile diabetes mellitus at a diabetes summer camp]. In F. Strian, R. Hölzl, & M. Halsbeck (Eds.), *Verhaltensmedizin und Diabetes mellitus. Psychobiologische und verhaltenspsychologische Ansätze in Diagnostik und Therapie* [Behavioral medicine and diabetes mellitus. Psychobiological and behavioral psychological approaches in diagnostics and therapy] (pp. 116–130). Berlin: Springer.

Rotter, J. I. (1981). The modes of inheritance of insulin-dependent diabetes mellitus or the genetics of IDDM, no longer a nightmare but still a headache. *American Journal of Human Genetics, 33*, 835–851.

Rovet, J. F., Ehrlich, R., & Hoppe, M. (1988). Specific intellectual deficits in children with early onset diabetes mellitus. *Child Development, 59*, 226–234.

Rozario, J., Kapur, M., & Kaliaperumal, D. (1990). An epidemiological survey of prevalence and pattern of psychological disturbance of school-going early adolescents. *Journal of Personality and Clinical Studies, 6,* 165–169.

Rutter, M., Graham, P., & Yule, W. (1970a). *A neuropsychiatric study in childhood.* London: Lavenham Press.

Rutter, M., Tizard, J., & Whitmore, K. (1970b). *Education, health, and behaviour.* London: Longman.

Rutter, M., Tizard, J., Yule, W., Graham, P., & Whitmore, K. (1977). Epidemiologie in der Kinderpsychiatrie – die Isle of Wight Studien 1964–1974 [Epidemiology in child psychiatry – the Isle of Wight studies 1964–1974]. *Zeitschrift für Kinder- und Jugendpsychiatrie, 5,* 238–279.

Ryan, C., Vega, A., & Drash, A. (1985). Cognitive defects in adolescents who developed diabetes early in life. *Pediatrics, 57,* 921–927.

Sanderson, C. A., & Cantor, N. (1995). Social dating in late adolescence: Implications for safer sexual activity. *Journal of Personality and Social Psychology, 68,* 1121–1134.

Sanger, M. S., Copeland, D. R., & Davidson, E. R. (1991). Psychosocial adjustment among pediatric cancer patients: A multidimensional assessment. *Journal of Pediatric Psychology, 26,* 463–474.

Sarason, G., Johnson, G., & Siegel, G. (1978). Assessing life change. *Journal of Consulting and Clinical Psychology, 46,* 947–952.

Sargent, J. (1985). Juvenile diabetes mellitus and the family. In P.I. Ahmed & N. Ahmed (Eds.), *Coping with juvenile diabetes* (pp. 205–233). Springfield, IL: Charles C Thomas.

Savin-Williams, R. C., & Berndt, T. (1990). Friendship and peer relations. In S. S. Feldman & G. R. Elliott (Eds.), *At the threshold: The developing adolescent* (pp. 277–307). Cambridge, MA: Harvard University Press.

Sayer, A. W., Hauser, S. T., Jacobson, A. M., & Bliss, R. (1993). The impact of the family on diabetes adjustment: A developmental perspective. *Child and Adolescent Social Work Journal, 10,* 123–140.

Sayer, A. G., Hauser, S. T., Jacobson, A. M., Willett, J. B., & Cole, C. F. (1995). Developmental influences on adolescent health. In J. L. Wallander & L. J. Siegel (Eds.), *Adolescent health problems: Behavioral perspectives. Advances in pediatric psychology* (pp. 22–51). New York: Guilford Press.

Schaetz, V., & Schaetz, A. (1986). Psychosomatische Einflüsse auf die "Einstellbarkeit" jugendlicher Diabetiker [Psychosomatic influence on the "adjustment" of adolescent diabetics]. In J. Sanner & G. Burmann (Eds.), *Klinische Psychosomatik von Kindern und Jugendlichen* [Clinical psychosomatics in children and adolescents] (pp. 23–50). Munich: Reinhardt.

Schafer, L. C., Glasgow, R. E., McCall, K. D., & Dreher, M. (1983). Adherence to IDDM regimens: Relationship to psychosocial variables and metabolic control. *Diabetes Care, 6,* 493–498.

Schellevis, F. G., van der Velden, J., van de Lisdonk, E., van Eijk, J. T. M., & van Weel, C. (1993). Comorbidity of chronic disease in general practice. *Journal of Clinical Epidemiology, 46,* 469–473.

Schernthaner, G. (1994). *Sekundäre Prävention* [Secondary prevention]. Paper presented at the 22nd Annual Meeting of the Austrian Society for Diabetes in Graz, Austria.

Schiefelbein, S. (1979). Children with cancer: New hope for survival. *Saturday Review, 14,* 11–16.

Schiff, H. S. (1972). *The bereaved parent.* New York: Crown.

Schmidt, G., Klusmann, D., Zeitzschel, U., & Lange, C. (1994). Changes in adolescents' sexuality between 1970 and 1990 in West-Germany. *Archives of Sexual Behavior, 23,* 489–513.

Schmidt, H. (1981). *Multidimensionaler Persönlichkeitstest für Jugendliche (MPT-J)* [Multidimensional Personality Test for Adolescents (MPT-A)]. Göttingen: Hogrefe.

Schmid-Tannwald, I., & Urdze, A. (1983). *Sexualität und Kontrazeption aus der Sicht der Jugendlichen und ihrer Eltern* [Sexuality and contraception as perceived by adolescents and their parents]. Stuttgart: Kohlhammer.

Schober, E. (1992). Wissen allein genügt nicht [Knowledge alone is not enough]. In R. Roth & M. Borkenstein (Eds.), *Psychosoziale Aspekte in der Betreuung von Kindern und Jugendlichen mit Diabetes* [Psychosocial aspects in the care of children and adolescents with diabetes] (pp. 41–44). Basel: Karger.

Schoenflug, K., & Jansen, X. (1995). Self-concept and coping with developmental demands in German and Polish adolescents. *International Journal of Behavioral Development, 18,* 385–405.

Schoenherr, S. J., Brown, R. T., Baldwin, K., & Kaslow, N. J. (1992). Attributional styles and psychopathology in pediatric chronic-illness groups. *Journal of Clinical Child Psychology, 21,* 380–382.

Schonfield, W. A. (1969). The body image in adolescents. In G. Caplan & S. Lebovici (Eds.), *Adolescence* (pp. 27–53). New York: Basic Books.

Schulenberg, J. M., Maggs, J. L., & Hurrelmann, K. (Eds.) (1997). Health risks and developmental transitions during adolescence. New York: Cambridge University Press.

Schulz, P., & Hellhammer, D. (1991). Psychologische Aspekte chronischer Krankheiten [Psychological aspects of chronic illness]. In H. Reineker (Ed.), *Lehrbuch der klinischen Psychologie* [Textbook of clinical psychology] (pp. 421–443). Göttingen: Hogrefe.

Schvanefeldt, J. D., & Ihinger, M. (1979). Sibling relationships in the family. In W. R. Burr, R. Hill, F. I. Nye, & I. L. Reiss (Eds.), *Contemporary theories about the family: Research-based theories* (pp. 453–467). New York: The Free Press.

Seiffge-Krenke, I. (1990). Developmental processes in self-concept and coping behavior. In S. Jackson & H. Bosma (Eds.), *Self-concept and coping in adolescence* (pp. 50–68). Heidelberg: Springer.

Seiffge-Krenke, I. (1992). Coping behavior of Finnish adolescents: Remarks on a cross-cultural comparison. *Scandinavian Journal of Psychology, 33*, 301–314.

Seiffge-Krenke, I. (1993a). Coping behavior in normal and clinical samples: More similarities than differences? *Journal of Adolescence, 16*, 285–304.

Seiffge-Krenke, I. (1993b). Close friendships and imaginary companions in adolescence. In B. Laursen (Ed.), *Close friendships in adolescence* (pp. 73–88). San Francisco: Jossey Bass.

Seiffge-Krenke, I. (1995). *Stress, coping, and relationships in adolescence.* Hillsdale, NJ: Lawrence Erlbaum Associates.

Seiffge-Krenke, I. (1997a). "One body for two": The problem of boundaries between chronically ill adolescents and their mothers. *Psychoanalytic Study of the Child, 52*, 340–355.

Seiffge-Krenke, I. (1997b). The capacity to balance intimacy and conflict: Differences in romantic relationships between healthy and diabetic adolescents. In S. Shulman & W. A. Collins (Eds.), *Romantic relationships in adolescence: Developmental perspectives* (pp. 53–68). San Francisco: Jossey-Bass.

Seiffge-Krenke, I. (1998a). *Adolescents' health: A developmental perspective.* Mahwah, NJ: Lawrence Erlbaum Associates.

Seiffge-Krenke, I. (1998b). The highly structured climate in families of adolescents with diabetes: Functional or dysfunctional for metabolic control? *Journal of Pediatric Psychology, 23*, 313–322.

Seiffge-Krenke, I. (1998c). Chronic disease and perceived developmental progression in adolescence. *Developmental Psychology 34*, 1073–1084.

Seiffge-Krenke, I. (1999). Families with daughters, families with sons: Different challenges for family relationships and marital satisfaction? *Journal of Youth and Adolescence, 3*, 325–342.

Seiffge-Krenke, I. (2000). Diversity in romantic relations of adolescents with varying health status: Links to intimacy in close friendships. *Journal of Adolescent Research, 15*, 611–636.

Seiffge-Krenke, I., & Brath, K. (1990). Krankheitsverarbeitung bei Kindern und Jugendlichen. Forschungstrends und Ergebnisse [Coping with illness in childhood and adolescence. Research trends and findings]. In I. Seiffge-Krenke (Ed.), *Krankheitsverarbeitung bei Kindern und Jugendlichen (Jahrbuch der medizinischen Psychologie, Bd.4)* [Coping with illness in children and adolescents (Yearbook of medical psychology, Vol. 4)] (pp. 3–22). Berlin: Springer.

Seiffge-Krenke, I., & Klessinger, N. (2000). Long-term effects of avoidant coping on adolescents' depressive symptoms. *Journal of Youth and Adolescence, 29*, 617–630.

Seiffge-Krenke, I., & Kollmar, F. (1996). Der jugendliche Diabetiker und sein Arzt: Diskrepanzen in der Einschätzung der Arzt-Patienten-Beziehung und der Compliance [The adolescent diabetic and the physician: Discrepancies in the evaluations of the patient-physician relationship and compliance]. *Kindheit und Entwicklung, 4,* 240–249.

Seiffge-Krenke, I., & Kollmar, F. (1998). Discrepancies between mothers' and fathers' perceptions of sons' and daughters' problem behaviour: A longitudinal analysis of parent-adolescent agreement on internalizing and externalizing problem behaviour. *Journal of Child Psychology and Psychiatry, 39,* 687–697.

Seiffge-Krenke, I., Moormann, D., Nilles, D., & Suckow, A. (1991). *Fragebogen zur Krankheitsverarbeitung für jugendliche Diabetiker* [Questionnaire on coping with illness for adolescent diabetics]. Unpublished manuscript. University of Bonn, Department of Psychology, Bonn, Germany.

Seiffge-Krenke, I., & Shulman, S. (1990). Coping style in adolescence: A cross-cultural study. *Journal of Cross-Cultural Psychology, 21,* 351–377.

Seigel, W. M., Golden, M. H., Gough, J. W., Lashley, M. S., & Sacker, I. M. (1990). Depression, self-esteem, and life events in adolescents with chronic disease. *Journal of Adolescent Health Care, 11,* 501–504.

Sells, C. W., & Blum, R. M. (1996). Morbidity and mortality among U.S. adolescents: An overview of data and trends. *American Journal of Public Health, 86,* 513–519.

Selman, R. L. (1980). *The growth of interpersonal understanding.* Orlando: Academic Press.

Sessa, F. M., & Steinberg, L. (1991). Family structure and the development of autonomy during adolescence. *Journal of Early Adolescence, 11,* 38–55.

Shulman, S. (1993). Close relationships and coping behavior in adolescence. *Journal of Adolescence, 16,* 267–283.

Shulman, S., & Seiffge-Krenke, I. (1997). *Fathers and adolescents: Developmental and clinical perspectives.* London: Routledge.

Shulman, S., Seiffge-Krenke, I., Levy-Shift, R., Fabian, B., & Rotenberg, S. (1995). Peer group and family relationships in early adolescence. *International Journal of Psychology, 30,* 573–590.

Siegal, M. (1987). Are sons and daughters treated more differently by fathers than by mothers? *Developmental Review, 7,* 183–209.

Sigusch, K., & Schmidt, G. (1973). *Jugendsexualität* [Adolescent sexuality]. Stuttgart: Enke.

Silbereisen, R. K., Noack, P., & von Eye, A. (1992). Adolescents' development of romantic friendship and change in favorite leisure contexts. *Journal of Adolescent Research, 7,* 80–93.

Silver, E. J., Bauman, L. J., Coupey, S. M., Doctors, S. R., & Boeck, M. A. (1990). Ego development and chronic illness in adolescents. *Journal of Personality and Social Psychology, 59,* 305–310.

Simeonsson, R. J., & McHale, S. M. (1981). Review: Research on handicapped children. Sibling relationships. *Child Care, Health and Development, 7,* 153–171.

Simmons, R. G., & Blyth, D. A. (1987). *Moving into adolescence: The impact of pubertal change and school context.* New York: de Gruyter.

Simmons, R. G., Burgeson, R., & Carlton-Ford, S. (1987). The impact of cumulative change in early adolescence. *Child Development, 58,* 1220–1234.

Simmons, R. J., Corey, M., Cowen, L., Keenan, N., Robertson, L., & Levison, H. (1985). Emotional adjustment in early adolescents with cystic fibrosis. *Psychosomatic Medicine, 47,* 111–122.

Simonds, J. F. (1976). Psychiatric status of diabetic youth with good and poor control. *International Journal of Psychiatry in Medicine, 7,* 133–151.

Simonds, J. F. (1977). Psychiatric status of diabetic youth matched with a control group. *Diabetes, 26,* 921–925.

Sinnema, G. (1986). The development of independence in chronically ill adolescents. *International Journal of Adolescent Medicine and Health, 2,* 1–14.

Sloper, P., & Turner, S. (1993). Risk and resistance factors in the adaptation of parents with children with severe physical disability. *Journal of Child Psychology and Child Psychiatry, 34,* 167–188.

Smith, M. S., Mauseth, R., Palmer, J. P., Pecoraro, R., & Wenet, G. (1991). Glycosylated hemoglobin and psychological adjustment in adolescents with diabetes. *Adolescence, 26,* 31–40.

Spirito, A., De Lawyer, D. D., & Stark, L. J. (1991). Peer relations and social adjustment of chronically ill children and adolescents. *Clinical Psychological Review, 11,* 538–564.

Spirito, A., Stark, L. J., Gil, K. M., & Tyc, V. L. (1995). Coping with everyday and disease-related stressors by chronically ill children and adolescents. *Journal of the American Academy of Child and Adolescent Psychiatry, 34,* 283–290.

Spurdle, E., & Giles, T. (1990). Bulimia complicated with diabetes mellitus: A clinical trial using exposure with response prevention. *Psychology and Health, 4,* 167–174.

Stabler, B., Surwit, R. S., Lane, J. D., Morris, M. A., Litton, J., & Feinglos, M. N. (1987). Type A behavior patterns and blood glucose control in diabetic children. *Psychosomatic Medicine, 49,* 313–316.

Statistisches Bundesamt (Ed.) (1991). *Fachserie Gesundheitswesen, 12, Reihe 3* [Special Series Nr. 12/3: Health Care Services]. Bonn, Germany: Statistisches Bundesamt.

Statistisches Bundesamt (Ed.) (1994). *Fachserie Todesursachen 12, Reihe 4* [Special Series Nr. 12/4: Causes of Death]. Bonn, Germany: Statistisches Bundesamt.

Stein, R. E. K., & Jessop, D. J. (1982). A noncategorical approach to chronic childhood illness. *Public Health Reports, 97,* 354–362.

Stein, R. E. K., & Jessop, D. J. (1984). General issues in the care of children with chronic physical conditions. *Pediatric Clinics of North America, 31,* 89–199.

Stein, S., & Charles, E. (1975). Emotional factors in juvenile diabetes mellitus: A study of early life experience of eight diabetic children. *Psychosomatic Medicine, 37,* 237–244.

Steinberg, L. D. (1989). Reciprocal relation between parent-child distance and pubertal maturation. *Developmental Psychology, 24,* 122–128.

Steinglass, P., Bennet, L. A., Wolin, S. J., & Reiss, D. (1987). The alcoholic family. New York: Basic Books.

Stern, M., & Zevon, M. A. (1990). Stress, coping, and family environment. *Journal of Adolescent Research, 5,* 290–305.

Stone, A. A., & Neale, J. M. (1984). A new measure of daily coping: Development and preliminary results. *Journal of Personality and Social Psychology, 46,* 892–906.

Streel, J. M., Young, R. J., Lloyd, G. G., & Macintyre, C. C. A. (1989). Abnormal eating attitudes in young insulin-dependent diabetics. *British Journal of Psychiatry, 155,* 515–521.

Strouse, J. S., & Fabes, R. A. (1987). A conceptualization of transition to nonvirginity in adolescent females. *Journal of Adolescent Research, 2,* 331–348.

Struwe, E. (1991). Diabetes mellitus [Diabetes mellitus]. In K. Betke, W. Künzer, & J. Schaub (Eds.), *Lehrbuch der Kinderheilkunde, 6. neu bearb. Aufl.* [Textbook of pediatric medicine, 6th ed., rev.]. (pp. 276–288). Stuttgart: Georg Thieme.

Sullivan, B.-J. (1979). Adjustment in diabetic adolescent girls: I. Development of the Diabetic Adjustment Scale. *Psychosomatic Medicine, 41* (2), 19–126.

Sullivan, H. S. (1953). *The interpersonal theory of psychiatry.* New York: Norton.

Sutton-Smith, B., & Rosenberg, B. G. (1968). Sibling consensus on power tactics. *Journal of Genetic Psychology, 112,* 63–72.

Swift, C. R., Seidman, F., & Stein, H. (1967). Adjustment problems in juvenile diabetes. *Psychosomatic Medicine, 29,* 555–571.

Tanner, J. M. (1972). Sequence, tempo, and individual variation in growth and development of boys and girls aged 12 to 16. In J. Kagan & R. Coles (Eds.), *12 to 16: Early adolescence* (pp. 1–24). New York: Norton.

Tavormina, J. B., Kastner, L. S., Slater, H. S., & Watt, S. L. (1976). Chronically ill children – a psychologically and emotionally deviant population? *Journal of Abnormal Child Psychology, 4,* 99–110.

Thompson, R. J., Hodges, K., & Hamlett, K. W. (1990). A matched comparison of adjustment in children with cystic fibrosis and psychiatrically referred and nonreferred children. *Journal of Pediatric Psychology, 14,* 559–575.

Thompson, R. J., Kronenberger, W., & Curry, J. F. (1989). Behavior classification system for children with developmental, psychiatric, and chronic medical problems. *Journal of Pediatric Psychology, 14,* 559–575.

Tobin-Richards, M. H., Boxer, A. M., & Petersen, A. C. (1983). The psychological significance of pubertal change. Sex differences in perception of self during early adolescence. In J. Brooks-Gunn & A. C. Petersen (Eds.), *Girls at puberty: Biological and psychological perspectives* (pp. 127–154). New York: Plenum.

Toeller, M. (1990). Diabetesschulung [Educating diabetics]. *Internist, 31,* 208–217.

Tolor, A., & Fehon, D. (1987). Coping with stress: A study of male adolescents' coping strategies as related to adjustment. *Journal of Adolescent Research, 2,* 33–42.

Tropauer, A., Franz, M., & Dilgard, V. (1970). Psychological aspects of the care of children with cystic fibrosis. *American Journal of Disease in Childhood, 119,* 424–432.

Trute, B., & Hauch, C. (1988). Building on family strength: A study of families with positive adjustment to the birth of a developmentally disabled child. *Journal of Marriage and Family Therapy, 14,* 185–193.

Tuomilehto, J., Rewers, M., Reunanaen, A., Lounamaa, P., Lounamaa, R., Tuomilehto-Wolf, E., & Akerblom, H. K. (1991). Increasing trends in type-I (insulin-dependent) diabetes mellitus in childhood in Finland. *Diabetologica, 34,* 282–287.

Udry, J. R., & Bill, J. O. (1987). Initiation of coitus in early adolescence. *American Sociological Review, 52,* 841–855.

Van Sciver, M. M., D'Angelo, E. J., Rappaport, L., & Woolf, A. D. (1995). Pediatric compliance and the roles of distinct treatment characteristics, treatment attitudes, and family stress: A preliminary report. *Journal of Developmental and Behavioral Pediatrics, 16,* 350–358.

Vernberg, E. M. (1989). Psychological adjustment and experiences with peers during early adolescence: Reciprocal, incidental, or unidirectional relationships? *Journal of Abnormal Child Psychology, 18* (2), 187–198.

Visher, E. B., & Visher, J. S. (1988). *Old loyalties, new ties.* New York: Brunner & Mazel.

Vonderach, G. (1989). Arbeitslosigkeit (Berufsnot) junger Menschen. [Unemployment in young people.] In M. Markefka & R. Nave-Herz (Eds.), *Handbuch der Familien- und Jugendforschung,* Bd. 2 [Handbook of research on the family and adolescence, Vol. 2] (pp. 699–716). Neuwied, Germany: Luchterhand.

Wagner, B. M., Compas, B. E., & Howell, D. C. (1988). Daily and major life events: A test of an integrative model of psychosocial stress. *American Journal of Community Psychology, 16,* 189–205.

Wallander, J. L., Varni, J. W., Babani, L., Banis, H. T., & Wilcox, K. T. (1988). Children with chronic physical disorders: Maternal reports of their psychological adjustment. *Journal of Pediatric Psychology, 13,* 197–212.

Weber, B. (1993). Diabetes mellitus [Diabetes mellitus]. In F. J. Schulte & J. Spranger (Eds.), *Lehrbuch der Kinderheilkunde, 27. neu bearb. Aufl.* [Textbook of Pediatrics, 27th ed., rev.] (pp. 234–244). Stuttgart: Gustav Fischer.

Weissman, J., & Appleton, C. (1995). The therapeutic aspects of acceptance. *Perspectives in Psychiatric Care, 31,* 19–23.

Weitzman, M. (1984). School and peer relations. *Pediatric Clinics of North America, 31,* 59–69.

Wertlieb, P. D., Hauser, S. T., & Jacobson, A. M. (1986). Adaptation to diabetes: Behavior symptoms and family context. *Journal of Pediatric Psychology, 11,* 463–479.

Westbom, L., & Kornfält, R. (1987). Chronic illness among children in a total population. *Scandinavian Journal of Social Medicine, 15,* 87–97.

Westbrook, L. E., & Stein, R. E. K. (1994). Epidemiology of chronic health conditions in adolescents. *Adolescent Medicine: State of the Art Reviews, 5,* 197–209.

White, K., Kolman, M. L., Wexler, P., Polin, G., & Winter, R. J. (1984). Unstable diabetes and unstable families: A psychosocial evaluation of diabetic children with recurrent ketoacidosis. *Pediatrics, 73,* 749–755.

Whiting, B. B., & Whiting, J. W. M. (1975). *Children of six cultures: A psychocultural analysis.* Cambridge, MA: Harvard University Press.

Wing, R. R., Lamparski, D. M., Zaslow, S., Betschart, J., Siminerio, L., & Becker, D. (1985). Frequency and accuracy of self-monitoring of blood glucose in children: Relationship to glycemic control. *Diabetes Care, 8,* 214–218.

Wittchen, H. U., Essau, C. A., von Zerssen, D., Krieg, J. C., & Zaudig, M. (1992). Lifetime and six-month prevalence of mental disorders in the Munich Follow-up Study. *European Archives of Psychiatry and Clinical Neuroscience, 241,* 247–258.

Wolman, C., Resnick, M. D., Harris, L. J., & Blum, R. (1994). Emotional well-being among adolescents with and without chronic conditions. *Journal of Adolescent Health, 15,* 199–204.

Wood, B., Watkins, J. B., Nogueira, J., Zimand, E., & Carrol, A. C. (1989). The "psychosomatic family": A theoretical and empirical analysis. *Family Process, 28,* 399–417.

Worchel, F. F., Copeland, D., & Barker, D. (1988). Control-related coping strategies in pediatric oncology patients. *Journal of Pediatric Psychology, 12,* 25–38.

Worchel, F. F., Nolan, B. F., Willson, V. L., Purser, J. S., Copeland, D. R., & Pfefferbaum, B. (1988). Assessment of depression in children with cancer. *Journal of Pediatric Psychology, 13,* 101–112.

World Health Organisation (WHO) (1946). *Constitution.* Geneva: World Health Organization.

Wysocki, T. (1993). Associations among teenager-parent relationships, metabolic control, and adjustment to diabetes in adolescents. *Journal of Pediatric Psychology, 18,* 441–452.

Youniss, J. (1983). Social construction of adolescence by adolescents and parents. In H. D. Grotevant & C. R. Cooper (Eds.), *Adolescent development in the family. New directions for child development* (pp. 93–109). San Francisco: Jossey Bass.

Youniss, J., & Smollar, J. (1985). Activities and communications of close friendships. In J. Youniss & J. Smollar (Eds.), *Adolescent relations with mothers, fathers, and friends* (pp. 94–109). Chicago: University of Chicago Press.

Index